Your HIGH-RISK Pregnancy

DEDICATION

To my family—
My husband of thirty-two years, Simon,
whose unrelenting love and support make everything possible;
my daughters, Rachel Miriam and Regine Anna;
and my son, Joshua Samuel—
who light up my life

and

to the loving memory of my father, Edward Marquise,
who lived long enough to witness the birth
of his three grandchildren.

Ordering
Trade bookstores in the U.S. and Canada please contact:

Publishers Group West
1700 Fourth Street, Berkeley CA 94710
Phone: (800) 788-3123   Fax: (800) 351-5073

Hunter House books are available at bulk discounts for textbook course
adoptions; to qualifying community, health-care, and government organizations;
and for special promotions and fund-raising.
For details please contact:

Special Sales Department
Hunter House Inc., PO Box 2914, Alameda CA 94501-0914
Phone: (510) 865-5282   Fax: (510) 865-4295
E-mail: ordering@hunterhouse.com

Individuals can order our books from most bookstores,
by calling (**800**) **266-5592**, or from our website at
www.hunterhouse.com

Your HIGH-RISK Pregnancy

A PRACTICAL AND SUPPORTIVE GUIDE

DIANA RAAB, MFA, RN

WITH ERROL NORWITZ, MD

Hunter House PUBLISHERS

Hunter House Inc., Publishers
PO Box 2914
Alameda CA 94501-0914

Acknowledgment is made for permission to reprint: "Passive Exercises for Bedrest," (p. 201) adapted from the Good Samaritan Medical Center, Phoenix, Arizona; chart (p. 149) from "Down Syndrome and Maternal Age," adapted from J. A. Roberts, and M. Pembray, *An Introduction to Genetics*, Oxford University Press, 1985; "Internal Female Reproductive Anatomy" illustration (p. 8) and "Fertilization and Implantation of the Egg" illustration (p. 12) adapted from *Natural Birth Control Made Simple* by B. Kass-Annese, RN, CNP, and H.C. Danzer, MD, Hunter House, 2003.

Library of Congress Cataloging-in-Publication Data
Raab, Diana, 1954–
Your high-risk pregnancy : a practical and supportive guide / Diana Raab,
with Errol Norwitz ; Norma Dvorsky, illustrator.
p. cm.
ISBN 978-0-89793-520-3 (pbk.)
1. Pregnancy—Complications. 2. Labor (Obstetrics)—Complications.
I. Norwitz, Errol R. II. Title.
RG571.R33 2009
618.2—dc22   2009024785

Project Credits

Cover Design: Amy King	Editorial Intern: Ashley Zeal
Book Production: John McKercher	Production Intern: Sara Hamling
Copy Editor: Mary Miller	Publicity Associate: Sean Harvey
Illustrator: Norma Dvorsky	Order Fulfillment: Washul Lakdhon
Proofreader: John David Marion	Administrator: Theresa Nelson
Indexer: Nancy D. Peterson	Computer Support: Peter Eichelberger
Editor: Alexandra Mummery	Rights Coordinator: Candace Groskreutz
Senior Marketing Associate: Reina Santana	
Customer Service Manager: Christina Sverdrup	
Publisher: Kiran S. Rana	

Printed and bound by Sheridan Books, Ann Arbor, Michigan

Manufactured in the United States of America

9 8 7 6 5 4 3 2 1   First Edition   09 10 11 12 13

Contents

Important Note

The material in this book is intended to provide a review of
resources and information related to high-risk pregnancies.
Every effort has been made to provide accurate and dependable
information. However, professionals in the field may have
differing opinions and change is always taking place. Any of
the treatments described herein should be undertaken only
under the guidance of a licensed health-care practitioner. The
authors, editors, and publishers cannot be held responsible
for any error, omission, professional disagreement, outdated
material, or adverse outcomes that derive from the use of any
of these treatments or information resources in this book,
either in a program of self-care or under the care of a licensed
practitioner.

Foreword

I will never forget my first delivery. I was nineteen years old, and it was the first day of my third year of medical school at the University of Cape Town. Even though I'd never seen a birth before, I'd made every effort to prepare myself for my first night on Labor and Delivery. I'd gone over my lecture notes and read a number of articles and textbooks, including a very readable and informative book I picked up in our local medical library called *Getting Pregnant & Staying Pregnant: Overcoming Infertility and High-Risk Pregnancy* by Diana Raab, RN, but no amount of reading could have prepared me for that first night.

I arrived for Labor and Delivery duty at 6:00 PM. Every delivery room was full, so women were also delivering on stretchers and chairs in the hallways. I soon discovered that this was just another night at Groote Schuur Hospital, whose labor unit is responsible for over thirty-three thousand deliveries each year. I was asked to go immediately to delivery room #3. An hour later, I emerged having assisted in the delivery of term breech-breech twins, supervised only by a nurse midwife. Over the next few years, much of the clinical obstetrics I learned was from midwives. Even today, when I get up at 3:00 AM to watch a chief resident help an intern take a medical student through a normal vaginal delivery (which probably could have happened safely at home), I still hear the midwives' voices in my head: "Errol, the best way to deliver a baby is with your hands in your pockets. Nature has been doing this well for thousands of years, so don't mess it up!"

Much has changed since I was a medical student. I have been fortunate to have trained and practiced in both obstetrics and gynecology and maternal-fetal medicine (high-risk pregnancy) at a number of outstanding institutions, including Oxford, Harvard, and Yale universities. My current clinical practice at Yale-New Haven Hospital is exclusively high-risk pregnancies. In my years of practice, the most important and rewarding development that I have witnessed has been the move away from paternalistic medicine (where the doctor or midwife knows best) to a partnership between the couple and their health-care provider.

Couples are no longer deferring their health-care decisions to their clinician, nor are they expected to do so. They are better informed, more engaged, and more involved in decision-making. The responsibility of the care provider now is to provide the couple with the most up-to-date information in a clear, objective, and nonjudgmental fashion that they can then use to make the best decision for themselves in a given situation. With this in mind, I was thrilled when Diana Raab asked if I would be willing to work with her to revise and update her book, with a particular focus on educating and supporting couples facing a high-risk pregnancy.

The term *high-risk pregnancy* is fraught with misconception. It conjures up images of women bleeding excessively during delivery or infants with disfiguring birth defects. Currently, one in five pregnancies is considered high-risk, and most of these pregnancies look very similar to low-risk pregnancies. *High-risk is not synonymous with a bad outcome.* Indeed, most women with a high-risk pregnancy have an uneventful course and a healthy baby. But a high-risk designation *does* mean that you need to be more vigilant, that you may need more frequent office visits, and that you may need to be referred to an obstetrician or maternal-fetal medicine specialist either for consultation or ongoing care.

Regardless of who follows your progress during your pregnancy, knowledge is power. It is the sincere hope of both Diana Raab and myself that the reader will find this book both informative and supportive. It is designed to help you determine whether or not your pregnancy is high-risk, to help you identify the most appropriate type of provider, and to point you toward important questions to ask your care provider. In this way, you can work alongside your care provider to optimize your pregnancy outcome, with the ultimate goal being a healthy mother and a healthy baby.

— Errol R. Norwitz, MD, PhD
Professor, Yale University School of Medicine
Co-Director, Division of Maternal-Fetal Medicine
Director, Maternal-Fetal Medicine Fellowship Program
Director, Obstetrics & Gynecology Residency Program

Acknowledgments

Anyone who has written a book understands the joy and despair that accompany the experience. It is an endeavor that demands an enormous amount of passion and devotion for both the subject and the art of writing. It is a task that dominates the author's life until the day of completion. In 2007, when my publisher, Kiran Rana, asked if I would be interested in updating my original manuscript in honor of the twenty-fifth anniversary of the first edition, called *Getting Pregnant and Staying Pregnant: Overcoming Infertility and High-Risk Pregnancy*, I had mixed emotions. I was honored by Kiran's request, and after all these years, I thought it would be wonderful to still have my book available to help women navigate through their high-risk pregnancies. I was thrilled to learn that there is still a demand for a book such as this one. It means that women continue to want to be both prepared and informed about what is happening to their bodies.

On the other hand, since the book's first edition, I have gone on to receive my MFA in writing, and my path has gone from primarily medical writing to the writing of a memoir, essays, and poetry. I have also become a journaling advocate and writing instructor.

I told Kiran I had to think about it and that the only way I would undertake such a project was if I could secure the assistance of a top-notch professional who works clinically with high-risk women. Because of the significant changes in medical science, I knew that I could not undertake this project alone. He urged me to do my research to find the right person to work with. Indeed, the Internet has made the world smaller, and because of it this book is possible.

Only moments after Googling an expert in high-risk pregnancies, Dr. Errol Norwitz's name came to the top of the list. Within hours, I contacted him and much to my surprise, he had heard of the original edition of this book and in fact it was on his bookshelf! Without any hesitation, he told me to e-mail him the details, and within a couple of days he embraced the idea of working on this project with me.

This is one of the highest acclaims a writer could ever receive. I wanted to give him a big hug, but because he was on the East Coast and I am on the West Coast, I thanked him deeply and hung up the phone. I stood both beaming and in shock that without any hesitation, he had agreed to undertake this enormous revision with me.

Since this book's first edition in the late 1980s, high-risk pregnancies have become much more common. As a result, I have decided to focus in this edition solely on difficult pregnancies and to omit the section on infertility.

As I mentioned in previous editions, a book of this kind is rarely, if ever, completed alone. Even though more than 60 percent of the book has been updated, the template and the core of the book is the same as the one first published in 1988. It is for this reason that I must continue to express gratitude to those who crossed my path back then, because their influence has ultimately affected its final form and led to its long-term success.

From the day this book was conceived more than twenty-five years ago, I owe much to many people who have offered their comments and criticism during the preparation of the original manuscript. In particular, I wish to acknowledge Andrew Mok, MD, for his dedicated commitment to being available when we needed him during all three of my difficult pregnancies and for his valuable review of the manuscript in its early stages.

Others whose assistance greatly contributed to this book are:

James E. Clark, MD; Hal C. Danzer, MD; Alan H. DeCherney, MD; Frederick Hoover, MD; George Huggins, MD; Pec Indman; Barbara Kass-Annese, RN, CNP; Mary Kostenbauder, MSN, RN; Ed Siegall, MD; and Diane Wind Wardell, PhD. Most importantly, I'd like to thank Barbara G. Ludman, MS, FNP-BC, for her enthusiastic spirit, insight, and expertise that helped bring this edition to fruition. I will be forever indebted to her.

and

Norma Dvorsky, whose creativity and amazing artwork made this book so unique, ever since its original publication in the 1980s. Her new illustrations in this edition bring a delightful tone and poignancy to the book.

As with any passage of time, we gain and lose friends. Since its original publication, I have lost three dear friends and I would like to honor them in this edition. They are gone, but never forgotten:

Barbara Provan, my dear friend who during my first pregnancy brought me lunch every day during my bed rest; my beloved nursing mentor, Lynda Percival Glickman, MSN, whose friendship I will miss forever; and Mehrnaz Sajedi, RD, who helped with the nutrition chapter and who left us much too early. May they all rest in peace.

and

Kiran Rana, my publisher, who twenty-five years ago recognized the intrinsic value of this book and has kept it in print all these years. A special thanks goes to Anita Levine-Goldberg, who prepared the revisions for the book's third edition. For this new book, I would also like to thank Barbara Moulton, the acquisitions editor; Alex Mummery, my editor at Hunter House; and Maggie Lang, my personal assistant, for her hard work and devotion. And of course, this edition would not have been possible without the dedication, medical input, and friendship of Errol Norwitz, MD, who in spite of a very busy schedule made time for our weekly phone calls to make this the most up-to-date book on the subject.

and

Last, but never least, Rachel (26), Regine (24), and Joshua (20), my children, who since the book's first edition have blossomed into three vivacious, hardworking, and loving young adults who are always interested in my work; my mother, Eva Klein Marquise, for her encouragement; my beloved father, Edward Marquise, for all his love and adoration; my husband's parents, Jeannine and Alexandre Raab, for their love and support throughout; and my grandparents, whom I wish my children could have known.

and

Most importantly, my husband, Simon, whose unrelenting love and support helped me survive three high-risk pregnancies and who stands by me in every way, during each one of my book projects.

— Diana M. Raab
Santa Barbara, CA, 2009

Introduction

The purpose of this book is to provide women, their partners, and concerned health-care professionals with a guide to difficult pregnancies. When the book was first released in the late 1980s, it was one of a kind. Today, many similar books are available. In addition, medical practice is continually changing, and by the time this book is actually published some of the information may be obsolete. It is for this reason that I urge you to check with your provider regarding any questions you may have.

My goal in each edition of this book has been to present sometimes complicated medical situations in a clear and concise manner, while trying to maintain a positive and supportive tone. I want the reader to be hopeful and optimistic about her outcome, just as I was. In addition, I hope that the anecdotes from other women will provide the much needed insight and courage to the couple experiencing a difficult pregnancy. The reader should never feel alone.

In this new edition, I focus less on infertility and more on the 20 to 30 percent of all pregnancies that fall into the high-risk category. To keep up with the times and to provide a more comprehensive overview of the pregnancy experience, I have also added some new chapters to replace the infertility chapters. These chapters are Chapter 1: Getting Pregnant; Chapter 2: Care During Your Pregnancy; Chapter 3: High-Risk Pregnancy: An Introduction; Chapter 10: Labor, Delivery, and Postpartum; and Chapter 13: Special Concerns During Pregnancy.

Furthermore, new subjects in already existing chapters also need to be addressed. These subjects include: conception via ART and IVF, the difference between a high-risk pregnancy and having high-risk factors, a month-by-month comprehensive of tests, a discussion on advanced-age pregnancy, eating disorders (obesity/anorexia), herbal and holistic care, travel and pregnancy, environmental toxins, choosing a provider, same-sex couples, single parenting, teenage pregnancy, rape/domestic violence, trauma during pregnancy, and circumcision.

Another valuable addition to this new millennium edition is the inclusion of journaling prompts at the end of each chapter. As a journaling advocate and instructor, I believe that it is important for women to chronicle their pregnancies, not only for themselves but for their children, who will one day enjoy reading what their mothers endured. For the high-risk mother, the exercise of writing can also be a cathartic one.

Appendices A and B have been completely updated and now also include Web addresses, something we did not have twenty-five years ago. The glossary is also updated to better explain medical and technical terms.

While sharing my professional knowledge is important, my goal is to offer personal encouragement and support. I have personally experienced the needs, the joys, the sorrows, the pains, and worst of all, the uncertainties of having a high-risk pregnancy. Even though all three of my pregnancies were difficult physically and emotionally, now that my eldest daughter has turned twenty-six, all of those problems seem insignificant, and I realize that every difficult moment I had to undergo for them to be born was something I would not have missed for anything in the world!

For those who are interested in knowing my inspiration for writing this book and the story behind my own pregnancy journey, I have summarized the key events below.

My Story

This book was born on a typewriter perched on a table built by my husband. That table was suspended above my expanding belly during my first pregnancy in 1983. It began as a written journey of my bed-rest experience. Over the course of a few years, my notes evolved to include information and anecdotes from other women also experiencing difficult pregnancies. Now, twenty-five years later, the book is an updated guide for women and their partners to help them navigate through their own high-risk pregnancy.

Even though I was a practicing nurse when I wrote the first edition, I was hungry for additional information. Friends and colleagues brought me books focusing on "normal" pregnancies, and I felt as if I did not fit into any of the categories described. I was not having a normal pregnancy. That was my impetus to write this book. My hope is that if women understand what is happening inside of them they will gain confidence in themselves, what they are going through, and the decisions they make. Many of the women interviewed for the anecdotes told me that my book had taken the mystery out of their problems. Often, our imagination is much worse than reality.

High-risk pregnancies are not fun. They seem to drag on forever. By sharing my story with you, I hope to help you see the light at the end of your tunnel. Today, my husband and I have three healthy children, two daughters and a son—the happy ending to our story. But reaching this point was far from easy.

My husband and I are both career professionals and worked for five years after we got married before deciding to start a family. Pregnancy was not an easy task for us. It took me over a year to become pregnant. When I found out I was pregnant I was ecstatic, and just like many inexperienced mothers-to-be, I saw no harm in spreading the good news. Within the first two months I was dressing in maternity clothes. Unfortunately, my enthusiasm was shattered by a miscarriage at only twelve weeks.

My obstetrician was away the weekend I miscarried and was very surprised the following Monday morning when I told him the news. It was all the more shocking for us because on the previous Friday, we had heard the baby's heartbeat during my routine prenatal visit and everything seemed perfect.

It took me a very long time to accept our loss, and I found it particularly difficult when I saw other women with their children. It seemed like a constant reminder of my failure. Over the next few months, the cause of my miscarriage was investigated. My first test, a hysterosalpingogram, showed I had a congenital uterine abnormality and a cervical condition, which meant that without proper intervention, I would be unable to carry a baby to term.

I learned that because of these congenital problems, the only way I would be able to carry a baby to term was to have major surgery. Perhaps because I was a nurse, I was afraid to have the surgery. I was aware of all the things that could possibly go wrong. I urged my obstetrician to take the most conservative approach. He told me that surgery was the only solution, and that if I were his wife, he would make the same recommendation.

We sought a second opinion from an obstetrician specializing in this type of surgery. He also recommended surgery. I was still uncomfortable with the idea, and so we sought yet another opinion. The third obstetrician had a different philosophy, one closer to mine. He claimed that with each pregnancy my double uterus would become stretched and I would be able to carry a fetus longer each time until I eventually carried to term. I already knew that I would have to have a cervical suture early in my pregnancy to solve the problem of my incompetent cervix (a.k.a incompetent cervix, cervical insufficiency).

Nine months later I received a positive pregnancy test, but I had problems right from the beginning. Around my sixth week I began spotting. Because it was the weekend (somehow all my problems occurred on holidays or weekends), we went to my hospital's emergency room and were told that there are two possible reasons for spotting early in pregnancy—impending miscarriage or low progesterone levels.

Because of my history of hormonal imbalances, it was decided that I needed two progesterone injections spaced two weeks apart. My obstetrician said that if the spotting were indeed due to a defective egg, I would abort during that two-week period. Luckily, that did not happen.

At twelve weeks, I was given a cervical suture to ensure that I would be able to carry my baby. I remained in the hospital for three days and was sent home on a medication intended to prevent premature contractions, which could have put the suture under stress. I took these pills for the remainder of my pregnancy.

Unfortunately, because the sutures were inserted after my cervix had begun dilating, I had to stay in bed for five months. I was tempted to write to Sophia Loren, who underwent the same ordeal. Because I really wanted that baby, I did everything my obstetrician recommended. I was advised not to climb stairs, and as a result, I had to stay on the upper level of our two-story home.

Each day was full of surprises. I had mild contractions a few times each day and visited the emergency room, as it turned out, once a month for the next five months. I spotted throughout the pregnancy and was told that my suture was being stressed and to take it easy. I never knew how long I would carry my baby. In my husband's words, "Every day was another blessing." It is impossible to describe the paradoxical passage of time—those days in bed that passed so quickly, yet also seemed to drag on for an eternity. I cannot begin to catalogue my emotions, which seemed to ricochet off the bedroom walls for those five long months.

Finally, at thirty-two weeks, approximately four weeks short of what is known as the term of pregnancy, I gave birth by cesarean to a beautiful 4½-pound baby girl. Although she did not cry at birth and was completely blue, it was the happiest moment of my life. Her first few moments of oxygen support were enough to give her the strength to carry on a life of her own.

The next happiest day of my life was two years later to the day, when I gave birth again, this time to a perfect 8-pound girl, Regine. She nursed right away and unlike my first, Rachel, who was a preemie, she did everything the books said she would do. This second pregnancy was much easier, partly because I knew what to expect. My husband and I breathed a sigh of relief, knowing that this baby was not premature—she was born both healthy and strong.

And at last, three years later, I gave birth to my son, Joshua. His was an easier pregnancy. I was much more active and confident that all would go well—and it did, as Joshua also did everything the books said he would do. I was now a proud parent of three children under the age of six and I vowed to look at the beauty and magic of bringing babies into the world and watching them grow into fine individuals.

Getting Pregnant

A grand adventure is about to begin. — Winnie the Pooh

Before discussing how pregnancy actually occurs and how many things must go right, it is important to provide a brief overview of both the female and male reproductive systems.

The Female Reproductive System

The female reproductive system is designed to carry out several functions. It produces female egg cells necessary for reproduction and transports the ova for fertilization in the uterus where the baby has a safe place to grow. Unlike the male reproductive system, which is primarily external, the female reproductive system is located entirely in the pelvis and is comprised of both internal and external organs.

The External Anatomy

When looking at the female external reproductive system (see Figure 1.1 on the next page), there is the vulva, which is a term that includes all the visible sexual parts. There are two sets of folds that protect the vagina— the labia majora (outer folds) and the labia minora (inner folds). When the folds are spread apart, there is the clitoris, urethra, vaginal opening, and two pairs of lubricating glands.

Labia Majora: These outer skin folds contain sebaceous glands that produce sweat and oil around the hair follicles that usually begin appearing in puberty. They also serve as a protective "door" to prevent infection and disease from entering the vagina and other internal organs. For some women, the color of this skin is darker than the inner folds, the labia minora.

Labia Minora: These inner skin folds are exposed when the labia majora are pulled back. They have no pubic hair and fold directly over the vagina. They are very sensitive to touch. During sexual arousal, the veins of

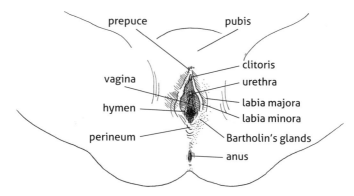

Figure 1.1: The external female reproductive anatomy

the labia minora become darker and constrict as they grip the penis. This is perhaps nature's way of keeping the male's semen inside.

The labia minora also secretes a white lubricant called smegma that should be washed away daily. The actual size of both labia can vary; they tend to become larger and more stretched out with childbirth.

The clitoris lies at the upper portion of the genitals where both skin folds meet. It is the most sensitive spot in the entire genital area and is highly erotic. The clitoris is comparable to the male penis in terms of its ability to enlarge with sexual excitement. Its size and shape may vary, and it may expand from ¾ inch to 1½ inches during sexual excitement.

Urethra: This is the tube, or duct, that carries urine from the bladder to the outside of the body. The tube is much shorter in women (about 1½ inches) than in men, and this is why women are more prone to urinary tract infections. Because the urethra is so close to the vagina, it is common for it to become irritated from prolonged or vigorous intercourse. Some women may feel discomfort during urination after intercourse. This may be alleviated by drinking one or two glasses of water before and after intercourse.

Lubricating Glands: Two ducts, known as Skene's glands, are located on either side of the urethra. During sexual arousal these glands secrete a lubricating fluid. Another set of glands, called Bartholin's glands, is located under the labia majora. If there is any infection in the vulva it will be easily transmitted to the glands and cause an inflammation, which sometimes may cause the gland to swell to the size of a golf ball. If the gland becomes infected with bacteria, a cyst may develop that will have to be removed. This is a common spot for the gonorrhea germ to thrive.

The Internal Anatomy

The vagina is a muscular canal lined with mucus membranes extending from the vulva to the uterus, and it is sometimes referred to as the birth canal (see Figure 1.2). It has many functions. It serves as the passage for menstrual flow, guides the penis, holds the semen near the cervix, and functions as the birth canal.

The vagina is usually 4 to 5 inches in length and very flexible. However, with age, sexual activity, and childbirth it tends to lose a lot of this flexibility. It secretes an odorless and watery discharge, sometimes clear and sometimes white. This lubricates the vaginal canal, keeps it clean, and helps maintain a slightly acidic environment to prevent infections. Some women find that their vagina may become very dry or very wet. Drier times usually occur before puberty, during breast-feeding, after menstruation, and after menopause. Wetter times occur during ovulation, during pregnancy, and during sexual arousal.

In young girls, the entrance to the vagina is partially closed off by the hymen. Hymens come in different sizes and shapes, and for some women they stretch easily. The first time the hymen is stretched by sexual activity, little folds of hymen tissue will remain around the vaginal opening. Occasionally these are large and may have to be surgically removed for comfort.

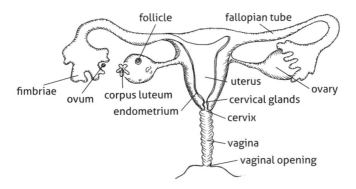

Figure 1.2: The internal female reproductive anatomy

Pelvic Floor Muscles: When you try to hold back your urine, you are contracting the pelvic floor muscles. These muscles also serve to hold the pelvic organs in place and provide support for your other organs. If these muscles are weak, you may have trouble reaching orgasm and controlling the flow of your urine (urinary incontinence).

Anus: This is the opening of the rectum, or large intestines, leading to the outside of the body. The skin around the anus is very smooth, but sometimes external hemorrhoids (small varicose veins) develop after childbirth. It is important to keep the anus clean and to wipe from front to back to avoid transporting fecal matter from the anus into the vagina.

Cervix: This small rounded opening, about 1½ inches across, separates the vagina from the uterus, or womb. It is sensitive to pressure, though it has no nerve endings. Discomfort during intercourse is usually due to the penis hitting the cervix, which pushes against the uterus. The cervix changes position, color, and shape during puberty, the menstrual cycle, sexual excitement, and menopause. No tampon, finger, or penis can go through it, although it is capable of incredible expansion during labor and delivery.

The cervix plays a vital role in fertility. To prevent the entry of foreign matter, the cervix is blocked by a plug of mucus, and it is this plug that is vital in fertility. During ovulation, when the egg is released from the ovary into the fallopian tube, the mucus thins to allow sperm to swim past and reach the uterus. When the cervix is not healthy because of disease or injury, it is unable to control the quality and quantity of mucus, and this can affect fertility.

The uterus or womb is a flat, pear-shaped organ suspended in the pelvic cavity by strong bands of ligaments. When you are not pregnant, your uterus is about the size of a fist. It has very thick muscular walls, some of the most powerful ones in the body. The top of the uterus is called the fundus and is the most contractile portion of the uterus. The uterine muscles are strongly influenced by hormones. During menstruation, the uterine contractions are strong, and they are, of course, even stronger during childbirth.

Each month, the inner layer of the uterus is shed during menstruation, unless of course you are pregnant! If pregnancy does occur, the embryo implants itself on the inner wall of the uterus (endometrium), which becomes a bed for the placenta.

The fallopian tubes, sometimes called oviducts or "egg tubes," extend outward and back from both sides of the upper end of the uterus (see Figure 1.3). They are about 4 inches long and look like ram's horns facing backward. Inside, the tubes are lined with brushlike tips called cilia, which propel the egg forward.

Each fallopian tube ends in the fimbria (see Figure 1.3), which are fingerlike extensions composed of many separate petals, each one a slightly different length and usually hanging down toward the ovary.

The fimbria are vital in transporting the egg from the ovary to the fallopian tube. There are various theories about how this occurs. One theory is that the egg drops onto one petal of the fimbria, which are covered with cilia cells that curl toward the inside of the tube. Another theory is that the fimbria sweep across the surface of the ovary and set up currents that wave the egg into the tube. In rare cases, when the egg is not "caught" by the tube, it may become fertilized outside the tube, resulting in an abdominal pregnancy.

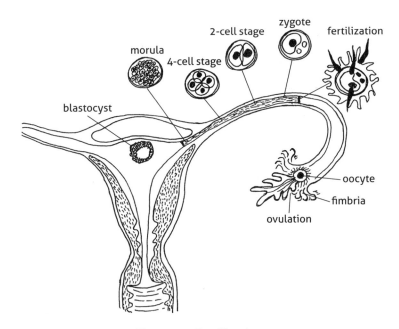

Figure 1.3: Fertilization

The fallopian tubes must be in optimum condition for fertilization to occur. They are extremely delicate, and this is why they are a major site of fertility problems.

The ovaries are two organs about the size and shape of unshelled almonds, located on either side of and somewhat below the uterus. This puts them about four or five inches below your waist. They are held in place by connective tissue and are protected by a surrounding mass of fat.

Ovaries have two functions: to produce germ cells (eggs) and to produce female sex hormones (estrogen, progesterone, and other hormones). When a baby girl is born, her ovaries contain about four hundred thousand immature ova; about four hundred of these will develop into mature eggs.

If for any reason a woman loses one ovary, the remaining ovary takes over the entire workload. This means it must produce one egg each month and double its hormone production. Ovarian disorders are also a common cause of infertility.

The Menstrual Cycle

Puberty is the time in a young girl's life when her reproductive organs mature. In general, puberty lasts about one and a half years, during which time the ovaries produce increasing amounts of the female sex hormone estrogen. This hormone is responsible for the female sex characteristics, such as breasts and body contours. It is also responsible for the uterus's development and helping the eggs to mature. Progesterone is also secreted and is responsible for the growth of pubic hair and the new intensity of erotic desire.

In combination, estrogen and progesterone cause the uterine lining to thicken and prepare for egg implantation—pregnancy (see Figure 1.4 on the next page). If pregnancy does not occur, the follicle dies, the progesterone level drops, and the uterine lining sheds. This shedding of the uterine lining is menstruation.

Menstruation usually begins between the ages of ten and sixteen. At this time, the girl is physically capable of becoming pregnant. The usual amount of menstrual flow amounts to about four to six tablespoons of vaginal and cervical secretions, tissues, and blood. The length of time for each menses varies from a few days to a week. In the beginning,

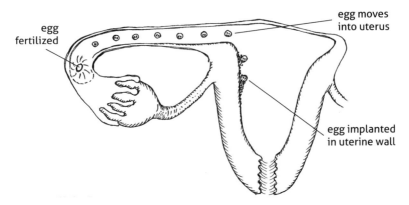

Figure 1.4: Fertilization and implantation of the egg

menstrual periods are very irregular while the body's hormones develop a pattern. After the first year or two, a pattern develops; some women may have a twenty-six–day cycle, while others may have a thirty-two–day cycle. Usually, the length of a woman's cycle remains the same, although this may be altered by stress, illness, a change in altitude, and so on.

The menstrual cycle has four phases: the bleeding phase—menstruation; the proliferative phase—the body prepares itself for pregnancy; the ovulation phase—the release of a ripe egg from the ovary; and the secretory phase—the secretion of progesterone and estrogen, which lasts for about fourteen days.

The growth and release of the egg and the growth and shedding of the endometrium are controlled by hormones. Understanding how hormones control fertility is important in understanding how fertility drugs help women to become pregnant.

The Male Reproductive System

The purpose of the male reproductive system is to produce sperm, to release sperm into the female during sex, and to produce and secrete male sex hormones. The male reproductive organs are located inside and outside the pelvis and include the penis, testicles, scrotum, glands, and ducts.

The External Anatomy

The penis has two functions: to provide an outside port for urination and to provide a means to move the sperm from the testes out of the penis into the vagina. The penis contains three cylinders of tissue surrounded by a tough fibrous covering. During sexual excitement, these tissues become engorged with blood, causing the penis to expand and become hard and erect. The most sensitive part of the penis is around the head, especially around the ridge that connects it to the shaft. During ejaculation, semen spurts out from the urethral opening at the tip of the penis.

The exact size of the penis is inherited. Large and small penises tend to run in families. Studies have shown that the size of the penis in no way affects sexual ability.

Some men are circumcised—the foreskin surrounding the penis (see Figure 1.5) is removed—while others are not. At one time, circumcision was done mainly for religious and/or cultural reasons, but over the years many have advocated the procedure for both hygienic and medical reasons. Some claim that the foreskin is a haven for bacteria, especially if proper hygiene is not practiced. If the circumcision is done at birth, it involves taking the fold of tissue (foreskin) over the tip of the penis and pulling, clamping, and cutting it. The incision is covered with antiseptic gauze and usually heals within ten days. The need for circumcision remains a matter of controversy.

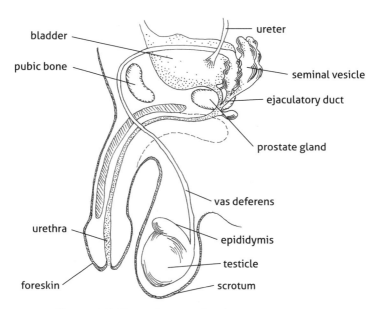

Figure 1.5: The male reproductive anatomy

Scrotum and Testicles: The scrotal sacs are located on both sides of the penis. Each protective sac contains one testicle, which is about 2 inches long and 1 inch in diameter. The primary functions of the testicles include the production of testosterone (male hormone) and the production of sperm. This is why it is important that the testicles remain free from injury. During sports or strenuous activities, it is recommended that men wear a jockstrap to provide the needed protection.

Perhaps nature's way of maximizing sperm production was to place the testes outside the body. To produce sperm, the testes prefer a cooler temperature. For some, fertility may increase in warmer weather, because when it is warm the muscles holding the testes relax and let the testicles drop away from the body. On the other hand, in colder climates the scrotal muscles contract and tend to bring the testes closer to the body.

The Internal Anatomy

The internal organs of the male reproductive system are sometimes referred to as the accessory organs and they include the epididymis, vas deferens, seminal vesicles, and prostate gland.

Epididymis: This long, hollow, and coiled structure is located just above the testicles, where sperm mature and are stored. The journey of the sperm through the epididymis takes three to twelve days, and by the end of the journey the sperm are completely matured. Mature sperm use the tail of the epididymis as a holding tank, and may remain here for as long as one month. Not all of the sperm will live that long, however, and a man who ejaculates only once a month may have a high concentration of dead sperm and therefore a lower fertility rate. The epididymis is prone to infections, such as chlamydia, which can cause scarring and thus block sperm passage through the epididymis.

The spermatic cord is comprised of the vas deferens and a network of veins and arteries.

Vas Deferens: These sperm ducts are two firm tubes that extend from the epididymis to the prostate. Mature sperm enter the vas deferens and are gently squeezed along by the tube's pulsating walls. The sperm travel through these tubes and are stored at their upper ends until they mix with the seminal fluid—secretions from the seminal vesicles and prostate—just prior to ejaculation.

The combination of seminal fluid (98 percent) and sperm (2 percent) make up the semen, or ejaculate.

Seminal Vesicles: These two glands store the sperm and contribute fluid to the ejaculate, secreting more than half of the ejaculate.

Prostate Gland: The prostate gland is slightly larger than a walnut. It surrounds the urethra and is located just below the urinary bladder. It secrets an important chemical that causes the semen to liquefy. The secretions from the prostate comprise most of the seminal fluid or ejaculate, and give the ejaculate its characteristic whitish color. This gland sometimes enlarges later in life, which may cause problems with urination. This can be detected by a physician during a rectal exam.

Cowper's glands are two tiny glands located just below and in front of the prostate gland. They secrete a small amount of clear, sticky fluid that holds the sperm together and is sometimes visible prior to ejaculation. This fluid sometimes contains sperm; which is why withdrawal from the vagina just prior to ejaculation is not a reliable means of birth control.

The urethra is the major channel of transport for both urine and sperm. It is a tube that runs from the bladder and down through the prostate gland where the ejaculatory duct empties into it, ending at the slit at the end of the penis. Both urine and seminal fluid travel through the urethra, but never at the same time. The body has an elaborate way of engaging the muscle that blocks urine flow during an erection.

Sperm Production (Spermatogenesis)

Sperm are not born—they are made. The process of spermatogenesis is coordinated by hormones produced by the testes and the hypothalamus, which is located above the pituitary gland. The hypothalamus initiates the process by releasing GnRH hormone to the pituitary, which secretes FSH and LH. These hormones encourage the release of testosterone.

The germ cells in the testes begin to mature and develop tails and are now capable of fertilizing an egg. For anywhere from ten to fourteen days, they are moved through the epididymis.

Ejaculation

Each man releases, on the average, 60 million or more sperm into the vagina with each ejaculation, each one carrying the necessary genetic information for the formation of a new person. Studies have shown that nearly 90 percent of these sperm are killed by vaginal secretions.

If intercourse occurs and the conditions are optimal, then within the next twelve to twenty-four hours the surviving sperm can swim through the cervical opening on their way to the uterus. Only a few hundred may actually reach the uterus, and many may go up the wrong fallopian tube. In the best situation, the union of the sperm and the egg occurs within thirty-five minutes of the time of ejaculation. If ovulation does not occur, some sperm may continue to live in niches inside the fallopian tubes and wait for the egg, which may or may not come. Many specialists claim that sperm can live under these conditions for as long as seventy-two hours, possibly longer.

How Pregnancy Occurs

Each month during the woman's reproductive years, about ten to twenty ovarian follicles (small sacs, each containing an egg) begin maturing under the influence of hormones such as FSH (follicle-stimulating hormone), which is produced by the pituitary gland in the brain in the early phase of the monthly cycle. Usually only one follicle develops fully to release a mature ovum ready for fertilization; the others degenerate.

A few days before the follicle has reached its maximum size, it secretes a large quantity of estrogen. This increased level of estrogen stimulates the cervix to produce a thinner mucus, which allows the sperm to enter the uterus. At the same time, this elevated estrogen stimulates the pituitary gland to release another hormone called LH (luteinizing hormone). The release of this hormone stimulates ovulation.

The follicle with the mature egg moves toward the surface of the ovary. At ovulation, the follicle disintegrates and the egg flows out. Some women may feel a twinge or cramp in the lower abdomen at this time.

The egg normally proceeds through the fallopian tubes, where fertilization occurs if sperm are present. If fertilization occurs, the fertilized egg travels down the fallopian tube for implantation in the uterus. The lining of the uterus must be both healthy and ready for implantation, and the body's hormones must be at an optimal balance for pregnancy to occur. In other words, the woman's body must be prepared for the pregnancy. There must also be both a healthy egg and a healthy sperm. If the egg is not fertilized, it is absorbed by the body and disappears, and menstruation begins.

Timing is very important for pregnancy to occur. It is important for the couple to have sex at the appropriate time in the menstrual cycle. Believe it or not, there are about 5 days each month when a fertile woman may become pregnant—the day she ovulates, about 3 days before, and 1 day after. In a 28-day menstrual cycle, ovulation usually occurs between day 14 and day 16. Regardless of the length of your cycle, if ovulation occurs, it will do so about 14 days before menstruation begins. For example, if you get your menses every 32 days, you will ovulate between day 16 and day 20 of that cycle.

After the egg leaves the ovary, it lives for about twenty-four hours. Sperm live in your reproductive system for about 3 days after intercourse. If ovulation occurs within that period of time, you may become pregnant.

Once fertilization occurs, the egg, barely visible to the naked eye, floats freely in the uterus. It then begins to implant itself in the uterine wall to grow and develop. The fertilized egg is called an embryo at first and later on in pregnancy is called a fetus.

Eggs carry genetic information called chromosomes. These twenty-three pairs of chromosomes, combined with the twenty-three pairs from the sperm, create the potential for a new person. The chromosomes carried by the female are called the X chromosomes and those carried by the male are called the Y chromosomes. If the embryo is XX, it will be a female; if it is XY, it will be a male. This is why people claim that it is the male who determines the sex of the child.

On an average, nine out of ten couples will get pregnant within a year of unprotected intercourse and one out of ten couples who do not have an underlying medical problem will take longer than a year to get pregnant.

If a woman is having difficulty getting pregnant, she should discuss this with her doctor. The doctor might recommend she take her basal body temperature (BBT) each day. The basal metabolic temperature is taken first thing in the morning, before getting up. It provides the information that helps determine if you are ovulating. A special thermometer may be purchased, which has an easy-to-read scale. These thermometers usually come with graph paper or sometimes specialists will give you a special chart.

Progesterone is the hormone responsible for an increase in your temperature, and it is released into your bloodstream only after you ovulate. In about 25 to 50 percent of women with normal ovulation, their BBT decreases slightly at ovulation and then rises as the progesterone levels increase. The rise may be indicated as a jump of about six-tenths of a degree (six lines on your graph).

If you are having difficulty becoming pregnant, your specialist may also suggest you use a LH dipstick to detect when ovulation occurs. These kits predict the day of ovulation based on urine samples. Some of these kits include Answer Ovulation Test, Clearplan Easy Ovulation Predictor (sometimes called Clearblue or Clear Plan Easy Ovulation Predictor), and First Response Ovulation Predictor Test. (Many of these kits are available on www.drugstore.com.)

Others that are now available include Answer Quick & Simple One Step Ovulation 7-Day Test Kit, Accu-Clear Ovulation Predictor, 5-Day Test Kit, and Early Detect Ovulation Home Test Kit. These urine tests measure the hormone LH in your urine, which reaches a high level in your bloodstream and urine about 24 hours prior to ovulation. If you do the urine dipstick each morning, the test will be negative until the day of your LH surge. If you do the test a day or two later, it will be negative. Ovulation should occur 36 to 46 hours after the LH starts to increase and about 24 hours after it reaches its peak. This method helps you pinpoint the day before ovulation, which will help you determine when you ovulate.

Before purchasing your kit, it is a good idea to find out when the urine sample should be collected. Some tests require a midday collection, which could be inconvenient for working women.

There are also now some saliva tests available. A couple of the more commonly used ones are Fertile-Focus Saliva Ovulation Fertility Test and Maybe MOM Mini-Ovulation Microscope.

Tips on Using Ovulation Predictors at Home

- Have all materials ready before beginning the test.
- Follow the directions on the label exactly as they are written.
- Do the test at the same time each day in the same room with the same lighting.
- Do not drink large quantities of water prior to the test (water dilutes urine and affects test results).
- Tell your physician about any medications you are taking (test results may be altered by certain medications).
- Do not use any contraceptives.
- Look for the first noticeable change in color, not the darkest.
- Remember that not all women ovulate each month.
- If you have any questions, ask your pharmacist or physician, or call the toll-free number included with your testing kit.

Assisted Reproductive Technologies (ART)

In spite of the techniques mentioned above, you still might have difficulty becoming pregnant. Do not despair, there are other modalities that might help you. Since this book's first edition, these techniques have been refined but still primarily include four methods: ovulation stimulation, artificial insemination (AI), in vitro insemination (IVF), and preimplantation genetic diagnosis (PGD).

Ovulation Stimulation: Your specialist will be able to easily identify ovulation problems by examining your temperature charts. If your temperature charts indicate that you are not ovulating, chances are you will be prescribed a fertility drug. Fertility drugs such as Clomid (clomiphene) stimulate the ovaries to produce eggs. It is a synthetic drug that signals the pituitary gland to produce hormones that stimulate ovulation. It is used when the woman's ovaries and hormonal networks are capable of working well, but simply need some "revving up." Even if the woman is menstruating regularly, Clomid helps develop follicles that are not reaching their normal size and helps immature follicles grow to maturity. Taking Clomid will increase your chance of having a multiple pregnancy.

Other medications used to stimulate ovulation include purified FSH, which is seen in medications such as Gonal-F and Perganol. Both Clomid and purified FSH injections may be used alone or in combination with other modalities such as intrauterine insemination (AI).

Artificial Insemination (AI): Artificial insemination (AI) is used primarily if there is a problem of male fertility whereby the sperm is borderline fertile, and if there has been little or no success after various attempts to increase the sperm count. It may also be recommended in certain cases of unexplained infertility or if the cervical mucus is hostile to sperm. The procedure involves the sperm being pushed through a catheter and deposited just outside or inside the cervix. The procedure is best timed to coincide with ovulation, which is detected through basal body temperature charts and changes in cervical mucus production. Sometimes fertility drugs such as Clomid will be used in conjunction with this alternative so that the actual time of ovulation is more predictable.

In Vitro Fertilization (IVF): In vitro fertilization (IVF), or the creation of "test-tube babies," is usually recommended when a woman has damaged or blocked fallopian tubes or severe pelvic adhesions. It may also be recommended for women with endometriosis or if her partner has infertility issues. This technique has been used more frequently, particularly with the advanced-age mother.

Basically, in vitro fertilization is a five-step process:

1. Monitor and stimulate the development of healthy eggs by taking Clomid.

2. Collect the eggs in a test tube.

3. Collect the sperm.

4. Combine the eggs and sperm together in the laboratory by providing an ideal environment for the embryo development.

5. Transfer the embryo into the uterus (usually two to three days after egg retrieval).

Preimplantation Genetic Diagnosis (PGD): Preimplantation genetic diagnosis, or embryo screening, is used to identify healthy embryos without genetic defects created through IVF prior to their implantation into the uterus. The primary advantage of this procedure is to avoid the difficult decision to have selective pregnancy termination of an abnormal embryo.

PGD might be suggested when one or both parents has a known genetic abnormality. This technique provides an early alternative to prenatal testings, such as amniocentesis or chorionic villus sampling (see page 177). Currently, this is the only technique available to those who want to avoid the risk of having a child with a genetic disorder. After the diagnostic test is performed, the healthy embryos are transferred to the uterus for implantation.

Getting Pregnant When Older

The current social trend is for women to wait longer than women did in previous generations before starting their families. When the couple finally decides to have children, it may be some time before they become pregnant. This is because most women are at their reproductive peak between the ages of twenty and twenty-five. As we get older, our reproductive system undergoes physiological changes that may affect fertility. In general, there is a reduction in the number of eggs that are capable of forming a viable embryo. The follicles that do ovulate may be less hardy than they were when the woman was in her twenties.

As a result, most women over the age of thirty-five have fewer viable eggs and may even ovulate less often. In addition, the incidence of endometriosis increases as women get older. Some clinicians suggest that women over the age of thirty-five have a blood test to check their levels of follicle-stimulating hormone (FSH). Performed on the second or third day of a woman's cycle, this test determines whether or not her eggs are still fertile.

Approximately four million American women have babies each year. Even though most are in their twenties and thirties, the number of pregnancies in those over the age of thirty-five has increased to more than 40 percent. In general, women have decided to wait longer to start families, either because they are pursuing educational or career goals or because they are getting married later.

One study that examined the experience of a first pregnancy after the age of thirty-five found that women in that age group want to find the "right time" to become pregnant. Having developed a career and attaining a certain amount of financial security gives women a sense of accomplishment before setting out on the road to motherhood.

Fertility rates tend to decline with age; therefore, the chance of conceiving decreases the longer a woman waits. For the most part, the quantity and quality of the eggs decline as we age. There are also hormone-related changes that could result in a delayed positive pregnancy test. If you are trying to get pregnant in your mid-thirties, studies show that your fertility rate could fall as much as between 25 and 50 percent. Concurrently, if you are trying to get pregnant in your mid-forties, your fertility rate may decrease as much as 95 percent.

In addition to taking longer to become pregnant, many professionals believe that being over the age of thirty-five places a woman in a high-risk category. Although there are certain exceptions, viewing the thirty-five-years-and-over category in this way simply alerts professionals that problems may occur.

Women who become pregnant after the age of thirty-five also tend to view pregnancy differently. They may be highly conscious about their pregnancy. Their mature outlook and experience have a definite positive effect on their pregnancy. According to Dr. George Huggins of Francis Scott Key Medical Center in Baltimore, "Today, the female consumer is much more savvy than she was years ago; most of those I see over the age of thirty-five have been very prepared for pregnancy. In addition, the thirty-seven-year-old, for example, is much more attuned, in contrast to the average twenty-year-old, who subconsciously makes the assumption that all will be well."

Studies indicate that mature mothers have a higher probability of having numerous health problems that may complicate their pregnancy. For example, a first-time mother over the age of thirty-five has a greater risk of pregnancy-related problems such as preeclampsia, labor difficulties, and genetic defects, such as Down syndrome (see Chapter 6).

If you have any preexisting medical problems, it is a good idea to alert your physician prior to your becoming pregnant. Decide with him or her what extra precautions, if any, you will need to take. Amniocentesis is sometimes recommended if you are over the age of thirty-five. If you would like to have this test and your physician does not mention it, you should ask. Chances are that your pregnancy will be uneventful, but it is a good idea to discuss any concerns you may have with your provider.

Fertility problems are not restricted to women. As men age, they may also be prone to decreased fertility. As a man gets older, his sperm might become slower to perform all the tasks necessary to survive the fertilization process. Some studies have also shown that smoking and some medications can possibly affect male fertility.

Conception Basics

Once you decide that you want to get pregnant, you should first stop all birth control and begin timed intercourse.

If you are using an intrauterine device (IUD) or oral contraceptive pill (OCP), you need to wait until they are removed or stopped before you can get pregnant. Typically, women ovulate fourteen days before their next menstrual cycle and fertilization occurs within twenty-four to forty-eight hours of ovulation, so that is why it is important for intercourse to be properly timed.

If your periods are irregular, you can find out when you are ovulating by following your basal body temperature. This is a less expensive way to monitor your ovulation. If money is not an issue, you might want to try the urinary LH kits to detect ovulation.

According to a workshop given by Dr. Norwitz on obesity during pregnancy, if you are trying to get pregnant and have had gastric bypass surgery, you should make sure to tell your physician. Sometimes this type of surgery may be associated with deficiencies in iron, vitamin B-12, folate, and calcium. Your physician may want to prescribe vitamin supplements prior to your becoming pregnant. Those women who are not attempting conception should be counseled about suitable contraception.

Preconception Counseling

Some women who are trying to become pregnant will choose to discuss their plans with their provider. If you already have a preexisting medical condition, such as diabetes, high blood pressure, kidney disease, lupus, or any other problem that might place you in the high-risk category, it is particularly important to meet with your physician before trying to get pregnant. During this meeting, your physician might suggest you set up an appointment with another provider who specializes in your type of condition.

Studies have shown that controlling any preexisting medical problem will result in the best pregnancy outcome. Your provider should discuss any medications you are taking. Some medications, such as those for thyroid problems, are important for you to continue taking for the duration of your pregnancy. Some providers might recommend that you stay off certain medications for three to six months before trying to conceive, so that your body can adapt to the change before the pregnancy. If this is not possible, some providers might recommend that early in pregnancy you wean off some medications. In other cases, they might recommend you stop taking a medication. For example, if you are taking an epileptic medication and have not had a seizure in a few years, your physician might decide to discontinue your medication and monitor the results.

It is also a good idea to discuss vaccinations. Most physicians will recommend that you get a flu shot at least one month before trying to get pregnant. In fact, the Centers for Disease Control and Prevention (CDC) now recommends that every pregnant woman receive a flu shot. In addition, most specialists will recommend that you avoid alcohol and live-attenuated vaccines, such as MMR or varicella, for at least one month before trying to conceive. Many providers suggest you start taking a supplement of folic acid three months before conception, if possible.

During your initial visit, your physician will mention the frequency of your prenatal visits. If you have just moved or plan on moving, it is a good idea to obtain copies of all your medical records so that you can present them to your new physician.

Tips on Promoting a Healthy Pregnancy

- Maintain a healthy weight and diet.
- Take 4 mg of folic acid every day.
- Avoid cigarettes, alcohol, and illicit drug use.
- Get the proper immunizations.
- Start early prenatal care.

Family Balancing (Sex Determination)

The male chromosome is the Y and the female is the X. To have a boy, there must be an X and a Y chromosome. To have a girl, two X chromosomes are united. Under ideal conditions, the male-producing, or Y sperm, have been identified as being smaller and often faster than the female-producing, or X sperm. The X sperm are also more resistant to various types of stress.

For centuries, people have used superstitions to predict the sex of an unborn child or have offered suggestions on how to predetermine the baby's sex.

Today, there are both medical and personal reasons why couples may want to choose the sex of their child. From a medical standpoint, they might want to avoid a rare genetic disorder manifested only in male infants. These are known as X-linked recessive disorders and include muscular dystrophy and hemophilia. In these instances, a male infant has a 50 percent chance of being affected by the disease, whereas a female infant has a 50 percent chance of being a carrier. However, for the most part, there is really no way to guarantee a female infant.

For those who have had infertility problems, the sex of their child may be irrelevant—a baby is what they want. But others believe that as long as the technology is available, why not use it?

The idea of family balancing or sex determination has always stirred a great deal of controversy. Dr. Roberta Steinbacher, a social psychologist, conducted a study at Cleveland State University and found that if a proven technique were available, about 25 percent of couples would take advantage of it. In the same study, 91 percent of the women and 94 percent of the men said they would prefer their firstborn to be a boy. Others say that sex selection would decrease population growth because couples often have more children than they want while trying to conceive the sex of their choice.

Several hundred children have been born in the United States using family balancing technology. There are two ways to choose the sex of your child. The first way is practiced by couples at home and the second way is performed in the confines of the laboratory.

Laboratory-Based Techniques

A number of techniques have been developed to "enrich" a woman's chances of conceiving the sex of choice. Typically, these methods improve the chances from a 51 percent chance of having a male child and 49 percent of having a female child to 80 percent for the desired gender.

Laboratory techniques for family balancing utilize the difference between the X and Y sperm. They are based on the separation of male- and female-producing sperm in the laboratory to produce the sex of choice. Typically, the male's semen is washed in a tissue medium and then run through two glass columns containing viscous layers of human serum albumen (protein medium). When the sperm have descended to the bottom, they are removed and separated from the liquids around them. The sperm of the chosen sex are then concentrated and injected into the woman's cervix shortly after ovulation.

Producing females in the laboratory is more difficult than producing males. The procedure costs from $200 to $300 and is offered in many clinics throughout the United States. The procedure is not 100 percent effective. One woman who had five girls visited a clinic, desperate to have a boy. To her surprise, she ended up nine months later with another girl.

Another similar procedure uses a centrifuge to separate X- and Y-bearing sperm. Since the female chromosome is heavier, it sinks to the bottom. The Y, or male, chromosome floats to the top. Doctors then perform artificial insemination using the isolated sperm, according to the parents' preference.

There are, however, less scientific techniques that have been advocated over the years and these are methods you can do yourself at home.

Techniques You Can Do at Home

There are other less proven methods, such as douching with a mild acid of two tablespoons of white vinegar to one quart of warm water prior to intercourse to increase the chances of having a girl. A douche of two tablespoons of baking soda in a quart of warm water may increase the chances of a boy. If you use these techniques, you are still taking your chances with probability.

Dr. Landrum Shettles, who is a pioneer in sex selection and coauthor of the book *How to Choose the Sex of Your Baby*, says that there are a number of factors couples should keep in mind when trying to determine the sex of their child. Shettles' theory is based on the fact that the male-producing sperm are faster than the female-producing sperm and therefore the timing of intercourse is critical in sex selection. In order to time intercourse, he recommends three home-based methods—taking morning basal body temperatures, monitoring cervical mucus, and using ovulation predictor kits, which are available online and at many pharmacies.

To have a girl, Shettles suggests you have sex two-and-a-half to three days before ovulation. Those with fertility problems will already be taking their basal body temperatures and therefore will know when they ovulate; however, the task is a little more complicated for other women. In his book, Shettles explains how to chart cervical mucus. After doing this for a couple of months, a woman will notice that her cervical secretions are watery and elastic just prior to ovulation.

He also believes there are other factors that come into play. He advocates that couples have sex every day from the end of the menstrual cycle until the few days before ovulation. A more controversial suggestion is to have sex in the missionary position with shallow penetration, allowing the sperm to be released into the more acidic vagina. He also recommends that when trying to have a girl, the woman should not reach orgasm.

To have a boy, Shettles suggests having sex twenty-four hours before ovulation and no more than twelve hours past ovulation. He says that having sex too far in advance of ovulation will decrease the chances of having a boy. In terms of positions during sex, he recommends deep penetration in the "doggy position" so that the sperm is deposited closest to the cervix. To have a boy, he claims that having an orgasm is important. He also recommends that the male have a caffeinated beverage prior to sex, which tends to make the Y sperm more active. Finally, he says men should wear boxers or loose fitting clothes to keep the testes cooler and thus increase the sperm count.

Pregnancy Tests

Whether you are a potential high-risk mother or not, the first step is to have a pregnancy test to ensure that you are pregnant. Over the years, there have been many types of pregnancy tests, some more accurate than others. The accuracy of the results depends on the test's sensitivity.

Pregnancy tests, whether blood or urine tests, check for the presence of human chorionic gonadotropin (hCG), a hormone produced by the developing placenta shortly after conception. The hormone hCG is detectable eight to ten days after conception. A positive test, in conjunction with other signs, will help confirm your pregnancy.

Some Early Signs of Pregnancy

- missed period
- fatigue
- nausea/vomiting
- increased vaginal secretions
- breast fullness
- darkened areola
- aching in lower abdomen
- increased urinary frequency

More recent tests can detect pregnancy a day or two after your missed period. Years ago, women would go to their physician if they suspected they were pregnant. Today, many women go to the nearest pharmacy and buy a home test. Others may choose to go to the health department or a midwife's office. Although the pharmaceutical industry is beginning to meet the needs of today's busy woman by improving the efficiency of the home pregnancy test, these home-based tests are generally not as accurate as the ones done in the laboratory or the hospital.

It is suggested that the home pregnancy test be done on the first to the third day after a missed period and onward. At this point, the pregnancy test is about 90 percent accurate and after a week of a missed period, it can be up to 97 percent accurate. It is important to check the expiration date on the kit prior to performing any tests.

If you are unable to perform the test right away, the urine should be covered and refrigerated. However, it is important that the urine is tested on the same day it was collected. For the most part, the urine test will detect the hCG whether it is concentrated or diluted. If you drink a lot of fluids on the day of your urine test and your urine is very, very diluted, there is a slim chance that the pregnancy test might not be positive the first time. It may take a longer time for the test to be positive, so you might want to repeat it. In general, false positive tests are extremely rare.

If you think you are pregnant but the test is negative, count again the number of days since your last period and repeat the test a few days later. There is a chance that not enough hCG has accumulated in your urine to provide a positive result. If your test remains negative and you still do not have a period, consult your physician, as there may be another reason for your missed period.

Another way to detect pregnancy is from a blood test, which is usually 100 percent accurate and can be done as early as one week after an assumed conception.

The earlier you know you are pregnant, the sooner you will be able to take care of yourself and the precious life inside of you. Your physician will be able to detect your pregnancy after your second missed period through other signs, such as your uterus being larger than usual, your breasts being more tender, and the color of your vagina changing to a purplish hue.

If your provider suspects an ectopic pregnancy, a hydatidiform mole, or a threatened miscarriage, he or she may recommend a pregnancy test called a B-hCG blood test. If you fall into any of these categories, your placenta will secrete either too much or too little of the hormone hCG. This test is the most sensitive pregnancy test available today because it is the only one that detects very minute levels of hCG. It is done either by a blood or a urine test; the blood test is often more accurate. Results are usually available from two to forty-eight hours later.

How Your Baby Grows

Being pregnant, and knowing that a baby is growing inside of you, is one of the most magical times of a woman's life. It can be equally exciting for the man who is soon to be a father. For the majority of women, pregnancy is a very natural process, but whether you are experiencing a normal or difficult pregnancy, babies typically grow in the same way—fertilization occurs, cells divide, brain synapses develop, body parts begin to form, and the heart begins to beat.

If you are like most expectant parents, you will also find this a special but also a scary time. You will be loaded with questions, such as how does my baby look? How is he or she changing from week to week? It is a good idea to have a general idea of your baby's growth stages and what is normal, so that if any abnormalities occur, you can identify them early.

First Month

During the early part of the first month fertilization occurs, marking the beginning of a new life that will be growing inside of you! At this time, the baby's sex is also determined. During your baby's earliest stage of development, cell division occurs. Within the first twelve hours after fertilization, your one-celled zygote divides into two cells and then those both split into two. This keeps happening, as the number of cells doubles every twelve hours and continues to do so until this zygote makes its way through the fallopian tube on its journey into the uterus. At this point, your growing baby looks like a tiny raspberry.

By the fifth day, your developing baby consists of about five hundred cells and is called a blastocyst. By the seventh day, this blastocyst implants itself in the uterine wall. When this happens, it is normal to have a little spotting or yellowish vaginal discharge. About twelve days after fertilization, the placenta begins to form and starts secreting large amounts of estrogen and progesterone, which is what will cause maternal physical changes in the endometrium, cervix, vagina, and breasts.

By the twenty-sixth day, the circulation between your uterus and the baby's placenta has begun and the amniotic fluid has formed. At this time, your body must begin producing more blood so that it can carry nutrients to your baby. In order to keep your baby well-nourished, your blood volume continues to increase throughout your pregnancy. In fact, by the time your baby is born, your blood volume will have increased by as much as 30 to 50 percent.

Early in your pregnancy, your provider may suggest that you increase your fluid intake. In addition, because of all these changes in the body, it is normal to feel somewhat more tired than usual. Listen to your body's demands and remember to set aside some time for rest.

By the twenty-eighth day, your baby will have formed a chorioamniotic sac around itself and it will measure about $\frac{1}{12}$ inches long.

During this first month, you might notice your breasts becoming more tender, tingly, or sore. These symptoms are all normal. You might also experience some morning sickness. As pregnancy progresses, some women find that the rings of brown or reddish-brown skin around their nipples and areolas begins to darken. Sometimes this goes away after pregnancy and other times it remains permanent.

Second Month
During this month, your baby's cells continue to multiply rapidly, and each one takes on a specific function.

Growth is most rapid during the sixth week of development. Your baby now triples in size and many of your baby's organs and fingers and toes begin to form. The embryo's chin now rests on its chest, and this may be easily detected on ultrasound. By eight weeks, your baby's total body size will amount to half the size of its head.

At this point, your baby is about half an inch long and your uterus is about the size of an orange.

Third Month

By the third month your baby has begun to grow fingernails and toenails, and the face begins to have some human elements, and in particular, the chin and nose become more refined. The bones have begun to form and the baby has small breathing movements. By the end of this month, your baby will measure about 3 inches long and your uterus will be about the size of a cantaloupe.

This marks the end of your first trimester.

Fourth Month

By this time your baby's genital organs may be identified and their scalp hair has begun to form.

On an ultrasound you may be able to see your baby sucking his or her thumb. You may begin to feel fetal movements at this time because the baby is moving about quite freely. Sometimes these movements may feel somewhat jerky and erratic. By now your baby is about 3 to 5 inches long and weighs less than 3 ounces.

This month marks the beginning of your second trimester.

Fifth Month

You are now halfway through your pregnancy and your uterus usually extends to your navel. Your baby's face is completely developed and the eyebrows and eyelashes begin to form. He or she develops body fat and the baby's breaths are more regular. In addition, your baby's hearing is fully developed and he or she can hear all sorts of sounds, but of course your voice will always be the most familiar. Sometimes loud sounds may startle your baby and he or she might react by moving around. This is an exciting moment for the expectant mother. This moving around or fluttering is sometimes called quickening. Some women say that it feels as if they have butterflies in their stomach, while others describe it as a growling feeling.

Sixth Month

By this month, your baby's skin is wrinkled and he or she has developed very fine hair, called lanugo, all over their body. The baby's muscles are also developing and the kicks can feel quite strong. These kicks help babies to develop their muscles. The baby gains up to an ounce of body fat and muscle each day. This helps them survive after birth. Their lungs are not fully developed, so babies born at this time may or may not survive, probably depending on their own health and the technology available to them after birth.

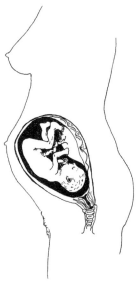

By the end of the sixth month, your baby will measure between 12 and 15 inches long and weigh about 1½ pounds (see Figure 1.6). If born at this time, your baby has a fifty-fifty chance of survival.

Seventh Month

By now, your baby's hands are fully developed. His or her skin is red and shiny and because of the increased body fat, it

Figure 1.6: Twenty-five weeks gestation

has lost some of the wrinkles. Your baby's eyes are beginning to open and close and he or she is beginning to develop sleeping and waking patterns. Most babies will sleep between 20 and 30 minutes at a time at this point in their development. However, this is not a reflection of how the baby's sleeping patterns will be after birth.

By the end of this month, your baby will measure about 10 inches long and will weigh about 2 pounds. If your baby is born at this time, thanks to modern technology, he or she will have a 75 percent chance of survival.

Eighth Month

During the eighth month, your baby continues to grow and you might notice less kicking because there is less available room inside your uterus. However, most providers believe that if you feel fewer than ten movements in two hours, you should inform your health-care provider.

Your baby now measures between 12 and 15 inches long and weighs between 3 and 4 pounds. If your baby is born now, he or she has about a 90 percent chance of survival.

Ninth Month

By the ninth month (see Figure 1.7), your baby's lanugo hairs have begun to disappear and their fingernails reach the ends of their fingers. In the male baby, the testes have started to descend into the scrotum. The next three weeks will mark your baby's most significant weight gain. Because your baby has little room to move, you may not feel any more movements, but you may feel some stretching and wiggles.

At this time, your baby should weigh at least 6 pounds and measure between 18 and 21 inches long, but these numbers vary

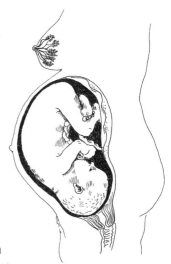

Figure 1.7: Thirty-eight weeks gestation

Journaling Your Pregnancy

Whether this is your first pregnancy, second pregnancy, or third, having a baby is a major milestone in a couple's life. Even though it seems while we are going through the experience we will remember all the details, that is rarely the case.

Journal writing is a powerful tool to document experiences, and it is also a way to create a keepsake for your child. Imagine reading about the day your mother felt the first kick inside! My own children have already experienced this magic and it is unmatched.

As I mentioned in the book's introduction, this book began as a journal of my bed-rest experience. As a writer, the process was intuitive, but for women who have never written before, their challenges may be greater. In either case, the rewards are guaranteed to be wonderful in the years to come.

Some journaling advocates, like Mae Respicio, believe that before setting out to write, you should first decide whom you're writing for. In her article "Write From the Start" (*Pregnancy*, 2008), she says, "Is this a journal for your eyes only or something to give to your child later? Maybe you'd like to write letters to your baby instead of a day-to-day chronicle." Respicio also states that there are many online blogs where you can post the details of your pregnancy.

Although it might be a good idea to decide who will be your audience beforehand, sometimes we just do not know. The important thing is to record everything that you would like to remember about your pregnancy—your sentiments, symptoms, hopes, dreams, memories, and milestones. Just getting the words down can be challenging enough!

It is also fun to give your journal a title. When I first began my journal I called it, "Another Day, Another Blessing," because I never knew how long I would carry my high-risk pregnancy. My initial intention was to either put together a book for publication and/or document my pregnancy for my future child. In my journal, I chronicled my physical and emotional sentiments, and I also spent time writing letters to my unborn child, which I hoped she would have the opportunity to read one day.

Some women do not have difficulty deciding what to write, but for those who need some guidelines, I have included journaling prompts at the end of each chapter in this book. The best thing to do is to transpose the questions into a journal of your liking, one that resonates with you. Then place it at your bedside table so that at the end of the day, before settling into sleep, you can jot down a few words. Some days there might not be too much to say, and that is fine. On other days, you might find the words pouring out of you.

Journaling Corner

What concerns or questions do you want to discuss with your physician at your next checkup?

What vaccinations or health care do you need to attend to prior to getting pregnant?

What are some other things you would like to do before you get pregnant?

Are there some habits you would like to change before you become pregnant (consider quitting smoking, changing eating habits, ceasing alcohol consumption, etc.)?

Why do you think this is a good time to have a baby?

How do you think your life will change after pregnancy (consider education, career, travel, goals, etc.)

2

Care During Your Pregnancy

Although different medical clinics and practices have various prenatal protocols, this chapter will provide you with general guidelines for your prenatal care. Be sure to check with your health-care provider about his or her recommendations for your care during your pregnancy.

The First Visit

On your first office visit, you should expect to have a complete physical examination, including a vaginal and breast examination, in addition to a blood and urine test. If you have not recently had a Pap smear, it might also be done at this time. During this visit, your physician or obstetrician will also help you determine your due date (see below).

If your examination goes well, you will be told to return every 4 to 6 weeks until your 28th week, then every 4 weeks until your 36th week. Then you will be asked to return for a visit every 1 to 2 weeks until the onset of labor. If yours is a high-risk pregnancy, these time intervals may be adjusted slightly.

Blood and Urine Tests

At the time of your first prenatal visit, your blood will be drawn for an array of blood tests. These tests are routine; you should not feel that your physician is suspicious of anything in particular.

A basic blood test always checks for a complete blood count (CBC), which is a broad screening test to check the red and white blood cells for anemia, infection, and other diseases. Your blood will also be checked for your blood group type and rhesus factor (discussed below).

In addition, your initial blood sample will be used to check for particular diseases. Details about these diseases will be discussed in subsequent chapters:

- rubella immunity
- gonorrhea
- syphilis

- thalassemia
- chlamydia
- hepatitis B

- sickle-cell disease
- HIV
- typhoid

Your urine sample will be checked for protein and possible signs of infection. The urine sample is sometimes taken from a midstream sample, which means that you urinate a little into the toilet, then urinate in the specimen cup, and then finish urinating in the toilet. On each prenatal visit you will be asked to provide a urine sample. This sample will be tested for sugar (glucose), protein, and signs of infection.

Rhesus-Factor Titers: Rh is a complex of three proteins (C, D, and E) found on the surface of the red blood cells. Individuals either have or do not have the Rhesus factor (Rh D antigen). Those who have the factor are considered to be Rh-positive. If you do not have this factor, then you are Rh-negative. There may be a problem of Rh incompatibility (see Chapter 5) if the mother is Rh-negative and the baby is Rh-positive. During their pregnancies, Rh-negative mothers are given a series of blood tests (Rh titers). If the blood tests show that the antibodies are increasing, the practitioner may decide to induce labor to prevent the fetus's blood from being destroyed.

Calculating Your Due Date

Today, due dates are usually calculated on a computer; however, in order to have the most accurate due date, it is important that you keep track of your cycles, particularly the first day of your period. Your due date will be calculated on one of your earliest prenatal visits. Knowing your approximate due date is of particular importance in high-risk pregnancies. Should your baby be in distress during your pregnancy, your physician's interventions will depend on your due date.

A full-term pregnancy lasts approximately 40 weeks and is composed of three trimesters, with 13 to 14 weeks in each one.

Because not all pregnancies are equal in duration, it is impossible to predict the exact date of your baby's arrival. Typically, pregnancies last between 37 and 42 weeks, and most babies are born between 39 and 41 weeks. Your due date is calculated based on the first day of your last menstrual period.

Here's how to do the calculation the old-fashioned way. The calculation is the easiest if you happen to know your exact date of conception. Simply add 38 weeks to that number. If you have regular cycles of twenty-eight days and know the first day of your last menstrual cycle, then just add 40 weeks to that date.

Women who have irregular periods or those who do not remember the date of their last period will have a more difficult time estimating their delivery date and will have to rely on ultrasound dating.

Even with all the calculations, only about 4 percent of all women deliver on their actual due dates. Keep in mind that this number is just an estimate. Statistics have shown that only about 66 percent of women will deliver within 2 weeks of their due date.

Exercise During Pregnancy

According to the American College of Obstetricians and Gynecologists (ACOG), unless there is a medical reason to avoid exercise, pregnant women should partake in moderate exercise, particularly if they did regular exercise prior to pregnancy. For the most part, exercise makes you feel better both physically and emotionally, plus it helps avoid excessive and unnecessary weight gain during pregnancy.

Normal weight gain during pregnancy is about 25 to 35 pounds. Pregnancy is not a time to exercise excessively in order to lose weight. If you eat normally and are losing weight while exercising, there is a chance that you are exercising too much.

Here is what one mother said about exercise during pregnancy:

> "Before I got pregnant, I used to workout every day, but when my doctor put me on bed rest due to complications of pregnancy, I had to forgo my entire exercise regime. I really missed my workouts and not only because of the extra weight, but I also found my morale declining. I got moodier because I was unable to work out. In the end, I gained more than 65 pounds with my pregnancy, and even with the help of a strict diet, it took me one year to take off the excess weight."

In addition to the obvious benefits of exercise for everyone, it is particularly important for the pregnant woman. For example, it can help prevent the incidence of gestational diabetes, relieve stress, and build stamina for labor and delivery. Exercise can also help minimize the effects of postpartum depression, which many women are prone to encounter after their baby is born.

It is important to pick exercises you enjoy. Brisk walking is often a good choice, and so is hiking, dancing, or swimming. Some women are reluctant to swim in fresh water because of the possible exposure to leptospirosis, a bacterial disease that has become endemic in certain parts of the United States. If bacteria carrying this infectious disease enters broken skin through a cut, it can result in miscarriage or preterm (premature) labor. Many women would not want to take the chance. Swimming in a pool is generally safe, as long as it is properly maintained.

It is a good idea to avoid sports that could potentially place you at a high risk for injury. These include sports such as skiing, horseback riding, rock climbing, kickboxing, basketball, and soccer. Scuba diving should also be avoided because of the issues with decompression. Many practitioners recommend that after the third month, you refrain from doing any exercises that require lying on your back, because doing so can restrict the blood flow to your baby.

The best advice is to listen to your body and to avoid any excessive exertion or overdoing any particular activity. Do not exercise to the point of exhaustion. If you become dizzy, have chest pain, bleed, or notice an increase or decrease in fetal movements, you should immediately call your doctor.

Before embarking on any exercise program, it is important to first speak with your health-care provider.

Nutrition and Pregnancy

During pregnancy—probably more than at any other time in your life—you need to eat well. Pregnancy is not a time for dieting. Dieting will deprive your fetus of the valuable nutritional support that it needs to grow. Severe dieting can have serious consequences. For example, when fat breaks down during dieting, toxic substances called ketone bodies are released. These can harm the fetus.

Eating a well-balanced diet with foods from the food pyramid formulated by the United States Department of Agriculture is a good general guideline (see Table 2.1 on the next page). The pyramid stresses the importance of eating foods from each of the six food groups.

Table 2.1: The Food Pyramid for a Healthy Pregnancy

Food	Daily Amount
Milk/Yogurt/Cheese	2–3 servings
Vegetables	3–5 servings
Fruits	2–4 servings
Meat/Fish/Eggs/Dry Beans/Nuts	2–3 servings
Oils/Fats	Sparingly
Breads/Cereals/Rice/Pasta	6–11 servings

Caloric requirements increase during pregnancy as the body strives to meet the needs of two persons. Women who are close to their ideal body weight do not need any additional calories during their first trimester. Beginning in the second trimester, it is usually recommended that pregnant women increase their daily caloric intake by three hundred calories. If you are exercising less or are on bed rest, you should speak with a nutritionist or dietitian about adjusting your intake accordingly.

Also, if you are pregnant and are nursing, it is important for you to see a nutritionist for a consultation. Sometimes breast-feeding during pregnancy is controversial, but it is generally accepted.

Weight Gain

During the first three months of pregnancy, a woman will normally gain between 4 and 6 pounds. From the beginning of the fourth month and until term, a steady gain of about 1 pound per week is desirable, although a spurt of 2 pounds is not unusual. There should be a steady weight increase. By the end of a normal pregnancy, a woman will have gained between 25 and 35 pounds (see Table 2.2 below).

Table 2.2: Approximate Weight Gain During Pregnancy

Fetus	7.5 pounds	Breasts	1.0–3.0 pounds
Placenta	1.5 pounds	Extra blood	4.0 pounds
Amniotic fluid	2.0 pounds	Body fluids	2.0 pounds
Uterus	2.5 pounds	Maternal store	4.0–8.0 pounds
	TOTAL: 24.5–30.5 pounds		

There are different parameters if you are underweight, overweight, or obese.

If you begin your pregnancy underweight, you should expect to gain between 28 and 40 pounds. If you are overweight, you should gain between 15 and 25 pounds. If you are obese, do not plan on gaining more than 15 pounds.

Certain changes in weight may indicate a problem. For example, a sudden weight gain in the second half of pregnancy that is accompanied by elevated blood pressure may be a warning sign of preeclampsia. Loss of weight or a failure to gain weight in the latter part of pregnancy is also a sign of a potential complication. When labor is imminent, some women experience a small weight loss. This is due to a decrease in fluid retention caused by a drop in progesterone, which usually promotes fluid retention.

Nutrient Supplementation

Nutrition in pregnancy is a delicate balance of taking the correct nutrients while maintaining a reasonable caloric intake. Although a well-balanced diet will provide all the required nutrients, there are certain nutrient supplements that may be required in special situations.

Iron: Iron is necessary for making hemoglobin, the protein in blood cells that carries oxygen to the other cells. A daily iron supplement providing 30 to 60 mg of iron might be prescribed for you. Iron is best absorbed on an empty stomach, but it can cause gastrointestinal discomfort and might even cause your stools to turn black. There is no need to worry.

Vitamin supplements fortified with iron often cause constipation. Instead of taking laxatives during pregnancy, it is advised that you eat foods with bulk and fiber, drink prune juice, and increase your daily water consumption. Some dietitians recommend drinking a cup of hot water on an empty stomach first thing in the morning to alleviate constipation.

Some women are at risk for iron deficiency, including those who become pregnant with low iron stores, those carrying twins, those who were underweight or malnourished when they became pregnant, adolescents, those with closely spaced pregnancies, those with a history of fertility problems, and those who have had previous gastric surgery. Iron-rich foods, in combination with an iron supplement, may be prescribed for these women.

Sources of Iron

• egg yolk	• almonds	• prunes, raisins
• beans	• kidneys	• bran (in moderation)
• liver	• oatmeal	• oysters
• fortified breads and cereals		

Calcium: Calcium is necessary for the developing the fetus's bones and teeth, and it is most needed in the second and third trimesters of pregnancy, when bone formation occurs. A total of 1,200 mg of calcium daily is recommended during pregnancy. Pregnant adolescents should add an additional 400 mg daily.

Women needing calcium supplementation are those with lactose intolerance or milk allergies, or those who simply do not like drinking milk. If you cannot tolerate any milk products, your physician may prescribe a calcium supplement of 1,000 mg. Some women use lactose tablets, which are perfectly safe during pregnancy.

Vitamin D: Vitamin D is essential for calcium's absorption in the body. It also plays a role in mineralizing the baby's skeletal system. Today, milk and margarine are fortified with vitamin D. However, those at most risk for vitamin D deficiency are those who dislike milk and those taking anticonvulsants. Exposure to sunlight also provides vitamin D, but if you are pregnant during the winter months, this exposure is often limited and you may be advised to take a vitamin supplement or to increase your dietary intake. Some dietary fiber tends to inhibit lactose absorption, while some sugars increase its absorption.

Folic Acid: Folic acid is in the vitamin B-complex group and is important for cell division and blood formation. It may help to prevent spina bifida and related birth defects that occur during the third week of gestation. Folic acid is very important during pregnancy because of the increased number of cells being produced by the mother. A pregnant woman will need about three to four times more folic acid than the nonpregnant woman.

For normal pregnancies or low-risk pregnancies, the daily folic acid recommendation is 400 to 600 mcg per day. For women having a high-risk pregnancy, the prescribed dosage is 4,000 mcg per day. High-risk women include those who have had a baby with a neural tube defect, those with a family history of neural tube defect, those taking certain medications (i.e., anticonvulsive medications), carrying multiple pregnancies, those with anemia, and the obese mother. These women are more likely to have a baby with neural tube defects. Some studies have shown that if women have been taking folic acid for more than a year, it can decrease the incidence of preterm birth.

For women who are at risk for developing folic acid deficiency and who are planning a pregnancy, it is often recommended that they start taking folic acid two months before conception and at least during the first month of pregnancy.

Folic acid is destroyed when cooked at high temperatures, so you should limit microwave cooking. When cooking vegetables, use smaller amounts of water. In addition, there is considerable loss of this vitamin due to oxidation when food has been stored for more than a few days, making it difficult to obtain through food sources alone.

Sources of Folic Acid

• meat	• asparagus	• kidney beans
• lima beans	• liver	• eggs
• nuts	• yeast	• fish
• enriched grains and cereals	• green leafy vegetables (spinach, romaine lettuce)	

Sodium: The volume of water in a woman's body increases during pregnancy. To maintain a good chemical balance, she needs to increase the total amount of sodium in proportion to her caloric intake. In the past, salt was not recommended for pregnant women. Theories have changed, however, and the current belief is that you should salt your foods to taste but avoid salting before tasting your food. Processed foods have large amounts of salt and should still be used in moderation.

Protein: Protein is essential for building fetal tissues and for metabolism. Protein provides the body with energy and is needed to manufacture hormones, antibodies, enzymes, and tissues. A pregnant woman should increase her protein intake to an average of 70 gm daily. Yogurt is an excellent source of protein and also contains vitamins A and D, as well as many B-complex vitamins.

Fluids: Water is important because it transports vital nutrients from one part of the body to another. It is also a necessary part of chemical reactions, such as in the breaking down of complex nutrients into smaller units. Our bodies are constantly losing water, through sweating, urinating, and breathing. We also lose water through vomiting and diarrhea.

Pregnant women need to drink more fluids. In addition to the milk requirement, it is important for them to drink 64 ounces of fluid daily.

Vitamin Supplementation: Vitamin supplementation during pregnancy is controversial. Some providers recommend supplementation in special situations, while others recommend it for all pregnant women. Whenever possible, nutritional deficiencies should be corrected by food rather than by supplementation. Discuss this carefully with your nutritionist or dietitian, keeping in mind that too much of some nutrients, such as vitamin A, may have the potential to cause serious birth defects.

Tips on Prenatal Vitamins

- Take the prescribed dose (usually one per day). Do not take megavitamins or begin any special vitamin program without supervision. Some nutrients may cause birth defects.
- If you find that taking your prenatal vitamin nauseates you, or if you feel like regurgitating it, take it with some food or try taking it at bedtime. If these measures do not help, consult with your provider. You may be told to stop taking it for a week or so. The other option is to take a chewable vitamin.
- Keep vitamins and other medications out of the reach of small children. In an attempt to "copy mommy," a toddler may think that pills are like candy. Iron pills can kill.

Food Cravings and Aversions

Some women may have food cravings, which some professionals believe is the body's way of saying you that you might be deficient in a certain vitamin. Some pregnant women crave citrus fruits because their body might need more vitamin C or if they have low blood sugar.

Food cravings for a particular food, though, are not a reliable detector of a deficiency. Pica is a craving for eating nonfood substances, such as paint, laundry starch, clay, dirt, or paper, and may be a sign of the need for iron in your diet. Some women have the classic craving for pickles and ice cream or a strong desire to eat other types of foods. Approximately 75 to 90 percent of pregnant women have food cravings during pregnancy that usually disappear in the beginning of the fourth month.

Food aversions are common during the first trimester. Studies have shown that between 50 and 85 percent of all pregnant women have some sort of food aversion during pregnancy. This aversion is often related to the huge hormonal changes inherent to pregnancy. Some believe that food aversions are nature's way to prevent women from eating certain exotic foods that might potentially harm their unborn child. Sometimes the mere smell of coffee or fried foods can send waves of nausea through pregnant woman. One woman said she could not eat enough ice cream, but on the other hand could not tolerate chicken, which was one of her favorite meals when not pregnant.

Fish and Pregnancy

Fish is a nutritious and healthy source of lean protein. It is also low in saturated fat and high in omega-3 fatty acids. Most dietitians or nutritionists suggest you eat two servings of fish each week, which amounts to about 12 ounces.

It is important to avoid eating large fishes (such as swordfish, shark, tuna, marlin, sea bass, mackerel, and pike) during pregnancy because they all contain mercury. Mercury accumulates in the atmosphere and then comes out in the rain. During the fish's life cycle, mercury accumulates in its body. Studies have shown that large amounts of mercury can damage your baby's developing nervous system, which might result in future learning disabilities and some other developmental delays.

Some fish have less mercury than others. Examples of fish safe to eat during pregnancy include salmon, sardines, farmed trout, catfish, flounder, and haddock. It is a good idea to stay away from fish sushi or any raw fish during pregnancy because most of the fish used to prepare sushi contain higher levels of mercury. Vegetable sushi is fine. Also, try to avoid freshwater fish caught by friends or family. The other option is to check with your local fish advisory.

In general, precaution should be taken when preparing fish. Try to keep the ten-minute rule in mind. This means finding the thickest part of the fish and cooking it for ten minutes per inch.

If you want to read more about the safety of fish, check out the EPA's website at http://www.epa.gov/waterscience/fishadvice/advice.html.

Listeria and Pregnancy

Listeria is a type of bacteria that can be found in certain contaminated foods. It originates in the water and/or the soil. Foods that have been exposed to this bacteria could cause problems for you and your baby and result in a disease called listeriosis.

Pregnant women are more susceptible to developing listeriosis because of their hormonal changes. According to the Centers for Disease Control and Prevention, pregnant women are about twenty times more likely than nonpregnant women for developing listeriosis.

The bacteria can be transmitted to the fetus through the placenta. This can lead to premature delivery, miscarriage, stillbirth, or serious health problems of the newborn, even if the mother has no symptoms. Actually, sometimes the symptoms can be mild and take a few days or weeks to appear. The symptoms are usually flulike with a sudden onset of fever, chills, muscle aches, and sometimes stomach upset. Listeriosis is diagnosed through a blood test and is treated with antibiotics.

Because symptoms are not always apparent, it is important for you to be diligent about what you eat. The USDA's Food and Safety and Inspection Service and the Food and Drug Administration provide the following advice for pregnant women and all high-risk consumers:

- Do not eat hot dogs, luncheon meats, or deli meats unless reheated until steamy hot.

- Do not eat soft cheeses such as feta, Brie, Camembert, blue-veined cheeses, and Mexican-style cheeses such as queso blanco fresco and soft, raw unpasteurized cheese slices and spreads.

- Do not drink raw (unpasteurized) milk or eat foods containing unpasteurized milk.

- Do not eat refrigerated pâté or meat spreads.

- Do not eat refrigerated smoked seafood (i.e., salmon, trout, white-fish, cod, tuna, or mackerel) unless it is an ingredient in a cooked dish or casserole.

Nutritional Guidelines for Special Situations

For the high-risk mother, setting nutritional guidelines is both challenging and often individualized. Below is a summary of nutritional guidelines for some of the special situations encountered by the high-risk mother. These are only suggestions, and you should consult your physician or registered dietitian before adhering to any specific dietary regime.

Anemia: Anemia is caused by a lowered hemoglobin level in the blood. Hemoglobin is the part of the red blood cells that carry your body's oxygen concentration. Therefore, it is important that its level be kept adequate. During pregnancy, your blood volume increases by 33 percent, which means that there are more red blood cells with less hemoglobin. As a result, many health-care professionals believe that vitamin supplements fortified with iron are necessary to meet this additional requirement.

There are various types of anemia, but iron-deficiency anemia is the one that most commonly affects pregnancy. There are a few reasons why women may be anemic. Those who tend to have anemia may have a history of heavy bleeding during menses, give blood three or more times a year, or follow a diet that is low in iron.

Iron supplements may be prescribed. If left untreated, severe anemia has risks for the unborn child, as it jeopardizes the baby's supply of oxygen and essential nutrients. It can affect the baby's growth and consequently his or her birth size.

Anorexia and Bulimia: Anorexia, the lack or loss of appetite, and bulimia, also known as binge-purge syndrome, are often lumped together under the term *eating disorders*. If you have either of these problems, they can adversely affect both you and your baby's health. If you are anorexic, you lose the benefit of all the unconsumed nutrients. If you are bulimic and vomiting, not only do you lose nutrients, but you also lose gastric chemicals and electrolytes that are used to digest food. This can also cause serious complications such as erosion to your esophagus, gastric ulcers, and dental decay.

It is important for you to know that if you suffer from either of these eating disorders and are actively binging or purging, or not eating the recommended calories required to sustain a pregnancy, you are putting both yourself and your baby at risk.

According to the American Pregnancy Association, women with eating disorders are more prone to miscarriage, depression, delayed fetal growth, gestational diabetes, preeclampsia, premature labor, low-birth-weight babies, increased chance of cesarean section, and complications during labor.

If you take laxatives, diuretics, and other medications during pregnancy, you should know that these may be harmful to your baby's development because they deplete your body of nutrients and water, which are essential for fetal growth and weight gain. Most women with eating disorders who are able to follow the recommended dietary guidelines do quite well during pregnancy without incurring any complications.

It is best that you let your obstetrical provider know about any eating disorders you currently have or have had in the past, so they can best advise you. It is also recommended that if you have a therapist who works with you to manage your problem, you should continue to see them regularly during your pregnancy. If you do not already have a therapist, this might be a good time to get one and you should ask for recommendations from your provider.

Obesity: In the last twenty-five years, the prevalence of obesity has doubled in the United States. For women of reproductive age, the actual prevalence of obesity is more than 30 percent and the prevalence of overweight women is from 55 to 60 percent. According to Susan Chu, an epidemiologist at the Centers for Disease Control and Prevention, one in five women who gives birth in the United States is obese.

Obesity is a serious risk factor for the pregnant woman and her unborn baby. Most of the complications that these women might incur are due to their preexisting obesity rather than to any extra weight they might gain during their pregnancy.

During prenatal visits, glucose levels are also frequently monitored because of the tendency to develop gestational diabetes. In addition, urine protein is measured because of the increased risk of developing pre-eclampsia.

If you are obese and are considering gastric surgery prior to becoming pregnant, the banding and ballooning procedures have been reported to be relatively safe because they are not considered major surgery. However, if you have had gastric bypass surgery, it is important for you to wait at least eighteen months before getting pregnant. In general, women who lose weight and are successful at doing so end up with fewer complications and risks during their pregnancies.

One risk of obesity is spontaneous abortion and an increased chance of structural fetal abnormalities, such as neural tube defects and cardiac problems. To prevent neural tube abnormalities, obese women are usually prescribed folic acid supplementation. Obese women are also at a greater risk of having a cesarean delivery. Sometimes an elective cesarean is recommended in order to minimize any risks to the mother and baby.

Obese women are more at risk for developing postoperative complications, such as excessive blood loss, wound infections, inflammation of the endometrial layer of the uterus (endometritis), and complications of anesthesia. They also have a tendency to have overweight babies, which could predispose them to long-term weight issues.

Bed Rest: In general, the pregnant woman on bed rest should consume the same number of calories per day as her more active counterparts. Because she is less active, it is important for her to consume nutritious foods from all the food groups, such as fruits, vegetables, low-fat proteins, and whole grains. It is best to avoid empty calorie foods such as cakes, cookies, candies, and chips. Whenever eating, especially sweets, the pancreas is stimulated to secrete insulin, which helps to metabolize the sugar and other foods. About one hour after eating, the blood glucose level falls rapidly. The fetus also experiences this drop. A relatively constant blood-sugar level is much better for fetal development. This is not to say that sweets should not be eaten during pregnancy, but they should be consumed in small amounts and ideally in conjunction with other high-protein foods.

Some women on bed rest will notice a decrease in appetite due to less activity, while others find that they are bored and eating is a time-filler.

Often the woman is unable to choose and prepare her favorite foods and therefore she loses her appetite. Being on bed rest may predispose some women to heartburn, which can further diminish appetite (see Chapter 8 for more information on bed rest).

Birth Interval: The optimal interval between pregnancies has not been established. However, there is a greater incidence of lags in fetal growth and prematurity if the birth interval is less than two years. Certain nutrients may not be adequately replenished within that time. If you have had more than one baby in two years, you should meet with a nutritionist to ensure that you and your baby are getting adequate nourishment. A vitamin supplement may be recommended.

Diabetes: Diet and/or insulin control of diabetes needs to be carefully monitored during pregnancy. Women who were diabetic prior to pregnancy have the highest chance of problems and need to be followed closely. The fetus has the greatest chance of developing birth defects during the first five to eight weeks of pregnancy, before most women even know they are pregnant. Whether you had diabetes prior to pregnancy or develop gestational diabetes, a dietician or nutritionist should plan your diet.

He or she will carefully consider the amount of energy you expend during a typical day and will measure this against your nutritional requirements and those of your baby. If you are diabetic and for some other reason must be on bed rest, this will also be taken into consideration, and your caloric intake will need to be slightly lower than that of an active nonpregnant woman.

Three meals a day, with midmorning, midafternoon, and evening snacks, will also be recommended. If you are on insulin, it is important to have regular and consistent meals. You may be taught to test your own blood-sugar level before and after meals. Certain medications, such as steroids, have the tendency to temporarily raise the blood-sugar level, which makes women using them more prone to diabetes in pregnancy if they have some of the other risk factors mentioned earlier. These women should be even more careful to restrict their total caloric intake. You should notify your physician if you have these symptoms so that a special diet can be formulated. Consuming smaller and more frequent meals is often recommended.

Complex carbohydrates, such as starches (whole-grain bread, pasta, cereals, corn, peas, and beans) and vegetables, will be recommended and should make up 40 to 50 percent of your diet. Recent research shows that juices are absorbed very quickly. The absorption rate also depends on the other foods being eaten at the same time.

Protein is also important for diabetics. Their diet should consist of 20 to 22 percent protein.

In addition to its benefits to the intestinal tract, fiber has been identified as a useful food in controlling diabetes, because it affects the body's general metabolism. If you are having a high-risk pregnancy with a risk of preterm labor, it is important to check with your provider before eating high-fiber foods. If you are not in the habit of eating high-fiber foods, it is important that they are added to your diet slowly. Sudden usage in large amounts can result in cramps and also stimulate uterine contractions.

Sources of Fiber

• raw vegetables	• raw fruits	• whole-grain cereals
• legumes	• nuts	• bran (in moderation)
• prunes		

Heart Disease: The nutritional alterations necessary for those with cardiac disease are similar to those for hypertension or preeclampsia (see below). Under supervision, you should maintain an appropriate weight and restrict sodium to 2 to 3 gm daily. Salty foods such as smoked meats, pickles, relishes, and condiments should be avoided. You should never be on a restrictive diet without the advice of your physician.

Lactose Intolerance: Lactose intolerance is a result of not producing enough of the enzyme lactase that is necessary to digest milk products. It is quite common and affects as much as 15 percent of the adult population. It is more common among African-American, American-Indian, and Asian-American populations.

Those with lactose intolerance have symptoms such as loose stools, diarrhea, gas, nausea, and abdominal bloating after consuming milk or milk products. This intolerance could be troublesome for the pregnant woman who needs to increase her calcium intake.

In some cases, the symptoms of lactose intolerance disappear during pregnancy. Some women claim they can tolerate only a small amount of calcium at any give time. Half a cup of whole milk is more often tolerable than skim or low-fat milk. Sometimes those with lactose intolerance find it easier to digest hard cheeses, unprocessed cheeses (e.g., cheddar, Swiss), yogurt, and canned fish with bones. Vegetables such as broccoli, spinach, and mustard greens also supply calcium, although calcium from vegetable sources is less easily absorbed by the body.

If you have lactose intolerance, you may want to check out this link from the American College of Gynecologists and Obstetricians: http://www.acog.org/publications/patient_education/bp0001.cfm.

Multiple Pregnancy: There are conflicting opinions about whether the mother's nutritional requirements should double or quadruple with a multiple pregnancy. The only way to assess adequate nutrition is via blood tests, fetal growth, and weight gain.

Those carrying multiple pregnancies should gain between 35 and 45 pounds (see Table 2.3 below). If you are carrying triplets, you should gain between 45 and 55 pounds. Studies have shown that those who gain weight within these ranges tend to have healthier babies. Those carrying multiple pregnancies will find that weight gain during the first trimester is a little more than for singleton pregnancies. In the second and third trimesters, the weight gain is about 1½ pounds per week.

Table 2.3: Weight Gain for Multiple Pregnancies

Pre-pregnancy weight	Twins	Triplets
Underweight	40–50 pounds	50–60 pounds
Average weight	34–45 pounds	45–55 pounds
Overweight	25–35 pounds	35–45 pounds

Check out this link for more information about multiple pregnancy: http://www.storknet.com/ip/reproductive_years/high_risk/multiple_pregnancy.html.

Hypertension and Preeclampsia: Preventing malnutrition in the pregnant woman has long been correlated with preventing hypertension or preeclampsia during pregnancy. Proper nutrition and increased protein intake when you have elevated blood pressure can help prevent more serious complications. Sodium or salt restriction is sometimes recommended in preeclampsia to minimize water retention and swelling.

Certain vitamins are of particular importance to the preeclampsic mother. Vitamins such as C, D, and B-complex are related to protein and energy metabolism. Studies have shown that placentas of toxemic women have about one-third the normal amount of vitamin B-6.

Vegetarians: Vegetarians can have healthy babies without compromising their dietary habits, as long as they receive proper nutritional counseling and do adequate meal planning. During counseling, you will learn to increase your total food intake and/or to include foods of a higher nutritional value.

Although vegetables contain protein, pregnant vegetarian women run the risk of not consuming enough protein. Those who eat eggs and milk products are usually able to meet their protein requirements. Vegans, on the other hand, who do not eat animal products such as milk, cheese, and eggs, run the risk of vitamin D and vitamin B-12 deficiency and therefore need supplementation and/or need to make sure to eat enough dried beans, peas, lentils, and other proteins.

According to Dr. Holly Roberts in her book *Your Vegetarian Pregnancy* (2003), "Like any pregnant woman, vegetarian women need to build a strong nutritional foundation to ensure their baby's health. One health issue unique to vegan women is the possibility of vitamin B-12 deficiency, though these cases are rare." This is the reason many doctors prescribe supplemental vitamin B-12 in addition to the standard prenatal vitamin.

In general, vegetarians tend to have smaller babies because their diets are lower in fat content. If you are a vegetarian and have an eating disorder, your chance of having a smaller baby is even greater.

Other Concerns and Lifestyle Issues

In addition to the recommended nutritional guidelines during pregnancy, there are certain concerns and lifestyle issues pertaining to the health of your unborn child that you should be aware of. Some of these issues include the use of alcohol, caffeine consumption, the use of recreational drugs, environmental hazards, the safety of X rays, and the safety of spa treatments.

Alcohol and Pregnancy

Alcohol is potentially dangerous to the unborn child because it is capable of crossing the placenta and entering the fetal bloodstream; therefore, concentrations found in the fetus are at least as high as those in the mother. If the pregnant woman is an alcoholic, there is a greater risk of having a complicated pregnancy, possible miscarriage, or fetal death.

No "safe" amount of alcohol consumption during pregnancy has been established, so it is recommended you simply avoid it. What researchers *do* know is that six drinks per day (3 ounces each) constitute a major risk. The timing of alcohol ingestion is also important. It appears that the most dangerous time to consume large amounts of alcohol are in the first and last trimesters. The reason for this is that during the first trimester there is rapid fetal cell growth, while in the last trimester there is rapid brain growth.

When more alcohol is ingested than the liver can process, the excess is released into the bloodstream. The alcohol then circulates in the blood until the body is able to detoxify it. When alcohol is present in a pregnant woman's body, it is distributed in the fetal liver, pancreas, kidney, thymus, heart, and brain. Alcohol has the ability to affect fetal growth because it interferes with carbohydrate, fat, and protein metabolism.

The most serious adverse effect of excessive alcohol consumption during pregnancy is fetal alcohol syndrome (FAS). Babies with this syndrome are born with a low birth weight and unusual facial features, such as small eyes, flat nose, and uncommon eye folds. Many also have various types of heart, skeletal, and genital problems. Death in the early newborn period is not uncommon, and those who survive have borderline to moderate mental retardation. According to the Centers for Disease Control and Prevention, the reported cases of FAS vary widely across the United States. It is believed, however, that the rates range from 0.2 to 1.5 cases per 1,000 live births each year.

Fetal alcohol effect (FAE) is the name given to alcohol-induced developmental impairment that entails anything less than FAS. It is often more difficult to diagnose and for this reason may be more widespread in the general population. Studies have shown that although children with FAE may appear normal, their learning ability is impaired. In a mild case of FAE, for example, the child may show a repeated failure to understand his or her multiplication tables, may also have difficulty mastering certain social skills, or may have poor judgment. These children may also have difficulty learning from their mistakes.

The subject of FAS was addressed in the 1989 book *The Broken Cord* by Michael Dorris. The story it tells about the dramatic effects of alcohol abuse on a pregnancy is both revealing and inspiring. The author presents the story of his adoption of a Sioux Indian who turns out to be afflicted by FAS. The trials, anger, and joy of raising such a child are all addressed.

If you drink wine or liquor every day and are contemplating pregnancy, it is a good idea to consider quitting or to seek help before jeopardizing the health of your future child. Remember that the damage of alcohol on your unborn baby is permanent.

Caffeine and Pregnancy

Caffeine encourages stress hormones such as epinephrine and norepinephrine to be released and this affects blood flow and the amount of oxygen available to the fetus. Many women make the wise choice to use decaffeinated beverages and substitute herbal teas for regular teas, but it is a good idea to check with your doctor before doing so. Green tea and regular tea are healthy for the pregnant woman because they are rich in anti-oxidants and contain less caffeine than coffee. In addition, more than one cup of coffee a day is not recommended during pregnancy, especially if you prefer drinking strong coffee.

To date, the exact effects of caffeine on pregnancy are unclear. Some studies have shown that caffeine can deplete the body's calcium levels. Some research has indicated that more than five cups of caffeine per day during pregnancy may be linked to miscarriage, stillbirth, low birth weight, and sudden infant death syndrome (SIDS).

Some practitioners may be vague in their recommendations; therefore, moderation is always the best choice. Table 2.4 on the next page provides an idea of the amount of caffeine in some popular items.

Table 2.4: Caffeine Amounts in Common Beverages

Coffee (1 cup)	120–150 mg
Decaf coffee (1 cup)	5 mg
Green tea (1 cup)	30 mg
Black tea (1 cup)	50 mg
Cola soda (1 cup)	30–65 mg
Milk chocolate (1 oz.)	10 mg

Recreational or Illicit Drugs

Recreational or illicit drugs are extremely dangerous for the pregnant woman. Smoking marijuana is not recommended during pregnancy for the same reason that you should stay away from environmental toxins. Recent studies have shown that if a pregnant woman uses marijuana, it may be associated with some neurological delay in her child. According to the March of Dimes (2006), "Pot and pregnancy don't mix." The organization says that marijuana may slow the baby's growth and may also increase the risk of premature delivery. Babies who were exposed to excessive marijuana during pregnancy may be born with withdrawal symptoms, meaning they may cry a lot or tremble.

The use of ecstasy and amphetamines has increased dramatically in recent years. There have not been many studies on the correlation between ecstasy and pregnancy; however, one small study showed an increase in congenital heart defects in female babies and a defect called clubfoot.

The use of methamphetamines (also known as "speed," "ice," "crank," or "crystal meth") has also been on the rise. Babies born to these mothers are three times more likely to grow poorly in utero and are often born early. The use of recreational drugs during pregnancy also increases the risk of complications having to do with the placenta.

The use of heroin during pregnancy also results in an increased chance of serious pregnancy complications and low-birth-weight babies. The use of cocaine during pregnancy can increase the chance of miscarriage, stillbirth, early labor, and abruptio placenta.

Other recreational drugs, such as crack, morphine, LSD, and PCP, should absolutely be avoided. Addiction to these illegal drugs can result in complications such as miscarriage, stillbirth, complications of labor, low birth weight, and failure of the baby to thrive. In addition, the use of these drugs during the later stages of pregnancy can cause addiction and/- or withdrawal symptoms in the newborn.

For further information, check out the National Clearinghouse for Alcohol and Drug Information. They may be reached at (800) 729-6686, or another good resource is the National Alcohol and Drug Hotline at (800) 622-6686.

Environmental Hazards

It is difficult to get through a day without being exposed to toxins that could inadvertently affect your growing baby, whether the toxins are in the air, water, environment, or food. You should not make yourself crazy about being careful, but there are a few precautions you should take.

In your home, the general consensus is that if it has an odor, do not use it. During pregnancy, it is not a good idea to use pesticides in your home because they have been linked to miscarriage. If you install new carpets, it is a good idea to keep the windows open during installation or simply leave the house. If you live in an area where fumigation is being performed, you might want to consider taking a trip for a few days, particularly if you are in your first trimester.

Studies have shown that mosquitoes really love snacking on pregnant women mainly because they are fond of carbon dioxide and pregnant women tend to take more breaths. Pregnant women also have a higher metabolism, and bugs usually like that. If you live in an area or travel to a mosquito-infested area, it is a good idea to use protection; however, avoid using any repellants containing DEET.

Lead exposure has been linked to low birth weight and impaired intelligence, speech, memory, and learning. Although there has been an increase in the use of unleaded fuel, it is recommended that pregnant women avoid rush hour and traffic jams to minimize any possible exposure to environmental toxins.

Some people choose to de-lead their homes. It is important not to do this during pregnancy because the dust contains lead, which can adversely affect the unborn child. Paint removed from buildings built prior to 1978 contain lead particles that may be very toxic.

Unfortunately, our diet is also a major source of lead. Food may be contaminated as a result of lead deposits from the atmosphere on crops. Studies have indicated that coffee and alcohol consumption is associated with increased maternal lead levels. It is known that dietary supplements of calcium, iron, and folic acid can lower blood lead levels. However, these should only be taken under medical supervision.

To date, there have not been any documented studies indicating that computers and cell phones can be detrimental to the unborn child. Also, there are no conclusive studies about the adverse effects of living in close proximity to power lines during pregnancy.

Recent studies have shown that the polyvinyl chloride (PVC plastic) often used in water bottles can be harmful. The truth is that if the plastic is heated it could release PVCs, although at the time of writing, there have not been any definitive studies.

X Rays

Pregnant women are advised to avoid routine chest and dental X rays to minimize the chances of causing any harm to the fetus.

Although the normal doses of a routine X ray (1 to 3 rads) do not necessarily cause harm to the fetus, the effect depends on the amount and time of exposure, and no amount of exposure to X rays can be considered safe. Some sources claim that exposure to more than 10 rads during the first three weeks of pregnancy can result in miscarriage or in a smaller-than-usual brain size. There is no statistical evidence of abnormalities occurring when the mother is exposed to less than 10 rads, but it is always recommended that her abdomen be shielded from radiation.

Hospital X-ray departments often have posters on the walls advising pregnant women against having unnecessary X rays. If you have any questions, ask about any diagnostic or treatment that is recommended for you.

Hair Dye and Hair Removal

Many experts recommend not getting your hair colored during the first trimester. After that time, some women opt for highlights instead of having a full head of coloring; this way the dye does not penetrate the scalp. Some hair stylists can also order plant-based products that are less toxic. These products are also frequently used with cancer patients. Although there have been no tests to prove the danger of hair dye to the unborn child, it is better to be safe than sorry.

In terms of hair removal, it is probably a good idea to stay away from depilatory creams, bleaching, lasers, and electrolysis. Of course, shaving, tweezing, and waxing are perfectly fine and will not harm your baby.

Spa Treatments

Some women have the luxury of receiving regular spa treatments, and in most cases, it is okay to continue most services during pregnancy. It is perfectly fine to continue with facials, manicures, pedicures, and body scrubs. Spa treatments involving high temperatures, however, should be avoided. These treatments include saunas, steam rooms, heat wraps, whirlpools, or tanning beds. Early studies in Europe have shown that the heat that is generated from sleeping blankets or Jacuzzis might also increase the chance of miscarriage and neural tube defects. However, there have been no further studies that support this finding.

It is important to check with your health-care provider whether you can have a massage during your pregnancy. If he or she says it is okay, it is important that you choose a well-trained therapist. You will probably be advised to avoid deep-tissue massages, particularly on your legs, because pregnant women are more prone to varicose veins and massaging that area could result in a blood clot becoming dislodged.

Positioning is important during a massage. Early in pregnancy, you might not be comfortable lying on your chest because your breasts will be tender. Later in pregnancy, lying on your back for long periods of time may be uncomfortable and might make you more prone to dizzy spells when you eventually stand up.

Medications and Pregnancy

In adults, the kidneys and the liver are responsible for facilitating the breakdown and excretion of medications in the body. Because the fetus's kidneys and liver are immature, the mother's liver and kidneys take on this task. Medications that might be normally considered mild, such as aspirin, may be potentially harmful to the fetus. In general, the most hazardous time to take any drugs—prescribed, over-the-counter, or recreational drugs—is during the first three months.

Probably two of the most publicized harmful and dangerous medications for the unborn child are thalidomide and diethylstilbestrol (DES). Thalidomide is now only used for Behçet's disease and also as a treatment for cancer. It is a known teratogen (agent causing malformation in the fetus), and its use during pregnancy has been associated with multiple deformities. DES, a drug given to many women between 1941 and 1971 to prevent miscarriage, has resulted in certain female-related cancers in the offspring of women treated with this drug. Its use has also been discontinued.

Any medication taken during a pregnancy should be administered with extreme caution. The best policy is not to take any drugs, prescription or nonprescription, unless you and your physician agree it is absolutely necessary and that the benefits outweigh the risks. During your first office visit, it is important that you give your physician the names of all your medications. You will probably be advised to remain on some of the prescription medications. According to *The Mayo Clinic's Guide to a Healthy Pregnancy* (2004), "A medication that was important for your health before pregnancy most likely will be important during pregnancy, too."

Principles of Medication Use in Pregnancy

- Only use medications if absolutely indicated.
- Avoid new medications during the first trimester (if possible).
- Use safer and preferably older medications rather than new ones.
- Use the lowest effective dose.
- Use one medication for each disorder, not multiples.
- Avoid the use of over-the-counter drugs (if possible).

Do not take any over-the-counter medications without first consulting your physician (for some simple guidelines, see Table 2.5). What may ordinarily be a harmless medication could be a potential hazard for you and/or your baby. For example, aspirin is not recommended for extensive use because it interferes with blood clotting. Your baby is most vulnerable during the first three months when the body's structures are formed and defects are likely to occur.

Table 2.5: Medications That May Be Hazardous to the Fetus

Medication Category	Example
Analgesics	Ibuprofen (Advil), aspirin
Antibiotics	Isotretinoin (Accutane), doxycycline, kanamycin, streptomycin, tetracycline
Antiblood-clotting	Warfarin (Coumadin)
Antidepressants	Lithium, imipramine, MAO inhibitors, paroxetine (Paxil)
Antihypertension	Benazepril, captopril, enalapril, lisinopril
Antiseizure	Phenytoin, carbamazepine (Tegretol), trimethadione, paramethadione, valproic acid
Antithyroid	Methimazole (Tapazole)
Cancer-fighting	Aminopterin, methotrexate, trimethadione
Hormones	Androgens, diethylstilbestrol (DES), synthetic progesterone, testosterone
Sedatives/hypnotics	Thalidomide
Tranquilizers	Diazepam (Valium)

Since the first edition of this book, the FDA has prepared some easy-to-follow and comprehensive guidelines for medication use during pregnancy. They have prepared what they call an FDA categorization. The list has five different categories of fetal risk for various medications. There are too many medications to be mentioned here; however, you can access the information on the following website: http://safefetus.com.

The following is a brief list of the categories of medications. On each page you will find the category of your selected medication. With each medication there will be the medication's indication and risk during pregnancy and breast-feeding.

Category A: Medications in this group have been shown to cause no harm to the unborn child.

Category B: Either animal-reproduction studies have not demonstrated a fetal risk but there are no controlled studies in pregnant women, or animal-reproduction studies have shown an adverse effect (other than a decrease in fertility) that was not confirmed in controlled studies in women in the first trimester (and there is no evidence of a risk in later trimesters).

Category C: Either studies in animals have revealed adverse effects on the fetus (teratogenic, embryocidal, or other) and there are no controlled studies in women, or studies in women and animals are not available. Medications should be given only if the potential benefit justifies the potential risk to the fetus.

Category D: There is positive evidence of human fetal risk, but the benefits from use in pregnant women may be acceptable despite the risk (e.g., if the medication is needed in a life-threatening situation or for a serious disease for which safer medications cannot be used or are ineffective).

Category X: Studies in animals or human beings have demonstrated fetal abnormalities, or there is evidence of fetal-risk in human experience or both, and the risk of the use of the medication in pregnant women clearly outweighs any benefit. The medication is contraindicated in women who are or may become pregnant.

Occupational Hazards

Certain work environments may also be hazardous to the unborn child. This is certainly true for hospital personnel. For the most part, the anesthetic gases used today are not harmful to the unborn child. However, if you work in an area with radiation, you should be quite careful, even if you wear a counter that keeps track of your rad exposure.

Ionized radiation exposure can be harmful to the unborn baby. The amount of exposure will determine its safety factor to your unborn child. The American College of Obstetricians and Gynecologists (ACOG) says that less than 5 rads is safe and more than 20 or 40 rads could result in miscarriage. One chest X ray is equal to 1 millirad. If you fly across the United States, the radiation exposure of being in an airplane is equivalent to having had three X rays and, according to the numbers above, it is quite safe. Radioactive dyes should not be used during pregnancy because they may damage the baby's thyroid.

An MRI is quite safe during pregnancy because it does not use ionizing radiation; it uses electron magnetic fields. However, an MRI is expensive to perform and tends to be loud. CAT (CT) scans, on the other hand, have some ionizing radiation, but they are not recommended during pregnancy. If they are absolutely necessary, the radiologist should protect your abdomen with a lead X-ray apron.

During pregnancy it is a good idea to avoid toxic fumes. You should avoid any areas where there are chemical or paint fumes. Benzene, for example, has been shown to cause cancer.

Alternative, Complementary, or Holistic Health Care

More and more women are turning to alternative and complementary care. The basis for this type of care is that good health stems from physical, emotional, and spiritual well-being. Those who practice holistic medicine believe strongly in the mind-body-spirit connection.

One of the basics of holistic care is healthy eating. This includes eating high-quality whole foods such as whole grains, organic fruits and vegetables, and good-quality proteins, like those found in seeds, beans, and organic meats (see the information earlier in this chapter).

Herbs

To complement good eating habits, alternative medical practitioners and holistic practitioners believe that some herbal supplements can benefit the pregnant mother. Natural herbs are often less expensive and healthier than prescription medications. Many practitioners trained only in Western medicine might be reluctant to prescribe a supplement that often has not undergone vigorous clinical research.

Although herbs are natural, not all of them are safe to use during pregnancy. Unlike prescription medications, herbal products are not regulated by the Federal Drug Administration (FDA) in the United States or the Natural Health Products Directorate (NHPD) in Canada. This means that they have not been widely tested for their safety or effectiveness. It is important to check with your practitioner before taking any herbal preparations. Today, many medical and nursing schools offer courses in alternative medicine, so practitioners are more well-versed than they were years ago.

The following herbs should definitely NOT be taken in pill form or via tea infusion during pregnancy because they can be unsafe for the fetus. However, these same herbs may be used in cooking because they are used in small amounts:

- aloe vera: shown to induce abortion in animals
- black cohosh: binds to estrogen receptors and can cause uterine contractions
- black haw tea: similar to aspirin in that it can cause bleeding
- blue cohosh: contains estrogen, a uterine stimulant that can cause miscarriage or preterm labor
- burdock: can stimulate uterine contractions
- calendula: can cause uterine bleeding
- chamomile: can induce miscarriage
- comfrey: can cause liver toxicity
- dong quai: can cause uterine bleeding and miscarriage
- ephedra: when used orally can stimulate the heart and raise blood pressure
- fennel: uterine stimulant that can cause miscarriage or preterm labor
- feverfew: uterine stimulant that can cause miscarriage or preterm labor
- flax seed: uterine stimulant that can cause miscarriage or preterm labor
- germander: can cause liver toxicity
- goldenseal: uterine stimulant that can cause miscarriage or preterm labor
- hops: has hormonal substances; relaxes uterine wall
- juniper: can cause uterine bleeding and possible miscarriage
- kava: can cause liver toxicity
- lavender: the essential oil can affect maternal hormones and/or harm the fetus
- licorice: can cause high blood pressure, headache, and uterine bleeding

- ma huang: contains ephedrine that may stimulate the uterus
- oregano: the essential oil can affect maternal hormones and/or harm the fetus
- passionflower: uterine stimulant that can cause miscarriage or preterm labor
- pau d'Arco: no evidence of its safety in pregnancy
- periwinkle: uterine stimulant that can cause miscarriage or preterm labor
- saffron: may cause uterine contractions and possible miscarriage
- saw palmetto: when used orally can cause hormonal activity
- senna: can cause intestinal cramps and diarrhea
- slippery elm: can cause miscarriage
- St. John's wort: may cause hormonal imbalances
- yohimbe: relaxes the uterus and may be toxic to the uterus

The following herbs have been identified as being safe or possibly safe during pregnancy:

- Cranberry: This herb has been used to treat or prevent urinary tract infections and has been shown to be safe in pregnancy.
- Dandelion root: This herb is sometimes used to treat some liver or bile conditions. It may also be recommended to treat gastric reflux and lack of appetite. It has also been suggested for carpal tunnel syndrome.
- Echinacea: This herb is often used to treat upper respiratory tract infections and it is safe to use during pregnancy. Sometimes goldenseal is used in conjunction with echinacea, but it is unsafe during pregnancy, so check the label before taking.
- Evening primrose: This herb has been used to treat eczema, premenstrual syndrome, menopause, endometritis, and some psychiatric conditions. You should limit your amount to less than 4 grams per day.
- Garlic: This herb has been used as a natural way to treat infections. It has also been suggested to decrease cholesterol and it is probably safe to use during pregnancy.

- Ginger root: Ginger root can help to relieve nausea and vomiting and can help relieve morning sickness.

- Peppermint and spearmint leaf: Peppermint and spearmint aid in digestion and also help to relieve nausea, flatulence, and morning sickness in some women.

- Red raspberry leaf: Raspberry leaf is rich in iron and it has been shown to decrease nausea, help uterine tone, increase milk production, and ease labor pains. It has also been recommended for leg cramps. After birth it can slow down bleeding and help the uterus regain its tone.

Mind-Body Connection

Pregnancy can be a joyous time, but for the high-risk mother it can be interspersed with stressful moments and fears of the unknown. Similar to other stressful times in your life, it is good to find a balance and minimize stressors for the optimal well-being of yourself and your unborn baby. In addition to the use of calming herbs, there are many things you can do while pregnant to help achieve a healthy balance between your mind and body.

First, it is important to find adequate support through your loved ones and/or community organizations. There are also special classes for pregnant women who want to keep in shape, whether it is through aerobics or swimming. However, for the high-risk mother, these might not be possible, and she will have to resort to other coping methods.

Everyone has their own ways of handling difficult times, whether it be through writing, reading, praying, deep breathing, yoga, or creative visualization. Whatever has worked for you in the past should continue to work for you during your pregnancy. The journaling prompts in this book will help you start to figure out what has been on your mind. There are many websites explaining how to do creative visualization. Relaxation and meditation techniques are good modalities to be used during pregnancy and beyond.

Relaxation: Entering a deep sense of relaxation involves a trust in yourself. You have to want to let go and believe in the benefits of bringing calm into your life. The two most common positions for relaxing are either lying down or sitting, whichever is more comfortable for you.

You will slowly begin to feel quite relaxed. Keep in mind that the body heals when both the mind and body are relaxed. The art of relaxation does not happen immediately, but rather, it needs to be practiced regularly.

Supine Position: The supine position involves lying on your back, which is generally okay until your twentieth week. After that point, it is not safe because your uterus will put pressure on your vena cava (a large blood vessel in back that carries blood to the heart), which could cause changes in your blood pressure.

Whether you are before or after your twentieth week, it is important to check with your provider. If you get the okay to lie on your back, then without using a pillow, extend your legs and spread your feet about 12 inches apart. Your arms should be outstretched from your body and your palms face up. Make sure you are dressed warmly because when you are relaxed, there is a tendency to become chilled.

Next, close your eyes. Take some long and deep breaths. Each time you exhale you should feel your body sinking into the ground or mattress. Begin by focusing on each part of your body, starting with your feet. With each breath, allow each part of your body to relax. Once you have made it all the way from your feet up to your head, continue the rhythmic breathing. Allow your mind to go blank. Do not allow yourself to become obsessed with any images or thoughts. You might find yourself drifting off into sleep and this is fine.

Seated Position: If you prefer the seated position for relaxation, you can sit on a cushion on the floor keeping your back as straight as possible. Some people prefer using meditation chairs. Rest your hands on your lap or place them palm down on your thighs. It is critical to keep your back straight. Follow the relaxation and breathing instructions suggested for the supine position (above).

Meditation: Meditation has been practiced for thousands of years. There are many different types of meditation practice. The type of meditation that has been advocated for wellness is called *mindful meditation*. It involves being conscious about what is going on, while paying attention to not reacting to your situation or the environment. When your body is in a state of relaxation, it becomes more connected with its core.

Meditation helps you learn how to accept what is going on, rather than reacting to it. It is the reaction segment that results in unnecessary stress on your body.

Some people choose to begin their meditation with a centering ritual, such as lighting a white candle. After your centering ritual, begin to meditate by closing your eyes. Become aware of your position and imagine your body as an envelope and that you are inside of it. Allow yourself to be inside your body. Remain in the moment. Begin to focus on your breaths. Notice which is the strongest part of your breath—the inhale or the exhale. You can figure this out by concentrating on your diaphragm and how it rises and falls. Some people exhale and imagine that they are blowing out a candle.

Continue to concentrate on your breath. If you feel your mind wanders to an image or thought, bring your attention back to your breath, mental focus, or mantra. Do not allow yourself to wander. Your breath should be the focus of your thoughts.

In the beginning, you can start with a five-minute meditation session, but soon, your 5 minutes may become 10, 15, or 20. You will find yourself looking forward to your quiet time and the sense of calm you feel afterward. You should practice meditation at least once each day, preferably at the same time each day. The more you can make the practice a habit, the better your results will be.

How to Meditate

- Find a centering ritual.
- Assume a comfortable position.
- Close your eyes.
- Focus on your breath, mental image, or mantra.
- Remain in the moment for 10 to 20 minutes.
- Stretch and slowly open your eyes.

Energy-Based Healing: Energy-based healing includes a variety of different forms and is based on the principle that there is a universal energy field that the practitioner can tap into to aid in creating harmony and balance within. By allowing the practitioner to facilitate your own natural ability to heal, you become an active participant in the process. If you are open and receptive to these modalities, it will enhance your healing process. There are many different types of energy-based healing, including healing touch, polarity therapy, sakara, therapeutic touch, and Reiki.

For example, healing touch is performed by a practitioner who places his or her hands on or near you to detect and work with the energy field that surrounds your body. Healing touch has been used successfully for pregnant women to promote relaxation and to prepare for childbirth. In fact, it has been used in some institutions for high-risk mothers, particularly those with symptoms such as elevated blood pressure, blurred vision, and headaches. The effects of healing touch can last anywhere from a few minutes to days or even weeks. Each person has his or her own unique response to energy work.

A full healing touch session, where the person receives a full sequence healing involving balancing the entire body, usually takes one hour. In the hospital setting, sometimes the session can be as short as a few minutes. During the shorter sessions, the practitioner usually works with a single issue or problem and uses "local" or specific techniques. For the most part, healing touch can be offered on a weekly basis or more frequently, but it can also be performed only once.

For most pregnant women, healing touch sessions create a deep sense of peace and unity. The sessions can also help the pregnant woman with the discomfort that occurs during and after delivery.

One healing touch professional recounts the following positive effect of the practice in one of her patients:

> "Colleen is a thirty-four-year-old woman who for years has been training to run her first marathon. She is pregnant for the first time. Even though she did not know she was pregnant at the time, at six weeks she successfully ran eighteen miles. During the previous year, she had an injury only four weeks before the marathon date and was unable to participate. This particular year she was extremely excited about running. However, she was concerned about being ten weeks pregnant. Her obstetrician wished her luck, but cautioned her not to increase her heart rate or get overheated.
>
> "As her family and friends cheered her on, Colleen successfully completed the marathon. That evening she was very sore and in tears because of severe hip and knee pain. She scheduled a healing

touch session and the practitioner found low energy throughout her energy centers. The practitioner then proceeded to balance all of her centers and used specific hands-on techniques over Colleen's painful joints. The following day, Colleen reported that she no longer had either stiffness or soreness and was able to enjoy all the accolades from her colleagues and friends at work."

Sexuality and Pregnancy

Humans are different from other species in that our desire for sexual contact continues throughout pregnancy. In fact, we are the only species that copulates during pregnancy. Our sexual relations are not reserved only for the purpose of procreating, as sex is also our way of expressing love. Sexuality, therefore, refers not only to the actual sexual act, but also to how we feel about ourselves. It is normal for pregnancy to cause changing attitudes toward sexuality in both the mother- and the father-to-be. Couples need to be open about their sexual needs and concerns among themselves and with their caregivers.

Sexual Desire

Changes in the desire for sexual contact are common during pregnancy and can be a result of many different factors—physiological and emotional well-being, cultural background, and attitudes toward pregnancy itself. Some women feel they are more attractive during pregnancy, while others are not at all overjoyed by their appearance. Some women take special care to always look and feel good throughout their pregnancy. Research has shown that women tend to experience a decrease in sexual desire in the first trimester, an increase in the second trimester, and a decline again in the third trimester.

Although these changes may be hormonal, it is clear that the normal complaints of early pregnancy, such as nausea and fatigue, can strongly affect sexual desire. Toward the end of pregnancy, when a woman has substantially increased in size, sex may not be as comfortable or as exciting. In addition, the latter part of pregnancy is accompanied by feelings that are more maternal than romantic. Fluctuations in sexual desire are normal during pregnancy, and therefore you should not be overly concerned if you alternate between feeling oversexed and undersexed.

Some couples, especially those encountering a high-risk pregnancy, may be afraid of hurting the fetus during sexual relations and therefore restrain or avoid intimacy completely. Many high-risk mothers are reluctant to ask their obstetricians about sexual activity and prefer the "better safe than sorry" approach.

Much of the literature focuses on the female sexual response during pregnancy. However, we must not forget the feelings of the male partner. The father-to-be also undergoes significant changes associated with pregnancy, and, although not physiologically based, these emotional issues may dramatically affect his sexual needs and desires. The new role of fatherhood brings with it many fears and uncertainties. The woman's bodily changes, such as increased breast size, swollen vagina, and protruding abdomen, may elicit varying responses in her partner. The man may feel unsure about sexual relations during pregnancy and may have difficulty expressing this fear. Feeling afraid is common among men and may be one reason for decreased sexual relations among some couples. If relations are resumed, the man may be unable to maintain an erection or to achieve orgasm because of the fear of injuring the unborn child. Other men may find the pregnant woman very attractive and feel an increase in sexual desire.

The Safety of Sex

Sexual contact is intimacy between two people. The type of intimacy depends on the individuals. While some couples are quite content cuddling and touching, the vast majority equate intimacy with the act of sexual intercourse.

It is important for you and your partner to voice your concerns about your sexual activity during pregnancy, because talking about it often relieves a great deal of tension. If you have any anxiety about the safety of sexual relations, you should discuss it with your physician. If you are advised to refrain from intercourse and/or orgasm, you can find alternative ways to express your love for each other.

For those who choose alternatives to sexual intercourse during pregnancy, it is important to know that there may be some risks. For example, because masturbation in women often provides a more intense orgasm than intercourse, your physician may recommend that you refrain from it. Those engaging in oral sex should note that air blown into the vagina may create the risk of an air embolism. This act should be carried out with caution during pregnancy.

More often than not, in normal pregnancies there is no evidence of orgasm or sexual intercourse adversely affecting the fetus or triggering bleeding, miscarriage, placenta previa, or preterm labor. If you are having a high-risk pregnancy, you should ask your caregiver if intercourse and/-or orgasm is recommended. Uterine fibroids, congenital uterine abnormalities, placenta previa, and cervical insufficiency are some situations in which your physician may advise you to refrain from sexual intercourse.

It is very common to experience some brief abdominal cramping following intercourse. If this continues or gets worse over a one-hour period, contact your physician, since it may be possible that your cervix is dilating. In general, intercourse is not advised during three specific times: if there is bleeding during pregnancy, for the first four weeks following vaginal childbirth, and for six weeks following cesarean birth.

For the most part, sexual intercourse during pregnancy is both appropriate and healthy for both partners. There are some positions that tend to be more safe than others for the pregnant woman and a few examples are given in Figure 2.2 below. These are taken from the pamphlet *Some Things About Sex and Pregnancy* by Ann Hager, RN.

Sometimes sex is not recommended during pregnancy, and those times include when there is bleeding or when there is premature rup-

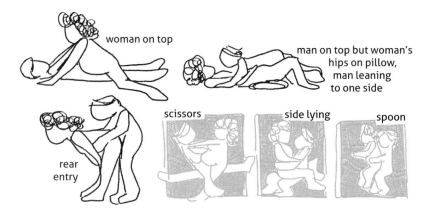

Figure 2.2: Alternative positions for high-risk couples

ture of the membranes. Whether bleeding is during the first, second, or third trimester, intercourse is not recommended. Bleeding during the early months can be indicative of impending miscarriage; if the miscarriage is due to a blighted ovum (an egg that does not develop properly), intercourse will not affect its outcome. Bleeding in the second and third trimesters may be due to uterine abnormalities or problems with the placenta, such as placenta previa and abruptio placenta. Your physician will probably recommend that you refrain from intercourse to prevent any problems.

Intercourse is not recommended once your membranes have ruptured, because it may result in a serious uterine infection. And if you ever feel a gush of fluid from your vagina, you should refrain from intercourse and immediately contact your health-care provider.

Tobacco and Pregnancy

In 1996, 13.6 percent of American women who gave birth were smokers. According to the Centers for Disease Control and Prevention, tobacco usage has fallen steadily since 1989, when about 20 percent of pregnant women smoked. Nevertheless, smoking remains a problem for the pregnant woman. Studies have shown a strong correlation between moderate to heavy smoking (one pack per day) and low birth weight and premature babies. Other problems that may be traced to smoking include premature rupture of the membranes, abruptio placenta, maternal hypertension, and miscarriage. Some studies also indicate that children born to smokers are more likely to suffer infections of the respiratory tract, such as bronchitis and colds, and may be more susceptible to SIDS.

If you already have a high-risk pregnancy and continue to smoke, you are exacerbating your situation. Recent studies have shown that not only is it harmful for smokers to smoke but it may be detrimental for nonsmokers to be in the presence of smokers. This is an important consideration for the pregnant woman.

Travel During Pregnancy

Unless your health-care provider indicates otherwise, there are no dangers to airplane travel during your pregnancy; however, if you need to take medications for motion sickness, you might want to delay your travels until the second trimester.

It is probably not recommended that you travel after thirty-four weeks, particularly if you want to deliver in the hospital of your choice. In the event of an emergency, most airlines will require a note from your physician giving you medical clearance to travel later in pregnancy.

When seated in the airplane, you should keep your seatbelt on for the duration of the flight. This is usually most comfortable when the belt is situated low around your hips or on your upper thighs (see Figure 2.3). In order to min-

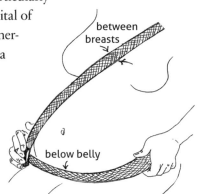

Figure 2.3: Proper seatbelt position

imize any swelling in your legs, it is a good idea to get up and stretch every hour or so. It is also a good idea to flex your calves while seated, just to keep the circulation in your lower legs moving.

Most pregnant women prefer the aisle seat, bulkhead, or emergency exit seats because they provide the most room and allow easy access to the bathroom. Remember to stay well-hydrated, because flying can be very dehydrating.

If you are traveling overseas, make sure to carry your medical records with you, and it is probably a good idea to obtain supplemental health insurance. While overseas, you should drink bottled water instead of tap water to minimize the chance of gastrointestinal problems or traveler's diarrhea.

Whether you are traveling by air, car, or sea, it is a good idea to have the address of the nearest hospital at your destination, in the event of any unexpected emergency.

For more information on traveling, here are some websites: Centers for Disease Control and Prevention: Traveler's Health at www.cdc.gov/travel and Obgyn.net: Country Pages at www.obgyn.net/country/country.asp.

Vaccinations and Pregnancy

In the Northern Hemisphere, the flu season usually falls between the months of November and March. The Centers for Disease Control and Prevention advocates the flu (influenza) vaccination during pregnancy. This is because during pregnancy the immune system is weaker and it cannot fight off infection as easily as it would normally. Although many studies indicate that having the flu shot is safe during any time of pregnancy, many women opt to wait until the second trimester before having the vaccine. This is because by this time the highest risk of miscarriage will be behind them.

Other vaccinations, such as live attenuated vaccinations, are not safe for the pregnant woman. If, however, you need a rubella vaccine, you should ideally get it one month before getting pregnant.

Even though there has been no documented case of an adverse reaction to most of these immunizations since 1975 when the United States began keeping a registry, most providers will still recommend that you avoid them. The good news is that these diseases are becoming rare because of the prevalence of childhood vaccination.

Here is a good link about vaccinations in pregnancy from the March of Dimes: http://www.marchofdimes.com/pnhec/159_16189.asp.

The Journaling Corner

What is the first thing you did when you found out you were pregnant?

How did your family react to your pregnancy?

What changes do you feel and what do you think they mean?

Has your mother spoken to you about her pregnancy, and if yes, what did she share?

How did you celebrate the news of your pregnancy?

What are your concerns, fears, or expectations about your pregnancy?

Write some notes to your unborn child. Start by writing a letter each month to your baby.

3

High-Risk Pregnancy: An Introduction

A high-risk pregnancy is one that endangers the health and possibly the lives of the mother and her unborn baby. About 15 to 20 percent of all pregnant women have some type of difficulty with their pregnancy. Although sophisticated medical technologies have helped, problem pregnancies are never easy for the mother, the baby-to-be, or the family. They are stressful, and the long road to a healthy birth may be strewn with numerous obstacles.

Your health-care provider may inform you either early or late in your pregnancy that you will have a problem pregnancy. The exact time when you are told this does not indicate the extent of your risk. For example, a woman over the age of thirty-five will probably be concerned throughout her pregnancy, although she may be at less risk than an obese younger woman, who is told in her thirty-fourth week that she has high blood pressure.

If you have a preexisting medical problem and there is a likelihood that yours will be a high-risk pregnancy, your physician will do a complete physical examination, record your medical history, and then inform you of your risk. Pregnancy may have an adverse effect on your preexisting problem and, conversely, the preexisting problem may affect your pregnancy and its outcome.

If you are a woman with a history of infertility problems, you will welcome your physician's special precautions. Holding on to the life of a baby is important to all expectant mothers, but it is especially important to you.

There are two types of high-risk pregnancies—those related to chronic or preexisting conditions of the mother and those stemming from complications with the pregnancy. Some women are considered high-risk in both categories. The two types of high-risk pregnancies will be discussed separately in Chapters 4 and 5.

Diagnosis of High-Risk Pregnancy

A woman with a high-risk pregnancy will need closer monitoring than the average pregnant woman. The type of monitoring may include, but not be limited to, more frequent visits with her practitioner, more tests to monitor her medical situation, blood tests to check medication levels, amniocentesis, numerous ultrasounds, and fetal monitoring. The results of all these tests are used to track the original medical condition, detect any complications, make sure the fetus is growing properly, and to help the practitioner make any decisions in regard to care.

High-Risk Pregnancy vs. Having High-Risk Factors

Some women are at a greater risk of having a high-risk pregnancy. These are women who have certain genetic backgrounds or a preexisting medical condition, or women who lead certain lifestyles or develop certain factors during their pregnancy.

Some risk factors may include, but are not limited to, the following preexisting factors:

- younger than eighteen years old
- given birth more than five times
- older than thirty-five years old
- low socioeconomic status
- previous pregnancy loss
- history of substance abuse
- being underweight or overweight
- anemia and/or poor nutritional status
- previous preterm birth (birth before thirty-seven weeks of gestation)
- previous birth of a very large or very small baby
- family history of genetic disorders or previous birth-defect baby
- preexisting medical conditions (i.e., diabetes, high blood pressure, and/or heart disease)
- use of infertility medications or treatments

Some external factors that might put a woman in a high-risk factor category include those living in extreme temperatures and high altitudes.

High-Risk Factors Before Pregnancy

- advanced age pregnancy
- advanced paternal age
- history of miscarriage
- asthma
- liver disease
- epilepsy
- diabetes
- kidney disease
- sickle-cell anemia
- depression
- eating disorder (obesity, anorexia)
- reproductive and female anatomy problems
- gastrointestinal problems (ulcers, Crohn's disease, ulcerative colitis)
- thyroid disease (hyperthyroidism, hypothyroidism)
- autoimmune diseases (SLE, rheumatoid arthritis, myasthenia gravis, ITP, APA)
- heart disease and high blood pressure

High-Risk Factors Related to Pregnancy

- hyperemesis gravidarum
- ectopic pregnancy
- hydatidiform mole
- ART/IVF
- hypertension
- gallstones
- appendicitis
- thromboembolism
- communicable diseases
- multiple pregnancy
- unusual fetal positions
- blood incompatibilities
- vaginal bleeding
- abruptio placenta
- placenta previa
- cancer in pregnancy
- sexually transmitted infections
- intrauterine growth restriction
- urinary and kidney tract infections
- preterm premature rupture of membranes (PPROM)
- postterm or prolonged pregnancy

Outcome and Prognosis of High-Risk Pregnancy

The positive outcome of a high-risk pregnancy depends to a large extent on the high-risk condition and the type of medical care the woman receives. Some maternal medical conditions present more problems than others. In some cases, women say that their problems have gotten better during pregnancy. Others might announce they feel worse. For example, some women with asthma claim they did not have to use their inhalers, while others say they needed to use them more frequently. Others might notice no change. Obviously, everyone is different.

Some medical conditions can have a huge impact on pregnancy and can result in poor fetal growth. Diabetes is a good example.

Choosing a Provider

If yours is a high-risk pregnancy, various types of providers may care for you during your pregnancy. Some women choose to be followed by their family doctor—a general practitioner—while others prefer to seek the attention of a physician specializing in obstetrics. Others may opt for the care of a nurse-midwife. Sometimes the decision depends on which provider is covered under your medical insurance policy. If you already have an obstetrician/gynecologist whom you like, unless he or she suggests otherwise, it is probably a good idea to stay with that provider. It is also important to consider the institution where your provider has delivery privileges.

Obstetricians/gynecologists (ob-gyns or OBs for short) are physicians who, following their graduation from medical school, have had three or more years of specialization in obstetrics and gynecology. Some choose to limit their practice to gynecology and do not deliver babies, but most often they do both. These practitioners are board certified.

Approximately 90 percent of pregnant women choose OBs to manage their care. Although a family practitioner is qualified to follow a woman through her pregnancy, if you are having a high-risk pregnancy, these practitioners should work in conjunction with an obstetrician who can help in the event of difficulties. In either case, an obstetrician would have to be called if a cesarean section were necessary.

Board-eligible physicians have finished their specialized training and are waiting to take their oral and written exams. During their first year after training, they must document all their deliveries in a special casebook that is later presented to the Board of Obstetricians and Gynecologists. They then have up to seven years to take their examination, although most of them take the exam within the first few years. It is important to know that these are obstetricians and gynecologists who can practice, but they have just not yet completed their exams. Board-certified ob-gyns have already completed their exams.

A *maternal-fetal medicine specialist (MFM)* is a new type of specialist. This is an ob-gyn who has also completed two or three additional years of postresidency fellowship in the area of caring for women with complicated or high-risk pregnancies.

Ob-gyn nurse practitioners are registered in advanced-practice nursing, and they have completed one or more years of postgraduate education. They often have a master's degree. These professionals specialize in women's health and are qualified to administer routine prenatal care for uncomplicated pregnancies; however, they are not licensed to deliver babies. Nurse practitioners tend to use a more holistic approach and work in consultation with a physician when problems arise.

A *certified nurse-midwife (CNM)* is a registered nurse who has completed one or more years of midwifery training after graduation and is then certified by the American College of Nurse-Midwives. Most have a master's degree. Midwives are capable of caring for uncomplicated pregnancies and births; however, they often work in consultation with a physician should any complications occur.

Professional labor assistants (PLAs), or doulas, are yet another addition to obstetric practice, since this book was originally published in 1989. These professionals are primarily trained in providing both emotional and physical support for women in labor. They often teach childbirth classes. Their focus is on making the pregnant woman comfortable during labor and helping to coach the couple through the journey. Doulas are not trained to deliver babies. More information on doulas may be found on their website at http://www.dona.org.

Childbirth educators work with the obstetrical team to teach couples about prenatal care, birth, and, in some cases, parenting. These professionals come from varied backgrounds, and in many cases, they are nurse-midwives. Childbirth educators believe in family-centered maternity care and freedom of choice based on knowledge of the alternatives. These professionals are often the ones who you will find teaching prenatal classes in your area.

Whether you decide to seek the care of a specialist or not, you need to understand your provider's plan. Here are some questions you may want to ask:

- How long will my typical office visit be?
- Do you recommend vitamin supplementation?
- How many births do you manage each month?
- How many cesareans do you perform each month?
- Do you believe in vaginal birth after cesarean (VBAC)?
- What happens if I have a problem at night or on the weekend?
- Who covers for you when you are unavailable?
- Are there medical students or residents who will be caring for me?
- If I go into preterm labor, what medications or interventions do you prescribe?
- Under what conditions do you induce labor?
- At what point in my labor do you arrive at the hospital?
- Will my partner be able to participate in the birth?
- How do you feel about pain relief during labor?
- How do you feel about fetal monitoring and epidurals?
- What percentage of your patients have an episiotomy?
- What are your fees? How are insurance claims handled?

Coping with High-Risk Pregnancy

Regardless of what categorizes your pregnancy as high-risk, the days ahead may not be easy. At times, you may feel scared and uncertain. One tip is to take one day at a time and to think of the stress of the situation as an opportunity for growth. There are many stages that high-risk mothers pass through that help them cope with their situation. First, you need to accept your pregnancy and the risks that it involves. Sometimes this is difficult, and women may find themselves denying there is problem. Chances are, the sooner you accept your high-risk pregnancy, the easier it will be for you to follow your practitioner's recommendations.

In some cases, women must give up certain activities or jobs. Having to take a leave of absence from work may be very stressful. Speaking with your employer about returning may help to relieve some pressure. If this is uncomfortable for you, it may be a good idea to speak with the social service department of your hospital, which may be able to serve as a liaison between you and your employer. You might even be eligible for disability insurance benefits. Seeking support from professionals, relatives, and friends is also important.

It is common to feel shocked when you are first told about your high-risk pregnancy. You may feel a sense of disbelief and may not actually hear the details of your physician's explanation. It is important to ask any questions that come to mind and to ask for further explanations at a later date. Keep a notepad in your purse, because concerns may come to you at the most unusual times!

It is normal to ask yourself, "Why me?" when faced with a problem pregnancy, but seeking the attention of specialists to find solutions to your problems is more productive than mulling over why it has happened. Understanding the reason for your problem will help you to cope with it. If your problem pregnancy may result in a child with disabilities, now is your chance to prepare for life after the birth. There are many excellent organizations that can help you (see Appendixes A and B).

High-risk pregnancies sometimes result in the death of a child. Understandably, couples facing a high-risk pregnancy always have this outcome in the back of their minds. Feelings of guilt are normal, but rarely justified. Couples need to remind themselves that everything was done in the baby-to-be's best interest and that medical science cannot perform miracles. Having the support of those around her is very important to a woman who is enduring a high-risk pregnancy. Having a supportive and understanding partner and family, in addition to a supportive and caring physician, is very important.

Feelings of hopelessness, discouragement, anxiety, and depression are all normal for the high-risk mother. It is natural to be bothered by women who are having "normal" pregnancies. It is not unusual to be envious of other mothers-to-be who can just get into their car and drive to the shopping center. High-risk mothers are often on edge. They learn to take one day at a time. This is what is unique about high-risk pregnancies. They are so dynamic. What may be okay today may not be okay tomorrow. For women in this situation, there is no reason to feel guilty. If you have questions about what is happening or what will happen, the best thing to do is ask your physician. Often, you will imagine your predicament to be much worse than it really is.

Dr. Robert Knuppel, an ob-gyn whose practice is primarily devoted to high-risk pregnancies, says that most of his high-risk patients have previously had complications and that "most women have been traumatized and sensitized." It is important to understand that in most cases you did nothing to cause your problem and that if you have any questions, you should ask them without hesitation. Most professionals will give you the answers you want to hear, but none will guarantee that "everything will be all right"—so try not to expect them to tell you that. The hours, days, and months may seem endless, but remember that it will not really be forever and that, after all, you are in bed not because you are sick but because you are awaiting one of life's happiest moments—bringing a child into the world!

Making Decisions

The first choice for a prospective mother-to-be is the decision to become pregnant. For some, especially those following career paths, this choice may have been the most difficult decision they have had to make. Making decisions involves much more than sitting down one evening and saying, "Okay, now I'm going to decide." For most people, it entails weeks or months of ongoing thought about the choice. It involves interactions and conversations with family, friends, and professionals. What you choose to do will depend on your ethical beliefs and principles as well as on your financial status.

After the decision to become pregnant has been made, you will need to choose a provider, a hospital, whether or not to have tests, whether to breast-feed, and so on. If you are at risk, you will continuously be making decisions concerning both your own and your baby's health. If you are over the age of thirty-five, you will need to decide whether you want to have an amniocentesis. If the results of the amniocentesis indicate problems, you will have to decide whether to have an abortion. This decision is probably the most difficult of all to make, since no one wants to terminate a potential life. Raising a child with disabilities, on the other hand, may be more than some women can contemplate.

The best decisions are educated and informed ones. When you must make a choice, it is important that you gather all the information you need. Sit down with a paper and pencil and write out the pros and cons. Consider all the facts. Make a list of all your alternatives. It is important to solicit the ideas and opinions of family, friends, and experts. Gathering and thinking over other people's viewpoints will help you come to your own, personal decision. Then you will know that you have made a truly caring and wise choice for yourself—and for your unborn child!

The Journaling Corner

How do you feel about your pregnancy?

How did you and your family respond to the news about your pregnancy?

How was your first meeting with your practitioner? What did he or she discuss or recommended for you?

Have you already been told that you are having a high-risk pregnancy? If yes, what type of high-risk pregnancy do you face and what did your practitioner tell you?

Describe the person who you will be able to lean on when you need emotional support.

4

High-Risk Factors Before Pregnancy

*It is said that the present is pregnant
with the future.* — Voltaire

This chapter will focus on maternal health problems, such as issues related to age, physical/emotional illnesses, and inherited abnormalities that may be passed down to the unborn child.

Advanced Age Pregnancy

Advanced maternal age is defined as a woman who is thirty-five or older on her expected due date. Not only do these women often have more difficulty getting pregnant, but as they age, the risk of having a baby with a chromosomal abnormality increases exponentially.

Years ago, the risk of losing a pregnancy as a result of amniocentesis was estimated to be one in two hundred and seventy births. Today, the risk of losing a baby with chromosomal abnormalities as a result of amniocentesis is about one in four hundred. The chance of losing a normal baby as a result of having an amniocentesis is probably much less—about one in a thousand.

Since the publication of the first edition of this book, amniocentesis and CVS are no longer routinely performed on those over the age of thirty-five. Instead, screening tests are first done and, if the risk is found to be high for an abnormality, then more invasive tests such as amniocentesis and CVS are recommended. These tests will be discussed in more detail in Chapter 7.

Women who are of advanced maternal age are at risk for developing more problems other than just chromosomal issues. They are at an increased risk for conditions such as gestational diabetes and high blood pressure. Also, for some unknown reason, they are also more at risk for having unexplained stillbirths. Some women of an advanced age are more likely to have underlying problems that were not apparent before they became pregnant. For example, their kidneys may be inefficient, and they might have not yet shown the signs and symptoms of high blood pressure. In other words, they might have underlying conditions, and in combination with the stress of pregnancy, an underlying condition may manifest itself.

"Pregnancy is a stress test for the woman's body to see how they cope with extra fluid or sugar load. Some women fail this stress test," Dr. Norwitz often tells his patients. Basically, the pregnancy sometimes unmasks an underlying, preexisting condition in the mother. Those women who fail the "stress test of pregnancy," might be at an increased risk of developing certain conditions, such as diabetes and hypertension, later in life.

Advanced-age women are also at an increased risk for having a cesarean delivery (see Chapter 11).

Advanced Paternal Age

To date, there has been no documentation that external factors relating to the father can cause a structural or genetic problem in the baby. However, a father's exposure to certain chemicals may diminish his sperm count and therefore his ability to get a woman pregnant. There has been some controversy as to whether advanced paternal age can affect the unborn child. Some studies have shown that fathers over the age of sixty-five are more likely to be fathers of babies with certain rare conditions—specifically, autosomal dominant disorders, such as dwarfism—but instances of this are extremely rare.

History of Miscarriage

Miscarriages occur in approximately 15 to 20 percent of all pregnancies and usually occur during the first five months of pregnancy—most often in the first three months. (See Chapter 9 for more details on miscarriage.)

Reproductive and Female Anatomy Problems

There are a number of reproductive and anatomical problems that could result in a high-risk pregnancy. These include conditions such as fibroids, cervical insufficiency, and septate uterus.

Fibroids

Fibroids, or leiomyomas, are common muscular tumors that grow in the wall of the uterus. They vary in number, size, and location and are found in approximately 25 to 35 percent of all women during the reproductive years. The presence of fibroids makes it difficult for the egg to implant itself in the uterus. However, once the woman becomes pregnant, studies have shown that the majority of uterine fibroids do not change in size during pregnancy, and those that do increase in size, tend to do so early in pregnancy.

The treatment for fibroids during pregnancy depends on their size and location in the uterus. If the fibroids are small and located outside the uterus, they do not usually cause problems for the pregnant woman. For most women, this is the case. However, if they are larger than 7 centimeters and are located inside the uterine lining, the placenta may not grow properly.

Women with large fibroids also run the risk of complications such as having breech babies, cesarean deliveries, preterm births, small babies because of growth restriction, preeclampsia, excessive bleeding, and/or failure of labor to progress.

Cervical Insufficiency

Cervical insufficiency (formerly called "incompetent cervix") is a rare condition characterized by weak cervical tissue that literally allows the baby to "fall" from the uterus during the second trimester. It is sometimes associated with a uterine abnormality called septate uterus (a uterus divided into two compartments), and a history of repeated miscarriages. If you have cervical insufficiency, chances are you will miscarry without noticeable pain. In fact, you probably will not know that you have cervical insufficiency until you miscarry once or twice. Only then will your physician suspect a problem. If a woman has had previous surgery to her cervix and a problem is already suspected, her physician may prescribe an ultrasound to measure the cervical length. This will determine if a stitch or cerclage will be necessary.

The treatment for cervical insufficiency is the surgical placement of a suture or cerclage (McDonald procedure) around the cervix to keep it closed (see Figure 4.1 on the next page). This procedure is usually done between the twelfth and the eighteenth week. Typically, the earlier the procedure is done during pregnancy, the higher the success rate.

The surgery is safely performed under regional anesthesia, although some physicians choose general anesthesia. Because the surgery does not take long, there is little risk of adverse effects of anesthesia to either the mother or the baby. Sometimes hospitalization is necessary for a few days after the procedure.

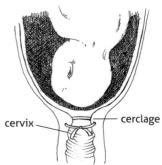

Figure 4.1:
Cervical suture

One woman describes her experience:

"I had three healthy children when I became pregnant with my fourth. Right from the start this pregnancy was quite different from the others. I was plagued with cramps, spotting, and nausea. By three months I was quite concerned, as it felt more like the end of pregnancy than the beginning. By four and a half months we were in real trouble. One day I phoned my husband at work because I was bleeding quite heavily and the cramping was more severe. I went to the emergency department and my ultrasound showed that the baby was alive and well. It was thought that the bleeding was caused by a polyp on my cervix, and in addition, my ligaments were bothering me.

"I went home and that night I awoke at 2:00 AM with intense cramping. I wasn't bleeding, but the cramping was so intense that I went to the hospital. I lost that baby and soon afterward it was determined I had developed cervical insufficiency. I was relieved to learn this, and very soon afterward I became pregnant once again and had a cervical suture placed at ten weeks. We didn't want to take any further chances."

Following the suture placement you will be advised to stay in bed, to avoid sexual relations, and to seek domestic assistance. A uterine relaxant may be prescribed in conjunction with bed rest. It is important for you not to lift anything heavy, since this may cause undue pressure on your cervix. Some women relieve mild pressure on the cervix by placing a pillow underneath the mattress, thus elevating the foot of the bed. My physician recommended that I elevate my feet above my pelvis to avoid any unnecessary pressure on the cervical suture line. I found this position to be very soothing and comfortable.

The suture usually remains in place until the thirty-seventh week or until labor begins, at which point your physician will arrange its removal in his office. If you have been taking a uterine relaxant, you will also be advised to discontinue it at this time. Some women become frightened when they discontinue their uterine relaxant, thinking that they will go into immediate labor. In most cases, however, labor does not ensue. In some cases, a cesarean may be scheduled for other reasons, while in other cases the woman may continue the pregnancy for anywhere from one or two days to three weeks.

Septate Uterus

A septate uterus is a rare congenital abnormality, in which a tissue membrane (septum) divides the uterus into two separate cavities. Sometimes the uterus is divided into two compartments (septate); sometimes it is forked (bicornuate). Some physicians recommend surgery to unite the two parts of the uterus; this increases the surface area of the uterus, thereby giving the fetus more room to grow. This surgery, however, has its risks, including hemorrhage, and in extreme cases, a hysterectomy will be necessary if the surgery fails. Some physicians may recommend repeated pregnancies in spite of the risk of miscarrying, in the hope that each pregnancy will stretch the uterus to make it adequate to carry a baby to term. Surgery is used as a last resort when the woman has had repeated miscarriages.

Diabetes

Diabetics have a metabolic disorder characterized by the inability to produce adequate amounts of insulin, which is an enzyme needed to help the body use glucose (sugar) for energy. Those with more severe diabetes are treated with insulin injections, while the milder forms are treated with a special diet and/or blood-sugar-reducing (diabetic) pills.

There are two types of diabetes that could affect the pregnant woman. The first is called *pregestational diabetes.* These women are diabetic before they get pregnant. Only about 1 percent of women of reproductive age are diabetic and some of them may already be taking blood-sugar-reducing pills or insulin. Women in this group have an increased risk of developing serious complications during pregnancy.

The second type is called *gestational diabetes,* or diabetes that only occurs during pregnancy. These women develop diabetes as a result of the hormones released during pregnancy. This type of diabetes is usually detected during routine blood tests at about twenty-four to forty-eight weeks. About 5 percent of pregnant women get gestational diabetes. Some risk factors for developing gestational diabetes include having had gestational diabetes in a previous pregnancy, having had a large baby, or a family history of diabetes and/or obesity.

Treatment for gestational diabetes usually involves dietary changes, and in some cases taking pills or insulin injections. If you have gestational diabetes, you will be put on a carefully structured diet, with six meals daily, including three regular meals and three snacks. A nurse specializing in diabetes will instruct you on how to test your own blood sugar. You should also expect to see your physician about every other week. Meeting with a nutritionist may also be recommended.

If you keep your regular prenatal appointments, chances are that your diabetes will remain under control. If you do not, however, you run the risk of having uncontrolled diabetes, which can lead to serious complications such as kidney problems, placental insufficiency, preeclampsia, and ketoacidosis. Diabetics are also more prone to having excessive amniotic fluid (polyhydramnios), vaginal infections, urinary tract infections, miscarriage, stillbirths, and babies born with congenital abnormalities. You should take careful note of your baby's movements and report anything out of the ordinary. After twenty-eight weeks of pregnancy, it is healthy to feel your baby kick ten times in the hour after eating.

Sometimes it is necessary for diabetic women to have a cesarean delivery, either because of complications related to diabetes or because their baby is too large to pass through the birth canal. If you are a diabetic, your baby will probably be carefully monitored after birth to ensure he or she remains in good health.

Risk Factors for Developing Diabetes in Pregnancy

- diabetes in the family
- preeclampsia with pregnancy
- previous delivery of a large baby
- diabetes in a previous pregnancy
- previous unexplained newborn death
- frequent urinary tract/vaginal infections
- previous stillbirth
- weighing over 200 pounds
- previous premature birth
- hypertension

Kidney Disease

Some maternal diseases affect proper kidney function, and these include recurrent urinary tract infections and underlying autoimmune disease. If you have an underlying condition such as lupus, then how your kidneys work is the most important indicator of how your pregnancy will progress. If your kidneys are damaged in any way, your pregnancy will be considered high-risk.

If you detect blood in your urine, you should immediately call your physician because it could mean you have a urinary tract infection. He or she will probably ask you to come into the office to have a midstream urine test done. Protein in the urine is usually indicative of a urinary tract infection. Your provider may also take blood to test for BUN and creatinine levels. The results of these two levels give the practitioner a general idea of how your kidneys are working. Sometimes a more detailed analysis will be prescribed and this involves a twenty-four-hour urine collection. This test is done in the laboratory and it determines the total amount of protein in your urine, which provides even more details about how your kidneys are working.

If all your tests are abnormal, there is a chance that you could develop high blood pressure and kidney infections during your pregnancy. This will put you into a high-risk category. Most likely you will be told to see a kidney specialist (nephrologist).

Gastrointestinal Problems

The most common gastrointestinal problems affecting pregnant women include peptic ulcers, and inflammatory bowel disease (Crohn's disease and ulcerative colitis).

Peptic Ulcers

Peptic ulcers are chronic sores that protrude through the lining of the gastrointestinal tract lining. Sometimes they penetrate the muscles of the duodenum, stomach, and/or esophagus. Studies have shown that approximately 44 percent of women with peptic ulcers say their symptoms improve during pregnancy. Researchers believe this may be due to the increased levels of blood progesterone.

Inflammatory Bowel Disease

Inflammatory bowel disease (IBD) causes a chronic inflammation in the digestive tract. The two most common types of IBD are ulcerative colitis and Crohn's disease.

Ulcerative colitis is an inflammation of the colon and rectum. The symptoms may include bloody stools, diarrhea, cramping, dehydration, abdominal pain, and serious weight loss. If a woman's colitis is relatively inactive at the time of conception, then chances are it will remain that way for the duration of her pregnancy. Problems occur if and when she requires emergency surgery to repair the problem, because this can result in premature labor and possible cesarean delivery to save the baby.

Crohn's disease is similar to ulcerative colitis, but it affects the entire gastrointestinal tract. If a woman has an active problem with Crohn's disease at the time of conception, she is at greater risk of having a miscarriage. However, if she is in remission at the time of conception, it is likely that she will have a normal pregnancy.

Both ulcerative colitis and Crohn's disease are diagnosed with sigmoidoscopy and colonoscopy, two safe procedures during pregnancy. Although there are no cures for these diseases, medications and other treatments are often prescribed and successfully used. Most of the medications used to treat IBD have been shown to be safe to the unborn baby.

Liver Disease

Many maternal conditions can affect liver function. If the liver has been damaged by drug use or alcohol, it can be quite serious. Infections such as hepatitis are the most common in the pregnant woman.

If you are having a problem with your liver, you will most likely be screened with liver function tests that will examine your bilirubin levels.

An increase in bilirubin indicates an obstruction in your liver, resulting in conditions such as gallbladder disease. The most frequently performed blood tests to determine if there has been any liver damage are the ALT and AST. These two enzymes are released when there is liver damage.

It is important to know that your baby has its own liver and is able to metabolize what yours cannot. Keep in mind that your baby's liver is relatively immature because it is one of the last organs to develop completely.

Hepatitis A and chronic hepatitis B and C are particularly dangerous because they can be transmitted from the mother's blood to the fetus's blood. At the present time, there is no treatment. Hepatitis B can be cleared by the liver, but in about one out of ten women it becomes chronic. In other words, the woman will have the disease for the rest of her life. Outside of pregnancy, hepatitis is treated with the medication interferon, but it is not considered a safe medication to be used during pregnancy.

If you have a liver infection, chances are your practitioner will avoid doing anything that could result in the virus being transmitted to your baby. Procedures such as amniocentesis, premature rupture of membranes, and putting a fetal scalp electrode on the baby's head are all contraindicated because all of them involve mixing both fetal and maternal blood.

To protect your baby from acquiring the hepatitis infection after birth, within an hour of delivery, he or she will receive a passive immunity vaccine (immunoglobulin), in addition to the first of a series of three hepatitis vaccines.

Hepatitis C is considered more dangerous and in about 5 to 10 percent of newborns it will be transmitted from the mother to her baby. For reasons not clearly understood, this number increases to 40 percent if the mother is HIV positive. Unfortunately, there is no way to prevent the baby from getting the virus, not even through cesarean delivery. If the mother has hepatitis C, her provider will also try to avoid the mixing of maternal and fetal blood.

There is controversy about breast-feeding and hepatitis. The American Academy of Pediatrics believes that it is safe; however, the consensus among obstetricians is that the virus is transmitted through breast milk and therefore it is *not* safe to breast-feed.

Thyroid Disease

The thyroid is an endocrine gland located at the front of the neck. It secretes hormones essential to a balanced metabolism. If the thyroid is not working properly, it may be either overactive (hyperthyroidism) or underactive (hypothyroidism).

Hyperthyroidism affects about 0.5 percent of pregnant women, and these women run the risk of having low-birth-weight babies. Hyperthyroidism must be treated with medication, and your physician will monitor you closely during your pregnancy.

Hypothyroidism rarely occurs in pregnant women because it tends to be associated with infertility. It is usually treated with thyroid replacements, such as synthroid. If untreated, a miscarriage may occur, because early in pregnancy, the fetus depends on the mother's thyroid activity.

Epilepsy

Epilepsy is characterized by recurrent seizures brought on by an abnormality of the neurological system. It is the most common preexisting neurological disorder among pregnant women. It is estimated that nearly one million American women of childbearing age have epilepsy.

Studies indicate that the hormonal and metabolic changes that occur during pregnancy predispose the epileptic woman to more seizures. The treatment for seizures is with antiepileptic medications, which are generally safe, but may sometimes result in fetal malformations. More than 90 percent of women taking antiseizure medications have normal babies. Most doctors recommend taking 4 mg of folic acid before conception to help reduce the risk of fetal malformations.

If you are epileptic and planning to get pregnant, you should discuss with your physician the best plan for you. If you have not had a seizure for a long time, your physician may try to stop your medications for a few months and monitor you closely. If you do have a seizure, your physician should be notified immediately. Seizures interfere with the fetal oxygen supply, which could jeopardize your baby's well-being. Your family and friends, or whomever is with you, should be prepared to answer certain questions, such as the date and time of your seizure, how long it lasted, what type of movements you had, if you were able to speak, and whether you slept afterward.

Autoimmune Diseases

Autoimmune disorders are five times more common among women and the incidence tends to peak during reproductive years. Below are some of the most common disorders in this group.

Systemic Lupus Erythematosus (SLE or Lupus)

Lupus is a chronic inflammatory disease of many systems in the body, occurring predominantly in young women. It affects approximately one in seven hundred women between the ages of fifteen and sixty-four, the onset usually occurring before menopause. The disease may begin abruptly, accompanied by fever and signs of infection, or it may exist unnoticed for months. Sensitivity to light, joint pain, a butterfly rash on the face, fatigue, and weight loss are common. The disease is characterized by flare-ups and is diagnosed by physical examination and blood tests.

Today, there is more hope for women with lupus who want to become pregnant. With optimal care and close supervision, these women can carry healthy babies. The best time for a woman with lupus to become pregnant is when the disease has been in remission for six months or more. This minimizes the stress on the pregnant woman while also minimizing the baby's exposure to medications.

In general, the effect of lupus on pregnancy is largely dependent on the phase in which pregnancy occurs (flare-up or remission). If you are in an active stage of lupus, it may flare up during pregnancy. Most symptoms, such as skin rashes and joint swelling, will rarely lead to any permanent damage to the fetus. However, the fetus should be closely monitored for any heart abnormalities, such as heart block, which is frequently associated with babies of mothers who have lupus. Babies born with heart block and no other heart problem will do well, but will require a pacemaker.

If you want to become pregnant and have lupus, your physician may prescribe the steroid prednisone and a low dosage of aspirin prior to conception to minimize the complications of lupus. Some pregnant women will be prescribed prednisone in addition to azathioprine (Imuran). At the present time, these are considered safe during pregnancy.

The incidence of miscarriage for women with lupus is about 25 percent, and for this reason, it is important for these women to be carefully monitored during their pregnancy.

One woman with eight pregnancy losses and one child describes her experience with lupus:

> "Had I known that I had lupus when I became pregnant, it would have been a lot easier. The doctors kept telling me that miscarriage is so common and that I should try again. Being the trusting person that I am, I followed their advice. It wasn't until I had miscarried the fifth time that I decided to change doctors. That doctor began doing tests on me because former autopsies of the fetuses showed that each time the placenta began to disintegrate. After many tests, I found out that I had a form of lupus that becomes very active during pregnancy. I was prescribed cortisone, which helped me. Now whenever I speak to women who miscarry, I encourage them to seek another medical opinion. I don't believe that there is such a thing as a miscarriage without a cause."

Rheumatoid Arthritis

Rheumatoid arthritis is a disease that causes chronic joint inflammation. The most common joints affected are the wrists, hands, feet, and ankles, but other joints may also be involved. Rheumatoid arthritis affects more than two million Americans, most often between the ages of twenty and fifty; however, it may begin during pregnancy or sometime in the postpartum period.

If you have rheumatoid arthritis prior to pregnancy, it might become less intense during pregnancy. Chances are that if you are on medications, they will have to be adjusted, because some of the medications used in the treatment of rheumatoid arthritis, such as aspirin, may cause excessive bleeding. In general, the fetus remains unaffected by rheumatoid arthritis; however, the woman may have some difficulty and/or pain during delivery because the hip joints and lumbar spine are usually affected.

Myasthenia Gravis

Myasthenia gravis is a serious muscle weakening that affects the skeletal muscles but not the smooth muscles, such as the heart and the uterus.

This autoimmune disease is caused by circulating antibodies that affect proper muscle contractions, which may or may not affect the pregnancy. Studies have shown that in 30 percent of women their pregnancy is unaffected; 40 percent of women claim that their symptoms become worse. The treatment is usually an anticholinesterase medication (i.e., neostigmine), which have some side effects, including abdominal discomfort, diarrhea, and vomiting.

Later in pregnancy, women with myasthenia gravis might have trouble with helping to push during labor; in other words, they have difficulty "bearing down."

There is a risk of premature delivery associated with this disease and in about 20 percent of women, the newborn baby also experiences some temporary muscle weakness within the first few days of birth.

Immune Thrombocytopenic Purpura (ITP)

Immune thrombocytopenic purpura (ITP) is a condition in which the blood does not clot properly. This is due to a low number of platelets (the part of the blood responsible for clotting). Those who have ITP usually have bruises on their skin or mucous membranes. The bleeding occurs in small blood vessels and looks like small dots on the skin. For some unknown reason, the immune system attacks and destroys its own platelets, and therefore blood clotting does not occur.

If you have any of the following symptoms, your physician will do a blood test to see if you have ITP:

- unexplained blood clots
- low platelet count
- recurrent miscarriages

Unfortunately, this condition often worsens during pregnancy and the extent depends on the mother's platelet count. ITP can be treated with corticosteroids, but they are not always successful. Obstetricians try to avoid cesareans deliveries with these women, but if a cesarean delivery is necessary, then a platelet transfusion may be necessary. This disease can cross the placenta causing similar problems in the fetus; however, studies have shown this to be rare.

For more assistance, you can contact the Platelet Disorder Support Association at (877) PLATELET (752-8353).

Antiphospholipid Antibody Syndrome (APLAS, APA, or APS)

Antiphospholipid antibody syndrome (APLAS) is an autoimmune disorder of blood coagulation that results in the formation of blood clots in the body's veins and arteries. The disease is caused by the mother producing antibodies against phospholipids (a substance found in membranes of every cell in the body). The pregnant woman's body sees the phospholipids as foreign material and as a result, it releases antibodies to attack them. In the end, the antibodies cause dangerous blood clots in the arteries or veins that prevent both mother and child from receiving proper nutrients.

APLAS is diagnosed by means of a blood test, and if diagnosed, it is considered extremely dangerous because it can lead to complications such as preeclampsia, miscarriage, growth restriction, or stillbirth. There is no cure for this condition, but the treatment is usually with aspirin and heparin. Sometimes prednisone is also given. For more information on the subject I recommend Triona Holden's book, *Positive Options for Antiphospholipid Syndrome (APS)*.

Asthma

Asthma is a chronic condition of the respiratory system causing airways, including the bronchial tubes and the lungs, to become temporarily inflamed and narrowed as a result of excessive mucus production, most often in response to environmental triggers. This narrowing, or constriction, results in the wheezing sound commonly made by asthmatics. Asthma often begins during childhood, but it can occur at any age.

If your asthma has been under control before your pregnancy, then chances are you will not have any problems during pregnancy. Most of the medications used for asthma, such as inhalers, bronchodilators, and steroids are perfectly safe to use during pregnancy. It is important that you take your medications, because if you are not getting enough oxygen, then neither is your baby. It is important to get your flu shot between the months of November to March to avoid getting the flu, which could predispose you to an asthma attack.

Heart Disease

Between 0.5 and 2 percent of pregnant women have underlying heart disease during pregnancy. A previous episode of rheumatic fever is responsible for about 50 percent of heart problems in pregnant women; however, this disease is now rare in the United States. Most heart problems are related to congenital factors. Other related ailments are heart-valve problems, congenital heart disease, and abnormal heartbeats.

The extra weight and water retention common in pregnancy make the heart work much harder, and for this reason, if you already have heart disease, you will be carefully monitored during pregnancy. On the other hand, if you are symptom-free, it is likely that your pregnancy will have no complications. However, if you have pain, discomfort, difficulty breathing at night or while lying down, and dizziness after activity—that is, symptoms arising after little or no exertion— you may have a difficult pregnancy.

Pulmonary hypertension (high blood pressure in the arteries of the lungs) is extremely dangerous, particularly during pregnancy. A woman with this type of heart disease is usually advised not to get pregnant. If a woman has heart valve problems, there is a 3 to 5 percent chance that her baby will inherit the problem. Usually, an echocardiogram is recommended between twenty to twenty-two weeks. Genetic testing may also be done.

Although the treatment varies depending on your situation, your physician will probably prescribe an iron and folic acid supplement (see Chapter 2). Medications such as furosemide, digoxin, propranolol, quinidine, heparin, or norpace are sometimes prescribed with caution. You may be advised to stay in bed to avoid unnecessary strain on your heart. Your physician will also probably refer you to a cardiologist for a more complete evaluation.

One of the main risks for the mother associated with heart disease can arise shortly after birth. What happens is that the body adjusts as a result of the hormonal and cardiovascular changes associated with pregnancy. If you have a history of heart disease or are predisposed to heart disease, your physician will continue to monitor you closely, even after your baby is born. Those who get short of breath, even while at rest or with little exertion, will obviously need to be monitored more closely.

Sickle-Cell Anemia

Sickle-cell anemia is an inherited hemoglobin disorder that primarily affects those of West-African origin. Children who receive abnormal genes from both parents have predominantly sickle-cell hemoglobin, which causes their red blood cells to become deformed when they are deprived of oxygen. As a result, they may suffer from anemia, which can range from mild to severe. They may have sickle-cell attacks, which are caused by the passage of these deformed red blood cells through the capillaries (the smallest blood vessels in the body). These people usually lead a healthy life, although they are at a greater risk for developing urinary tract infections.

Every African-American couple is screened for sickle-cell disease. There is no cure, and death may occur during an acute crisis due to a severe infection or health problem. Sickle-cell anemia may be detected prenatally. Those with a family history of this disorder should seek genetic counseling prior to considering pregnancy (see Chapter 6).

Depression

Over the years, the incidence of depression has increased, and in severe cases, it can interfere with normal day-to-day functioning. The hormonal changes associated with pregnancy, such as elevated progesterone, can sometimes lead women to feel "blue." Individuals predisposed to depression are those who have low self-esteem, those who tend to be very self-critical, and those who tend to be pessimistic. Although depression runs in families, stress can also be a trigger. Depression crosses all socioeconomic groups and ages. Studies have shown that women who experience postpartum depression tend to display early signs of depression during pregnancy.

The treatment for depression usually begins with counseling and/or psychotherapy. Sometimes antidepressant medications are given to supplement these modalities and they are usually safe to use during pregnancy. The only medication that has shown to cause problems is paroxetine hydrochloride (Paxil), which studies have indicated can cause a two-fold increase in fetal heart defects.

Other treatments for depression include moderate exercise, such as walking, yoga, Pilates, or qigong. To treat depression holistically, some practitioners may recommend omega-3 essential fatty acid supplements (3,000 mg per day), with food. Also, treatments such as acupuncture and massage can help alleviate stressors that sometimes lead to depression.

Some women make the independent decision to stop their medications when they get pregnant, but this is not advised. If you feel good on your antidepressants, it usually means that they are working for you and your body needs them. It is dangerous to wean yourself without medical supervision. Antidepressant medications sometimes take three to six months to work and if you stop them too quickly, your symptoms may return and you may feel even worse than you did prior to beginning the medication. In order to minimize the effects of stopping antidepressants, most practitioners will suggest decreasing the dosage slowly. If you have a history of depression, you are at high-risk of developing postpartum depression after your baby is born (see Chapter 10).

Other Problems

You may have a history of other medical problems not listed in this chapter that may place your pregnancy in a high-risk category. If you have a special condition, remember to ask your physician how your pregnancy will be affected and what he or she recommends for you. Physicians have many patients and many things on their minds, and they cannot be expected to remember everything. Reminding your physician of your important medical details and history is your responsibility—and always remember to mention any medications you are taking, whether they are prescribed or over-the-counter.

One last comment. If you are changing health-care providers or have moved, it is important that you bring all the records of your previous pregnancies with you to the appointment with your specialist so that he or she can provide the best care possible.

Journaling Corner

What concerns do you have about your pregnancy right now?

What books have you found most helpful, and why?

Describe any trips you've taken during your pregnancy and how you felt during those trips.

Do you have any particular food likes or dislikes?

What is the best advice anyone gave you about being pregnant?

Have you experienced any feelings of depression with this pregnancy or previous pregnancies? What goes through your mind when you are "blue"?

5

High-Risk Factors Related to Pregnancy

Life shrinks or expands in proportion to one's courage. — ANAÏS NIN

In addition to some of the chronic problems discussed in Chapter 4, there are a number of conditions that can cause complications during your pregnancy. The most common ones are discussed below.

Hyperemesis Gravidarum (HEG)

Many women experience occasional morning sickness (nausea and vomiting) during their first trimester. Having small, frequent meals is usually helpful to alleviate these symptoms. However, if the symptoms go beyond mild nausea, hyperemesis gravidarum is usually suspected. Severe vomiting and nausea in pregnancy have also been associated with hydatidiform mole (discussed later).

The symptoms of hyperemesis gravidarum include weight loss, dehydration, and imbalances of the body's electrolytes, such as potassium and sodium. Hospitalization is often necessary to provide intravenous nourishment and psychological support. Some sources indicate that this condition may be associated with increased levels of chorionic gonadotropin hormones, the hormones secreted by the placenta during pregnancy and present in the urine of pregnant women. In fact, these hormones are the indicators of pregnancy in pregnancy tests. They alter the body's metabolism, which may result in a slowing down of digestion.

It is important to understand that if you are diagnosed with this condition, it does not mean that something is wrong with your pregnancy; indeed, it may be a sign that your pregnancy is healthy and progressing well. Some experts believe that it may be nature's way to protect both you and your baby.

If you need more information or support in coping with morning sickness, a wonderful resource that Dr. Norwitz frequently recommends to his patients is a book called *Managing Morning Sickness: A Survival Guide for Pregnant Women* by Miriam Erick.

Ectopic Pregnancy

An ectopic pregnancy is one where the egg implants itself outside of the uterine cavity. About 98 percent of ectopic pregnancies occur in the fallopian tube, although implantation can also occur in the ovary, the cervix, or abdominal cavity (see Figure 5.1). Any previous injury or obstruction to the fallopian tube may have resulted in scarring that could affect the egg's journey to the uterus for implantation. An embryo that implants itself outside the uterus usually cannot develop normally.

The incidence of ectopic pregnancies has risen over the years and, according to the *New England Journal of Medicine* (1997), approximately one hundred thousand cases are reported each year. Despite this increase, mortality rates have decreased dramatically because of new diagnostic medical and surgical techniques.

Early diagnosis of an ectopic pregnancy is critical to save a woman's life and safeguard her future ability to bear children. If you have an ectopic pregnancy, you might have some of the telltale signs, such as fainting, a missed period, abdominal pain (mild at first, then becoming severe), vaginal bleeding, and a mass felt in your abdomen. The first sign is usually pain in the lower abdomen. Some women complain of a dull,

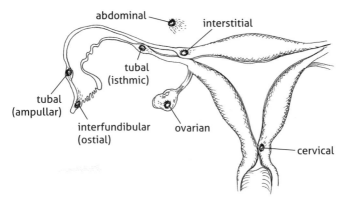

Figure 5.1: Common sites for ectopic pregnancy

aching pain, while others may experience excruciating pain. One woman said that she had such intense pain she thought her appendix had ruptured. If you have any of these symptoms, you should immediately call your physician.

An ectopic pregnancy is usually diagnosed by ultrasound, blood tests, and a pelvic examination. The reason for the ultrasound is to detect a normal pregnancy inside the uterus. If you have a high hcG blood level and a fetus is not located in your uterus, your obstetrician will assume that you have an ectopic pregnancy. When an ectopic pregnancy is confirmed, a decision will be made about what to do.

If the pregnancy is early and you are not bleeding, medications such as methotrexate, an anticancer medication, will be prescribed. This medication dissolves the placental and embryonic tissue. It also eliminates the risk of surgical damage to the fallopian tubes and subsequent infertility.

Some women may not require any medication because their ectopic pregnancy will be reabsorbed by their body. In some instances, microsurgery needs to be performed to remove the products of conception and to save the fallopian tube. On the other hand, if you are having excruciating pain, it usually means that your tube has ruptured and emergency surgery will have to be done to remove the products of conception and your fallopian tube.

Waiting for surgery may be very uncomfortable for you. It is best to remain calm and to stay in a comfortable position. Sitting or standing usually intensifies the discomfort in the rectal area, and for some women lying down intensifies shoulder pain, especially if bleeding has occurred in their abdomen because of the ruptured fallopian tube.

Facing surgery for an ectopic pregnancy is difficult. You will be dealing with the normal fear of the surgical procedure, as well as the possible loss of fertility. Ectopic surgery may decrease your chances of being able to conceive again, but it does not entirely eliminate the possibility of a future pregnancy. Chances are that you will experience all the anger and concerns that accompany loss (see Chapter 9). Speaking with other women who have been through a similar experience may help you cope, and certainly journaling your feelings cannot be overemphasized.

Fortunately, because of early diagnostics and proactive care, women today with a history of having had an ectopic pregnancy have a good chance of a successful future pregnancy. Also, you should know that you only need one healthy fallopian tube to get pregnant.

Sometimes developing an ectopic pregnancy is a random event, but in other instances there are certain risk factors that might predispose some women to an ectopic pregnancy. These include the following:

- endometriosis
- a history of tubal adhesions
- a previous ectopic pregnancy
- DES exposure
- a history of pelvic inflammatory disease (PID)
- a previous surgery to the fallopian tubes or pelvic cavity
- a history of excessive tobacco usage

Hydatidiform Mole

A hydatidiform mole, or molar pregnancy, is an abnormal development of the placenta that results in a benign or malignant tumor. In this rare condition, a developing pregnancy degenerates and the placental tissue forms a grapelike mass called a hydatidiform mole. It occurs in about one in fifteen hundred pregnancies in the United States and is eight times more common in East Asia. It is also more common in women under the age of twenty and over the age of forty. The causes are unknown, although it has been associated with nutritional deficiency, chromosomal abnormalities, and hormonal imbalance.

The symptoms of a hydatidiform mole include signs of preeclampsia, extreme nausea, bleeding, an unusually large uterus for the stage of pregnancy, and the absence of fetal heart sounds. It is usually detected late in the first trimester or early in the second trimester. The diagnosis is made by ultrasound.

The treatment options include vacuum aspiration, similar to the procedure used in abortion, oxytocin or prostaglandin induction to expel the contents of the uterus, or hysterectomy. If you have a hydatidiform mole and your childbearing years are nearing an end, hysterectomy may be recommended.

The loss that a woman feels following this procedure is often similar to that of a miscarriage, since she thought she was having a baby up until the time the diagnosis was made. Some women may have odd feelings, such as feeling like a "freak" or feeling less feminine and desirable. It is important that you continue to look after yourself and be good to yourself. (See Chapter 9 for more information on dealing with loss.)

Assisted Reproductive Technologies (ART) and In Vitro Fertilization (IVF) Pregnancies

A growing number of women who have difficulty becoming pregnant turn to assisted reproductive technologies (ART). According to the Centers for Disease Control and Prevention, the number of ART cycles performed in the United States increased 54 percent during the years 1996 to 2000.

Although the idea of finally being able to bring a baby into the world is an exciting one, most of these women end up having a high-risk pregnancy. This is because many tend to be older and sometimes there are the risks equated with advanced age pregnancy. In addition, there is a higher incidence of multiple pregnancies in ART pregnancies. For example, in the year 2000, 35 percent of all live births from ART were multiples, as compared to 3 percent in the general population.

These women are also at a greater risk of having low-birth-weight babies and possibly babies with birth defects. The increased incidence of high-risk issues does not necessarily mean you will need to be monitored by a high-risk specialist, but you should be aware of the risks.

Hypertension

Hypertension is a condition in which blood pressure is higher than normal for your age and weight. It is more common in women who are pregnant for the first time and those who are over the age of thirty-five or under the age of eighteen. Other factors may contribute to your risk for having high blood pressure during pregnancy, such as having a family history of hypertension, diabetes, being overweight, having kidney disease, a history of hypertension in a previous pregnancy, or carrying multiple fetuses.

If blood pressure is not maintained at normal levels, it may result in intrauterine growth restriction, premature birth, placental separation (the placenta ages more quickly with hypertension), or fetal death. Today, if detected early, hypertension can be successfully treated and managed. It is important that when you have your blood pressure taken, that it is done in both the seated and lying positions.

There are two types of hypertension that can have an effect on pregnancy: chronic hypertension and gestational hypertension. Chronic hypertension develops over a period of many years and gestational hypertension usually develops after twenty weeks of pregnancy. The symptoms and treatments are different, although both have similar effects on the woman and her baby.

Chronic Hypertension

Most women who have chronic hypertension can have healthy babies. It might be a good idea to meet with your physician prior to becoming pregnant so that he or she can effectively manage your blood pressure and medications. By the time you arrive in your second trimester, your provider will have probably performed baseline liver and kidney blood tests. Beginning at thirty-two weeks a nonstress test will be performed every week (see Chapter 7). In most cases, your provider will recommend that induction of labor is done at about thirty-nine or forty weeks.

When not pregnant, chronic hypertension is often treated with angiotensin-converting enzymes (ACE inhibitors) such as enalapril or captopril; however, these medications are not safe during pregnancy. The American College of Obstetricians and Gynecologists (ACOG) recommends pregnant women take methyldopa (Aldomet) to treat chronic hypertension. Some physicians suggest calcium blockers such as nifedipine (Adalat, Procardia) and beta blockers such as labetalol (Normodyne, Trandate). These are all quite safe during pregnancy.

Other providers believe that the treatment for chronic hypertension should primarily involve keeping blood pressure down without the use of medications. You will be told to lie on your side whenever possible and to limit salt products in your diet. Water retention can cause blood pressure to rise and therefore should be avoided. It is important to avoid foods that encourage the body to retain water, such as potato chips, pickles, smoked meats, and carbonated beverages. A high-protein diet may also be recommended to replace protein lost in the urine. You will probably be told to stop working at this point.

Bed rest (see Chapter 8) is sometimes prescribed, in addition to having at least eight to twelve hours of sleep each night. An afternoon nap will also help you relax and minimizes the chances of overworking your heart.

Gestational Hypertension

Gestational hypertension is a condition characterized by an increase in blood pressure during pregnancy. It usually occurs after twenty weeks of gestation when you tend to gain extra weight.

There are two types of gestational hypertension: gestational hypertension non-proteinuria (without protein in the urine) and gestational hypertension proteinuria (with protein in the urine), also known as preeclampsia.

Gestational Non-Proteinuric Hypertension: This type of hypertension was formerly called pregnancy-induced hypertension and refers to high blood pressure at the end of pregnancy without protein in the urine and with no symptoms of preeclampsia. Typically, this type of hypertension does *not* cause any harm to either the mother or baby.

Preeclampsia (Formerly Toxemia): Preeclampsia is a disease that affects approximately 7 percent of pregnant women. It is characterized by:

- protein in the urine (proteinuria)
- elevated blood pressure
- swelling of the face, hands, and feet

Additional symptoms may include headaches, blurred vision, and epigastric (upper abdomen) pain. Some women complain that their hands feel as if they are ballooning. Preeclampsia can be either mild or severe. Treatment for preeclampsia depends on its severity. Bed rest is often recommended in the later stages of pregnancy, as well as lying on your side, which helps to increase the blood supply to the fetus. Dietary changes, such as those mentioned earlier for hypertension, may also be prescribed. You will be closely monitored by your physician and in some cases hospitalization may be necessary.

One mother recalls her preeclampsia in the latter part of her pregnancy:

"I'll never forget how swollen my hands were. I had been married for five years and my wedding ring grew so tight that I had to have it cut off—it was causing my finger to turn blue. I couldn't even open the door to get the newspaper from outside. I often wondered what I would do if we had a fire in the duplex—how would I escape? My doctor treated my problem by putting me on bed rest for the last two months of my pregnancy. It managed to keep my blood pressure down without the use of medications. I was also very strict about my diet. The hardest part, however, was just after waking up in the morning. My hands and feet were so stiff that I had to wait an hour before I was even able to dress myself...when I finally did, gee, did I look funny in my husband's running pants and size 12 slippers! Anyway, it was all worthwhile because I had two healthy 7-pound boys at thirty-six weeks."

Eclampsia: Some women with preeclampsia will develop a severe complication called eclampsia. Eclampsia refers to seizures or coma during pregnancy in the setting of preeclampsia and in the absence of other neurological problems. The diagnosis is confirmed when a woman has protein in her urine, high blood pressure, and seizures. There are often no warnings for eclampsia. There is a possibility of death for both mother and baby, so early delivery is usually recommended.

HELLP Syndrome: HELLP syndrome is sometimes used to describe one of the life-threatening manifestations of severe preeclampsia. It is an acronym that stands for hemolysis, elevated liver enzymes, and low platelets. Some women with severe preeclampsia get symptoms such as headaches and seizures (eclampsia), and some get HELLP syndrome.

Researchers do not know why women manifest severe preeclampsia in different ways. Some studies have shown that it may have to do with their ethnic background. For example, African-American women are more likely to get seizures, whereas Caucasian women are more like to get HELLP syndrome.

Gallstones

The gallbladder is a sac located under the edge of the liver. Its role is to store bile, which aids in digestion. Those who develop gallstones are frequently overweight, and they tend to consume large amounts of fatty or highly seasoned foods. Gallstones (cholelithiasis) are more common in pregnant women, and pregnancy may also exacerbate the problem, leading to an inflammation of the gallbladder (cholecystitis).

The symptoms of gallstones include a sudden aching pain in the upper right part of the abdomen, sometimes radiating to the back and shoulder. It usually occurs after eating, especially after eating fatty foods. The pain or sense of fullness lasts fifteen to sixty seconds. If you have gallstones, your physician may simply suggest a diet change and pain-relieving medications, such as meperidine or morphine. In certain situations, surgery may be necessary.

Cholestasis During Pregnancy

Cholestasis during pregnancy usually occurs in the last trimester and is caused by a slowing of bile through the gallbladder as a result of the changing hormones of pregnancy. This slowing of bile acids through the gallbladder and backup of bile acids into the bloodstream is usually characterized by extreme generalized body itching, which sometimes becomes worse at night.

Approximately one or two pregnant women in a thousand will develop cholestasis. It is more common in women with multiples (twins, triplets, etc.), women whose mothers or sisters had the disease, women who have had liver disease in the past, or women who have had cholestasis in previous pregnancies.

Some women may notice, in addition to the extreme itching, a loss of appetite, fatigue, light-colored bowel movements, depression, or dark urine. Less-common symptoms include pain in the upper-right side of your abdomen or mild jaundice. The diagnosis is confirmed by a blood test that shows an elevated bile acid level. Treatment is usually with a medication called ursodeoxycholic acid, topical creams such as Sarna lotion, or antihistamines.

Cholestasis can cause fetal distress, premature labor, or stillbirth. Your provider will monitor your baby closely. To prevent any fetal complications, your provider may decide to induce your labor and deliver your baby several weeks before your due date. Typically, cholestasis resolves spontaneously a few days after your baby is born.

Appendicitis

Inflammation of the appendix occurs in approximately one in every one thousand pregnancies. Most cases of sudden appendicitis occur within the first six months of pregnancy. The problem with having appendicitis during pregnancy is that it may be difficult to diagnose in a timely matter and it may be challenging for the provider to perform a proper physical examination.

The most common symptoms of appendicitis are fever and abdominal pain. Initially, the pain may be generalized, but eventually it becomes localized to the lower right quadrant. Usually the pain is accompanied by fever, loss of appetite, and a change in bowel habits, either constipation or diarrhea.

If you have sharp pain in the lower right part of your abdomen, you should see your provider immediately. He or she will perform an examination and also do a blood test. If you have appendicitis, your white blood count will be elevated. In pregnant women, the pain may also be felt in the right upper part of the abdomen because the uterus has pushed the abdominal contents upward. Sometimes this pain can be confused with gallbladder pain.

There is a chance of the appendix rupturing, which in some cases can be life-threatening. For unknown reasons, pregnant women are two to three times more likely to suffer a ruptured appendix than their nonpregnant counterparts. Ruptured or not, the treatment for appendicitis is immediate surgery. Surgery is necessary because a ruptured appendix is very dangerous. It can spread the infection throughout the abdominal cavity, then to the uterus, and then to the baby, which could have grave ramifications.

Thromboembolism

This is a condition whereby a blood vessel becomes blocked by a clot. There are two types: a deep vein thrombosis and a pulmonary embolism. A deep vein thrombosis is a blood clot formation in a deep vein, usually in the legs or pelvis. A pulmonary embolism is a blood clot that has formed in the pulmonary artery.

It is thought that pregnancy hormones can affect blood clotting factors and make women more susceptible to thromboembolisms. The condition is more common in those who are relatively immobile. What happens is that blood pools in the lower legs, making a perfect environment for blood clot formation. This is one good reason to do the passive exercises described in Chapter 8 during bed rest. Other high-risk situations may predispose a woman to thromboembolism, such as abortion, cesarean birth, air travel, long car trips, or infections following delivery.

In the nonpregnant woman, oral antiblood-clotting medications such as warfarin (Coumadin) are prescribed to thin the blood; however, these medications are unsafe during pregnancy. Heparin, another anticoagulant, can be safely given to the expectant mother (either subcutaneously or intravenously) because it is unable to cross the placenta. If you are not hospitalized, you may be taught how to give yourself heparin injections at home. Minor cases of thromboembolism are usually treated medically and sometimes low-dose aspirin will be prescribed to thin the blood. Surgery is only performed in the event of a life-or-death situation.

Infections

An infection that you may have ignored before pregnancy could be a real danger when you are expecting. All infections pose a potential risk to mother and child. Some common types of infection include kidney/urinary infections, sexually transmitted infections (syphilis, gonorrhea, herpes, cytomegalovirus, chlamydia), HIV virus, toxoplasmosis, rubella, and chicken pox.

Bacteria in the Urine

At each of your prenatal visits, you will be asked to provide a urine sample. Sometimes the urine analysis shows bacteria. If there are no other signs of infection, your condition is called asymptomatic bacteruria.

Some women are more prone to having bacteria or protein in their urine. Typically, these are diabetics or women with neurological problems who need to catheterize themselves. The urine of these high-risk women must be checked on a monthly basis.

Urinary Tract Infections (UTIs)

The typical signs of a urinary tract infection include feeling like you have to urinate frequently—and when you do so, it turns out to be in small amounts, accompanied by a stinging or burning sensation while you void, discomfort in the kidney region or the lower back, and sometimes blood in the urine (hematuria).

If you have any of these symptoms, you should immediately contact your practitioner. If your urine test shows you have a urinary tract infection, you will be treated with oral antibiotics such as sulfonamides, ampicillin, or macrodantin. Some women find that regular use of cranberry juice and/or vitamin C helps to acidify the urine and prevent recurrent urinary tract infections. Whole grains, nuts, and fresh fruits also help to acidify the urine. Some herbal teas such as uva ursi, horsetail, shavegrass, cornsilk cleavers, and lemon balm are also beneficial for the bladder. However, if you are pregnant, you should speak with an herbalist about the safety of using these teas during pregnancy.

Some women are more prone to urinary tract infections than others. The tips below can help decrease your chances of getting a urinary tract infection:

Preventing Urinary Tract Infections

- Wipe front to back after urinating.
- Have a urine test every trimester.
- Wash after intercourse.
- Urinate at the first urge.
- Drink six to eight glasses of water daily.
- Avoid perfumed toilet papers, soaps, and bubble baths.
- Avoid feminine hygiene sprays and douches.
- After intercourse, try urinating and then drink a glass of water.
- Treat vaginal infections as soon as symptoms occur.

Your health-care provider might also take some actions to prevent urinary tract infections during your pregnancy. Some may choose to do a urine test every trimester. High-risk women may be given a small daily dose of antibiotic.

It is important that urinary tract infections are treated immediately. If left untreated, a urinary tract infection could lead to a kidney infection (pyelonephritis), which is sometimes more difficult to treat but is not harmful to mother or baby. A kidney infections may also be due to other illnesses, such as diabetes and lupus.

Pyelonephritis is an inflammation of the kidney usually caused by bacteria that has ascended from the bladder after entering through the urethra. It may be caused by an untreated urinary tract infection. If left untreated, it can lead to preterm labor.

The symptoms of pyelonephritis include fever, chills, aching lower back pain, loss of appetite, and nausea/vomiting. Treatment is with intravenous antibiotics in the hospital.

Sexually Transmitted Infections (STIs)

There are a number of sexually transmitted infections that could affect your pregnancy and its outcome. They include syphilis, gonorrhea, genital herpes, cytomegalovirus, chlamydia, HIV, and tricomonas.

Syphilis: Syphilis is a sexually transmitted infection caused by the bacterium *Treponema pallidum.* It has been called the "great imitator" because many of the signs and symptoms are difficult to distinguish from other diseases. The incidence has increased over the years and in 2006 over 36,000 reported cases were documented in the United States. The highest incidence of the disease is in women between the ages of twenty and twenty-four. Pregnant women can transmit the infection to their babies. The incidence among newborns has also increased from 339 cases in 2005 to 349 cases in 2006.

The first stage of syphilis is characterized by a painless chancre (ulceration) that appears between ten and ninety days after exposure and heals within forty days of its appearance. The second stage is characterized by a rash, accompanied by malaise, fever, and aching bones. Syphilis is very contagious during this stage, which lasts about three months. The third stage is characterized by latency (no symptoms) as the organism invades other parts of the body. During this stage, a woman can continue to infect her unborn children for up to four years after she initially contracted the disease.

If diagnosed early, treatment with the antibiotic penicillin is used. If treated prior to sixteen weeks of pregnancy, the mother will be completely cured and the infant will be unaffected. It is critical that both the mother-to-be and her partner are both treated for syphilis.

According to the Centers for Disease Control and Prevention (CDC), depending on how long a pregnant woman has been infected, she may be at risk of having a stillbirth or giving birth to a baby who dies after birth. The infected baby will be born with symptoms of the disease and if not treated immediately, the baby may develop serious problems quickly after birth.

Gonorrhea: Gonorrhea is a very common disease in the United States today. It is estimated that seven hundred thousand people are affected annually, although many cases go unreported. Today, gonorrhea is typically detected during prepregnancy and prenatal screening. Gonorrhea is transmitted through sexual contact. In men, the main symptom is a disturbing burning of the penis, with a pus discharge. Women may be free of symptoms and may carry the organism for years without knowing it. Eventually, a woman who has the disease develops pelvic inflammatory disease, an inflammation of the uterus, fallopian tubes, and ovaries that often leads to scar tissue in nearby organs. It can sometimes be a causative factor in infertility. Gonorrhea is usually detected when the woman develops otherwise unexplainable arthritis.

If a woman with gonorrhea becomes pregnant, the risks to the fetus include preterm labor, growth impairment, blood infection, blindness, and newborn conjunctivitis between two and seven days after birth. To prevent the latter, the standard practice in North American hospitals is to administer silver nitrate or erythromycin eye drops to newborns within an hour after birth. For adults, penicillin is the most common treatment for gonorrhea. Erythromycin is sometimes given because of the increased chance of chlamydia being present with gonorrhea.

Genital Herpes: Herpes is a contagious infection caused by the herpes simplex virus and it is the most prevalent sexually transmitted disease in the United States. Researchers have found that both Type I and Type II can cause genital infections, even though historically, genital infections were associated with Type II. Today, 20 to 30 percent of genital infections are Type I. Although the incidence has decreased slightly in the past decade, it can be identified in one out of five adolescents and adults combined, although most do not develop symptoms. In women, genital herpes is characterized by blisters or ulcers on the genitals lasting one to three weeks, and on an average about twenty days. When the ulcers are present, herpes is very contagious. Its most serious aspect, however, is that the disease organism remains dormant between outbreaks. People who come into sexual contact with someone with herpes may unknowingly be infected as well.

It is rare for herpes to be transmitted through the placenta to the fetus. Those who are infected with genital herpes early in pregnancy, during critical periods of fetal development, may have a higher incidence of miscarriage or stillbirth than others. Those infected with herpes after twenty weeks of gestation have a higher incidence of preterm labor and transmission of the virus to the newborn baby. The baby can contract the herpes virus through the birth canal, creating the risk of brain damage, blindness, and death. If there are no lesions, the risk to the baby is low.

If there are no apparent lesions and the woman goes into labor, the baby will be delivered vaginally. However, if lesions or symptoms are present at the time of labor, a cesarean will be recommended because the herpes virus can pass from mother to baby when the membranes rupture in labor and/or during vaginal delivery.

If a woman has herpes during pregnancy (or has a history of herpes), her physician will usually prescribe antiviral medications, such as acyclovir (Zovirax) at about thirty-six weeks to suppress the infection and minimize the chances of lesions occurring during labor. This intervention is completely optional and should be discussed with the provider.

Cytomegalovirus (CMV): Cytomegalovirus is a common virus that infects people of all ages and it is the most common type of uterine viral infection. CMV is spread by intimate contact with infected body fluids, such as breast milk, cervical mucus, semen, saliva, and urine. For most adults there are no symptoms. For others the symptoms are flulike and similar to those of mononucleosis.

Pregnant women can catch CMV through contact with other children in a day-care setting, particularly those between the ages of one and two-and-a-half. The risk of acquiring CMV may be minimized by good hand washing and personal hygiene. The CDC suggests washing for at least fifteen to twenty seconds. The CDC also suggests not kissing children under the age of five or six on the lips or sharing drinks with them.

In the United States each year, about one in five hundred children is born with or develops disabilities as a result of a CMV infection. The types of disabilities include mental disabilities, hearing loss, vision loss, growth problems, lung problems, bleeding problems, and spleen and liver problems. If the virus is contracted by the baby during delivery, the symptoms may not appear for a number of years. Parents may notice hearing difficulties, learning problems, and a high susceptibility to infections during their first two years of life. Most babies born with CMV never develop symptoms or disabilities.

CMV is detected through a maternal blood test. Unfortunately, these tests are not good indicators as to whether the unborn child will be at risk. Some institutions do routine blood tests on newborns. Although the brain damage is not reversible, the parents can make long-term decisions concerning the child's care and/or prepare for the early treatment of learning and hearing problems.

There is no treatment for CMV, although researchers are working on a future vaccine. It is important to know that there are many strains of CMV, which is why you can contract it over and over again.

Chlamydia: Chlamydia is the most reported STI in the United States today. About four million new cases occur each year. In 2006, the Centers for Disease Control and Prevention reported 1,030,911 cases of chlamydial infections. The incidence is probably greater because as much as 75 percent of women do not show symptoms; therefore, the cases go unreported.

If symptoms do occur, they do so approximately one to three weeks after exposure. Most often males complain of inflammation of the urethra (urethritis). Women generally complain of having an abnormal vaginal discharge, a burning sensation during urination, pain during sexual intercourse, and malaise.

Unfortunately, those who don't have symptoms are often the ones who spread this bacteria. If you do have any of these symptoms, it is important to see your physician so that treatment can be initiated immediately. Chylamydia is diagnosed by examining the bacteria in the urine and also by examining vaginal and urethral discharges. If treatment is necessary, amoxicillin or azithromycin is prescribed.

Recent research indicates that pregnant women with untreated chlamydia are more likely to have premature delivery. During vaginal delivery the bacteria is passed on to the fetus, resulting in newborns with eye and respiratory infections. The eye infections are treated with antibiotic eye ointment.

For more information on sexually transmitted diseases, visit the following links: the Centers for Disease Control and Prevention at http://www.cdc.gov/std/ and the American Social Health Association at www.ashastd.org.

Human Immunodeficiency Virus (HIV): The human immunodeficiency virus (HIV) is the virus that causes acquired immunodeficiency syndrome (AIDS), and during pregnancy it may be passed from mother to child. AIDS is a chronic disease that destroys the body's ability to fight infection. When this book was first published in the 1980s, this disease in North America was confined mainly to homosexual men; however, today the major transmission rate in the United States is among heterosexuals, which means that it can affect the pregnant woman and her unborn baby. The risk of heterosexual transmission is one in three hundred.

HIV infections are transmitted via body fluids, such as semen and blood. Those at risk include those having blood transfusions, hemophiliacs, intravenous drug users, prostitutes, homosexuals, and heterosexuals who have multiple partners. There is still no cure and a vaccine is still several years away.

According to a recent study done by the Centers for Disease Control and Prevention, AIDS is the third leading cause of death among women ages twenty-five to forty-four. Approximately eighty thousand new infections occur each year, and women account for more than 22 percent of those cases. The U.S. Department of Health and Human Services and the CDC claim that 80 percent of the cases of AIDS in women are found among women of childbearing age (fifteen to forty-four years of age).

Today, all pregnant women should be screened for the HIV virus during their first prenatal visit. If the virus is found, it is usually treated with AZT in combination with antiretroviral therapy (HAART).

Prenatal screening has virtually eliminated the incidence of mother-to-child transmission (vertical transmission). However, the risk of vertical transmission with untreated HIV is 25 to 33 percent. Treatment during pregnancy, during labor, and for the first six weeks of the baby's life will decrease the vertical transmission rate to 5 to 8 percent.

Interestingly, the risk to the fetus appears to be related to the amount of virus in the mother's blood, which is known as the "viral load" and is measured as HIV RNA copies per mL of blood. If the viral load is <400, the risk of vertical transmission is very low (estimated at <2 percent) and there is no proven benefit to cesarean delivery in this setting. If the viral load is >1,000, elective cesarean delivery at thirty-eight weeks gestation prior to labor or ruptured membranes has been shown to significantly decrease the risk of vertical transmission.

Breastfeeding is strongly discouraged in women with HIV, because the virus is excreted in breast milk. In untreated women, the risk of vertical transmission with breastfeeding may be as high as 18 percent. The risk in treated women is not well-defined.

Beginning in 1991, the CDC, in collaboration with state and local health organizations, began to strengthen programs to prevent HIV transmission in women. For more information on AIDS in pregnancy, call the National AIDS Information Clearinghouse at (800) 458-5231. (For other resource groups and associations, see Resources.)

Trichomonas: Trichomonas is a sexually transmitted infection. The symptoms vary widely; however, many women notice a thin, greenish-yellow, odorous vaginal discharge. Sometimes this is accompanied by vaginal itching or irritation while urinating. Some women have no symptoms. The infection is easily treated with a medication called metronidazole that is considered safe to use during pregnancy. It is important that both partners are treated for this infection before resuming intercourse.

In pregnancy, untreated trichomonas infection can increase the risk of preterm delivery and low-birth-weight babies.

Communicable Diseases

A communicable disease is one that is carried by a microorganism and transmitted through people, animals, surfaces, food, and the air. Having a communicable disease such as rubella, chicken pox, or toxoplasmosis could affect the health of both you and your baby.

Rubella: Rubella, or German measles, is a contagious infection characterized by fever, swollen lymph nodes, aching muscles and joints, and a generalized skin rash. The virus multiplies in the upper respiratory tract and after seven to ten days it enters the bloodstream. Rubella is relatively rare in the United States, mainly because by two years of age, nearly 93 percent of the nation's children have been vaccinated against the virus. In 2004, there were only nine reported cases in the United States, which is the lowest rate since 1966.

During your first prenatal visit, you will be screened to determine if you have immunity. If you are not immune, you will be immunized after your baby is born and before you are discharged from the hospital.

If you have *not* had rubella and are *not* pregnant, it is a good idea to get immunized. The best time to do this is immediately after the start of your menstrual period, so that you can be sure you are not pregnant. You should wait at least three months before trying to conceive. If, however, you are pregnant and are not immune, it would be a good idea to be immunized after your pregnancy to avoid problems in future pregnancies.

If you were not immunized and contract rubella during pregnancy, the fetus is quite vulnerable. Today, researchers estimate that one in every one hundred thousand babies contracts rubella and the most dangerous time for the mother to contract the virus is during the first trimester.

There is no treatment for rubella. Routine prenatal blood tests done early in pregnancy indicate a woman's rubella antibody level. If a woman is susceptible to infection and has been exposed, genetic counseling (see Chapter 6) will provide an option for an elective abortion. If you are pregnant and have never had rubella, but are exposed to a child with the disease, you should notify your physician.

Chicken Pox: Chicken pox, or the varicella-zoster virus, is a childhood illness that can pose risks to the unborn baby if contracted during pregnancy. It is characterized by feelings of fatigue, headache, fever, and an itchy, blistering rash on the skin. Typically, the symptoms occur about fourteen to sixteen days after exposure.

According to the March of Dimes, more than 90 percent of pregnant women are immune to chicken pox either because they had the disease prior to pregnancy or they were vaccinated as children. Women who are immune to chicken pox cannot become infected; therefore, they do not need to worry about it causing problems during their pregnancy.

Today, about one in two thousand women contracts chicken pox during pregnancy. If contracted during pregnancy, chicken pox may have detrimental effects on the developing fetus, especially during the first trimester or in the last few days before birth. About 10 percent of women will suffer complications like pneumonitis (lung infection) and meningitis (brain membrane infection). The mortality rate for these complications is about 50 percent in pregnancy.

Chicken pox during pregnancy can also affect the baby. Birth defects include muscle and bone problems, blindness, seizures, malformed limbs, and/or mental retardation. Some physicians give a solution of immunoglobulin, which contains disease-fighting antibodies, to women exposed to chicken pox in the first or second trimester. If a mother develops chicken pox during delivery, the baby may develop a rash one to two weeks after the mother's sores appear.

Toxoplasmosis: Toxoplasmosis is caused by a parasite found in domestic cat feces, soil, and raw meat. It occurs most frequently in tropical climates. The CDC estimates that about 15 percent of women of childbearing age are immune to toxoplasmosis. Fetal blood sampling is sometimes done between twenty and twenty-four weeks to detect the presence of toxoplasmosis.

Each year, ten thousand babies in the United States contract the disease. If you are infected with toxoplasmosis during the first trimester, the risk of your baby becoming infected is about 15 percent. If you become infected in the second trimester, the risk increases to about 30 percent, and if infected during the third trimester, the risk increases to 60 percent. The earlier in the pregnancy that this disease occurs, the more severe the damage will be to your baby.

Preventing Toxoplasmosis

- Eat only well-cooked meat.
- Wash fruits and vegetables well.
- Wear gloves when gardening.
- Practice meticulous hand washing during pregnancy, especially after handling cats.
- Carefully clean counters and utensils after preparing meat.
- Have another family member change the cat litter box. (Daily cleaning is recommended.)

Toxoplasmosis during pregnancy may cause miscarriage, prematurity, stillbirth, or neonatal death. The maternal treatment is with folinic acid (leucovorin), sulfadiazine, or pyrimethamine, which can reduce the risk of fetal infection by about 50 percent.

Multiple Pregnancy

Multiple pregnancies occur once in every eighty pregnancies. According to the American College of Obstetricians and Gynecologists (ACOG), in the past decade, the number of twins being born has increased about 33 percent. The number of triplets, quadruplets, and other high-order births has gone up 178 percent.

There are two types of twins. Those formed from either one egg (identical twins) or two eggs (nonidentical or fraternal twins). The incidence of identical twins is random and occurs in one in three hundred pregnancies. This number increases to one in one hundred for those who have had in vitro fertilization (IVF).

Nonidentical twins are more common and can be either of the same sex or different sexes. The incidence is one in eighty pregnancies. If there is a history of twins in your family, your chance of having nonidentical twins is increased. If you have been taking fertility medications, your chance of multiple pregnancy is also increased. Others who may also be prone to having twins include those who have recently been on the contraceptive pill, those who have undergone IVF or GIFT (gamete intrafallopian transfer), those who are over the age of forty, and those who have had four or more children.

Detection of Multiple Pregnancy

Your practitioner will suspect a multiple pregnancy if you have excessive nausea and vomiting and your uterus is larger than normal. Carrying more than one baby will usually be confirmed by ultrasound early in pregnancy. Two sacs may be seen on the ultrasound as early as six to eight weeks. Your physician may also suspect a multiple pregnancy because of your weight gain or because two heartbeats are heard.

In about 15 percent of all multiple pregnancies, vanishing twin syndrome occurs. In this situation, one of the twins is reabsorbed by the mother's body. This usually occurs before the sixteenth week.

Care During Multiple Pregnancy

Many women feel perfectly fine during their multiple pregnancy. However, your physician will carefully monitor your progress. Most professionals recommend checkups twice a month for the first half of the pregnancy and weekly checkups thereafter. In addition, you may be advised to increase your nutritional and vitamin intake. You may also be told to curtail strenuous sports and to plan several rest periods during the day. If you have a stressful and tiring job, you might be well-advised to take a leave of absence or to decrease your hours to ensure that you get adequate rest.

As soon as your physician ascertains you are having a multiple pregnancy, he or she will want to determine the arrangement of the fetuses' placenta and the membranes. This is called the chorionicity. This is critical in determining the outcome of the pregnancy. Nonidentical twins always have a separate placenta and membrane. Identical twins may have a separate or shared placenta and membranes. This first arrangement has the best outcome, whereas the second scenario is more risky. What might happen is that the umbilical cords can become tangled, resulting in a higher incidence of stillbirth. Unfortunately, if one baby dies, the other one will almost always also die or survive with major neurological problems.

Fifty percent of identical twins share a placenta and have separate membranes. About 20 percent have separate membranes and a separate placenta. In order to prevent early labor and delivery, bed rest is sometimes (but not always) prescribed for those carrying more than one baby. Physicians have varying opinions about this recommendation.

The most common recommendation while carrying more than one baby is bed rest at about the thirtieth week (see Chapter 8). Even though bed rest may not be prescribed early, it is especially important that all mothers of multiples receive plenty of rest. Ideally, you should rest in a semi-recumbent position or lying down on the left side, because this takes the pressure off the vena cava, the principal vein in the back, which drains blood from the upper part of the body. These rest periods should occur two or three times daily.

Today, the risks associated with multiple pregnancies are much lower than they were years ago. Some possible problems include hypertension, anemia, unusual fetal positions, gestational diabetes, stillbirths, smaller babies, and early delivery. Early blood-sugar tests may be performed to detect diabetes, and your blood pressure will also be carefully monitored. Expect repeat ultrasounds to check the babies' growth, cervical checks, and nonstress tests as part of the standard procedure for monitoring multiple pregnancies. Premature birth is the single most important risk with multiple pregnancies, occurring ten times more often in multiple pregnancies. Approximately 80 percent of all twins and three-quarters of triplets are born before the thirty-seventh week.

Multifetal Pregnancy Reduction (MFPR)

This procedure is done to reduce the number of fetuses in a pregnancy consisting of three or more fetuses. It is a selective and elective procedure done after careful evaluation and examination with a qualified specialist.

The goal of MFPR is usually to end up with two fetuses, because doing so increases the chances of a successful pregnancy. Multifetal pregnancy reduction is a viable option for many couples. Studies have shown that on the average, for every extra fetus in the uterus during the first trimester, the woman loses about three and a half weeks of pregnancy. For every fetus that is lost, you gain three weeks.

The procedure is usually done at about thirteen or fourteen weeks and tends to minimize the complications often associated with carrying a multiple pregnancy. The procedure is done during an ultrasound. A needle is inserted into the uterus and the embryo is given potassium chloride until the heart stops pumping. In most cases, the specialist performs the procedure on the fetus situated higher up in the uterus to minimize the possibility of miscarriage. After the procedure, the embryo is absorbed into the body.

Selective Reduction

Selective reduction is reducing the number of fetuses in a multiple pregnancy because of congenital abnormalities in one or more of the fetuses. It is usually performed after the first trimester screening tests. In this case, the specialist targets a specific fetus, whereas in multifetal pregnancy reduction, it is more or less a random choice. Selective reduction is performed in the same way as MFPR.

Twin to Twin Transfusion Syndrome (TTTS)

Twin to twin transfusion syndrome (TTTS) is a high-risk condition of identical twins who share the same placenta. One placenta is supplying two fetuses, and they are obtaining unequal amounts of blood. In other words, one baby gets more blood than the other. The result is that one fetus becomes the donor and the other is the recipient. As a result, the donor ends up being smaller and risks having anemia, while the recipient thrives, is larger, and has an excess of blood.

The signs of twin to twin transfusion syndrome include the mother becoming quite large in a two- or three-week period, because of the excessive urination by one twin, and also one twin being very small and the other being very large.

TTTS is detected early in pregnancy and is likely to be fatal to one or both of the fetuses. Sometimes lasers are used to disrupt blood vessels. At other times, pulling some of the extra amniotic fluid from the twin with more fluid can help balance the amount of fluid and stabilize the situation.

Coping with Multiple Pregnancy

Coping emotionally with a multiple pregnancy may not be easy, especially if there are other children at home or if a multiple pregnancy is discovered late in the pregnancy. Some women react with excitement:

> "I was absolutely ecstatic when I heard that I was having twins. I already had a three-year-old at home and this did not bother me. I knew when I was only six weeks pregnant that there was a possibility that I would have twins. At three months, the ultrasound showed that there were two amniotic sacs. I was warned about the possibility of having premature babies but was confident that everything would be all right. It sure was—at thirty-eight weeks, I gave birth to two healthy 7-pound twins, one girl and one boy."

Other women react with fear and anger:

> "After two years of infertility workups, you'd think I would be happy. However, I encountered the opposite reaction. I suddenly did not want to be pregnant anymore. I cried an awful lot. For financial and

emotional reasons, I felt I would be unable to offer my children the best. I always dreamt about cuddling one baby. I never felt happy about having twins—but it was something I grew to accept. My husband, on the other hand, felt the opposite. He was delighted that he too could have the one-on-one relationship with a baby at the same time as I would."

The actual adjustment to a multiple pregnancy depends on the individual woman and other factors, including the woman's partner, family, age, economic status, health, and personal philosophy. A common concern for the couple is the effect on their relationship after two or more babies are born. They may have feelings of inadequacy, of being unable to cope with more than one child. For the most part, extra babies are not planned, although with the advent of ultrasound they may at least be expected. This gives the couple time to prepare as well as to seek outside assistance. Sometimes husbands look forward to the multiple births, because they know they will be more involved in the early stages, when the woman has to juggle two or more crying babies.

Many couples, however, find themselves underestimating the workload involved in caring for more than one baby at a time. The stress may lead to marital problems, depression, and child abuse. If you find you are overstressed, it is important to seek counseling to avoid any of these potential side effects of multiple births.

Learning how to ask for help is very important for the mother who is having a multiple pregnancy. You will need your strength, and a few hours of assistance during the day from a mother's helper or a relative may help you conserve that needed energy. Speaking with other mothers who have had multiple pregnancies may help you gain much-needed perspective. Some local twins clubs have telephone committees that help minimize the sense of isolation experienced by so many new mothers. These women may also be able to advise you on other resources, such as where to get used furniture, strollers, and clothes, because you will have to have double, if not more, of everything. A strong support system is important during these times. At a later date, you might be interested in helping other new mothers having multiple births.

Unusual Fetal Positions

Most babies move around in the uterus for the first six months but settle into the head-down position by the seventh or eighth month. Their position is called their "presentation." Sometimes babies may be positioned in the breech presentation, where their head is up, as though they were sitting inside of you. This occurs in approximately 3 to 4 percent of all deliveries at term. Some other, rarer positions include shoulder presentation, face presentation, and transverse position.

A breech presentation may be suspected during your routine prenatal visit when your baby's heartbeat is heard above your navel rather than below it. It can also be detected during an ultrasound. Women who have a baby in this position say that it feels like the baby's kicks are lower in their abdomen. It may be difficult to have a breech baby vaginally. The safest position for the baby's head is for it to be tucked into its chest. If the baby's head is extended backward and he or she is delivered vaginally, there is a real risk of damaging the neck and spine.

Management of Breech Presentation

There are a variety of ways to manage a breech presentation. Some turning techniques are recommended because the mother can do them herself. These are called the "positioning methods." The following method is performed during the last month of pregnancy: The woman lies on her back on a firm surface with her hips elevated about 9 to 12 inches, with the use of pillows. She does this twice a day and stays in this position for ten minutes. This should be done on an empty stomach. If you perform this technique and feel that your baby has turned, you should stop and notify your health-care provider about the new position change. Keep in mind that this technique is not always effective in turning the fetus.

Some women try unusual yoga positions or standing on their head to get their baby to turn. Others advocate maintaining a head-down position, crouching on hands and knees with your head down and buttocks up, for fifteen minutes twice daily. You should check with your physician prior to performing any of these techniques; they are advised only under careful supervision.

Moxibustion: Since the first edition of this book, another method of rotating the baby has been used successfully in the United States called moxibustion. This is a traditional Chinese medicine technique involving acupuncture and the burning of mugwort (a small, spongy herb). It has been used in Asia for thousands of years and like most forms of Chinese medicine, the idea is to strengthen the blood and stimulate the flow of *qi* (pronounced "chi") for good health. A study published in the *Journal of the American Medical Association* in 1998 found that up to 75 percent of women with breech presentations before childbirth had fetuses that rotated to the normal position after receiving the moxibustion treatment.

The treatment involves applying heat from a burning moxibustion stick to an acupuncture site on the bladder meridian, which is located on the outside corner of the fifth toe. The stick is left in place for five to ten minutes. A practitioner then warms one toe for five or ten minutes and then moves on to the other toes. Sometimes a few treatments per week are recommended. Some centers send the woman home with a stick to perform the procedure herself. Most often the treatment is started at about thirty-four weeks.

There are no contraindications for this technique, although some women with respiratory problems may find the smoke and pungent odor to be bothersome.

External Rotation: External rotation, or "version," is another way to turn a baby. This medical procedure involves the practitioner physically turning the baby by pressing on the mother's abdomen. This is a learned skill and some practitioners have more experience than others. It is important to check with your provider to ensure he or she is well-experienced in performing this procedure. The success rate of this procedure is about 50 percent.

The procedure begins with your baby's position being verified by ultrasound. A medication such as terbutaline may be given either by injection or in the form of an epidural. The physician then places one hand on your abdomen over the baby's head and the other hand over its buttocks. The hands are moved in opposite directions and the baby is gently stroked to encourage it to change positions. The procedure takes about thirty minutes and you will be monitored, before, during, and after the procedure, mainly because there is a risk of the umbilical cord becoming wrapped around the fetus's neck. Sometimes the procedure is painful because of the amount of pressure that needs to be applied.

Natural Rotation: Opinions vary as to how late in pregnancy the fetus can turn itself. Some claim that the baby may turn itself even after thirty-eight weeks. Timing is important, because if the rotation is done too far in advance, the baby may revert to the breech position by the time of delivery. In addition, if a complication such as abruptio placenta or a change in the baby's heart rate should occur, an emergency cesarean would be necessary, resulting in the delivery of a premature baby. If you have a breech presentation and want to have a vaginal delivery, speak with your physician. He or she may consent with the understanding that you might have to have an emergency cesarean in the event of problems.

This outcome may also depend on the hospital's policy. Many hospitals are unwilling to take the risk of a vaginal breech delivery.

Blood Incompatibilities

There are many kinds of blood incompatibilities. In order to understand what can happen, it is important to understand about blood types. There are four different blood types: A, B, AB, and O. Babies inherit their blood type from both of their parents. Sometimes a baby has a different blood type than their mother but the same one as their father.

ABO Incompatibility

ABO blood incompatibility is the most common blood incompatibility and the most dangerous type. It affects between 20 and 25 percent of all pregnancies.

When there is an ABO blood incompatibility problem, the mother makes antibodies against her baby's blood. (The only time this does not happen is if the mother and baby have the same blood type or if the baby is type O.) Before the baby is born, the mother's antibodies cross the placenta and break down the baby's red blood cells. This results in the baby becoming anemic or jaundiced, which is seen on ultrasound. There are two treatment choices. The baby can be delivered if the pregnancy is past twenty-four weeks' gestation. Otherwise, a series of blood transfusions can be done in the uterus during pregnancy and after delivery.

Rh Incompatibility

A problem with Rh incompatibility occurs when a pregnant woman and her baby have different Rh blood types. Each blood group is classified with the presence of another protein on the surface of the red blood cells that indicates the Rh factor. If you have this protein on your red blood cells, you are Rh-positive. Approximately 85 percent of the population is Rh-positive.

Throughout pregnancy, there is constant trafficking of fetal cells to the maternal circulation and visa versa. If the mother is Rh-negative and is exposed to the fetus's Rh-positive red blood cells, her body may make antibodies against the Rh protein on the fetus's red blood cells. The reason that this does not affect the current pregnancy is because the initial antibodies made by the mother are IgM which is an antibody in the B cells that is the primary antibody against A and B antigens. These antibodies are large and do not cross the placenta, so they cannot break down the fetus's red blood cells, which could lead to anemia and heart failure. If exposed for a second time, however, the mother will make IgG antibodies. These antibodies do cross the placenta and can therefore harm the fetus.

Years ago, this incompatibility was quite serious, but it has become less of a problem since the advent of the immunizing agent Rh(D), also known as RhoGAM. This immunoglobulin is given to the mother near or around her twenty-eighth week through a muscular injection. This injection prevents her from producing dangerous antibodies that could adversely affect her newborn or future pregnancies.

Rh(D) may also be given if you have vaginal bleeding at any time during your pregnancy and if you have had any type of invasive procedure such as an amniocentesis or CVS. All Rh-negative mothers receive this injection after each pregnancy, whether it goes to full term or is terminated by abortion or miscarriage.

If you have a negative Rh (rhesus) factor, your physician will monitor you closely during your pregnancy. If both you and your baby's father are Rh-negative, you will not need Rh(D). Most providers will want to be provided with documentation of the father's blood type, in writing, to confirm this.

In your second pregnancy, if you are Rh-negative and your baby is Rh-positive, there will be a problem unless the situation is detected. As the fetus grows, some of the red blood cells that it produces pass through the placenta into the mother's blood, and her system produces antibodies to the Rh factor. These antibodies recross the placenta and destroy the fetus's red blood cells. The baby will be born with abnormal blood cells, a condition called erythroblastosis, which may lead to anemia, jaundice, or both. In very severe cases it may cause stillbirth.

Years ago, physicians prescribed amniocentesis to detect blood incompatibilities. Today, a doppler ultrasound is used to examine the blood flow in a major artery in the baby's brain. If the baby is becoming anemic because of an incompatibility, it will affect the blood flow and appear on an ultrasound.

Vaginal Bleeding

Bleeding during pregnancy can be a very frightening and uncertain experience. Between 25 to 50 percent of pregnant women spot at some time during their pregnancy. The spotting most often occurs during the first two months of pregnancy, most often between the ninth and twelfth weeks. Spotting does not necessarily mean that your pregnancy is at risk, but it is always better to be safe rather than sorry; thus, it is important to call your physician or go to the emergency room at your local hospital.

Some causes of vaginal bleeding include:

- egg implantation in the uterus
- infection of the cervix
- diminished progesterone
- imminent miscarriage
- cervical insufficiency
- placenta previa
- abruptio placenta
- cervical polyps
- trauma to the cervix as a result of intercourse

Some women become concerned when they discover blood after wiping themselves in the bathroom. Sometimes the blood is due to hemorrhoids, which are common during pregnancy. Before calling your physician, make sure that the blood is coming from your vagina.

What is done about your bleeding depends on your trimester. With caution, you may have an internal examination. Sometimes a speculum is inserted to determine whether the source of bleeding is the cervix, the uterus, or the vagina. If your physician believes that it is inevitable that a miscarriage will occur, he or she may choose to take a wait-and-see approach. In either case, an ultrasound will be done to detect your baby's status.

What to Do If You Bleed

- Phone your physician or nurse-midwife.
- Document the amount of bleeding, color of the blood (bright, brownish), and the type of pain (constant, intermittent).
- Recall any associated symptoms, such as fever or cramping.
- Recall what you were doing when the bleeding began.
- If the bleeding is severe and painful, go to the emergency room immediately.

The incidence of significant vaginal bleeding in the last half of pregnancy is about 3 percent, most often due to abnormalities of the placenta. This bleeding is usually intermittent and painless. If you have any bleeding in the last half of your pregnancy, it is important to go immediately to the hospital. You will be seen by a physician and an ultrasound will probably be performed to identify the source of your bleeding and to make sure you do not have a low-lying placenta or placenta previa.

Abruptio Placenta

Abruptio placenta is characterized by premature separation of the placenta from the uterus. The separation may be partial or complete. It is the leading cause of mortality among newborns and may require an emergency cesarean delivery. Abruptio placenta occurs once in every twenty to eighty-five pregnancies (studies vary). The exact cause is unknown, but some possible related factors include a prior placental abruptio, inherited bleeding disorder, smoking, cocaine use, trauma to the abdomen, short umbilical cord, uterine abnormalities, hypertension, and more than five previous pregnancies.

If you have abruptio placenta, you will know that something strange is happening. You may have any of the following symptoms: vaginal bleeding after the twentieth week, decreased fetal movement, and sudden and severe abdominal pain. Sometimes there will be no bleeding. There may be tenderness when your abdomen is palpated.

Because of the threat to both you and your baby, you will be closely monitored. If you have a partial separation, you will be placed on complete bed rest in the hospital. Your heart rate and your baby's heart rate will be continuously monitored. If you go into premature labor, you will need a medication to stop labor. If you have a more severe abruptio placenta, delivery by cesarean section may be the only option to save both of your lives. One of the risks of a complete abruptio placenta is a possible need for a hysterectomy.

Placenta Previa

Placenta previa, which occurs in approximately one in 200 to 250 pregnancies, is a condition in which the placenta is placed abnormally in the uterus in such a way that it covers the cervical opening (see Figures 5.2 and 5.3). Often placenta previa is detected during a routine ultrasound. In other cases, women begin bleeding painlessly in the last trimester of pregnancy. Most women with placenta previa experience their first bleeding after their thirtieth week, although some women do not bleed. Many studies have been conducted to determine the causes of placenta previa. Some report that it is due to previous uterine surgery, while others say it is due to advanced age, a history of many pregnancies, inadequate uterine lining, or congenital uterine abnormalities.

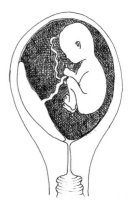

Figure 5.2:
Partial placenta
previa

Treatment depends on the severity of your condition, but it most often includes bed rest to prevent early delivery. Sometimes women are able to rest at home; in other cases, hospitalization may be recommended. You will be advised to avoid sexual intercourse, douching, and straining to pass a stool. Stool softeners may be prescribed. A repeat ultrasound will be performed later in pregnancy to monitor the status of the placenta. Sometimes placenta previa found in an early ultrasound may not persist as the pregnancy progresses. In most instances, the placenta moves out of the way of the cervical opening and only in 5 percent of women is it present at term.

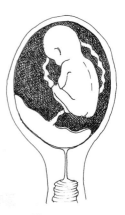

Figure 5.3:
Complete
placenta previa

If you are not yet at thirty-eight weeks or at term, lung maturity tests (see Chapter 7) may be performed in the event of possible preterm labor. A cesarean is often the delivery of choice, usually at about thirty-six weeks.

Prolapsed Umbilical Cord

This emergency situation is most often seen when the baby is in an unusual position or if the membranes rupture prematurely. When the water breaks, the baby's umbilical cord descends through the cervix into the vagina while the baby remains inside the uterus. It is an emergency, because if the fetus's umbilical cord is pinched or kinked, or if it goes into spasm, the baby will not receive an adequate supply of oxygen.

It will be difficult for you to know if you have a prolapsed umbilical cord. Some women say they feel as if there is something in their vagina. A prolapsed cord may be detected by your physician after your membranes have ruptured.

Treatment involves an emergency cesarean delivery. In the meantime, you may be told to get on your hands and knees, put your chest on the ground, and put your rear into the air. This will keep the pressure off the umbilical cord. Another option is to elevate your hips above your shoulders by lying down and placing a pillow underneath your hips. If you are already in the hospital, your physician will place his or her hand inside of you to hold the umbilical cord in place and then will rush you off to the operating room for an emergency cesarean section. You should not be surprised that his or her hand will have to remain inside of you until the baby is born!

Intrauterine Growth Restriction (IUGR)

The term "intrauterine growth restriction" (IUGR) is used to describe a condition whereby the fetus is smaller than it should be for the number of weeks of pregnancy. Typically, the fetus weighs less than 90 percent of all other fetuses of the same gestational age. A baby that is small for his or her age often has a small placenta.

There are many reasons why some babies do not grow as well as others. Some reasons are due to chromosomal abnormalities, multiple gestation (less room inside the uterus for the baby to grow), poor maternal weight gain, maternal hypertension, maternal infection, smoking, and alcohol usage. Many of the causes of IUGR are preventable.

IUGR occurs in approximately 5 to 10 percent of all pregnancies, and these babies are at great risk during the first few weeks of life. Ultrasound has helped to diagnose IUGR early. Resting on one's side has been recommended to increase blood flow to the placenta.

Treatment for IUGR varies. Repeated ultrasounds are usually done to monitor the baby's status. Other tests, such as biophysical profiles and nonstress tests, may also be performed (see Chapter 7). IUGR babies are usually delivered before the thirty-sixth week by cesarean to avoid the chance of death, which may occur between the thirty-sixth and fortieth week. The exact timing of the cesarean delivery is a highly individualized decision.

Preterm Premature Rupture of Membranes (PPROM)

Preterm premature rupture of the membranes (PPROM) is the rupture of the amniotic sac surrounding the fetus before labor begins. It occurs in approximately 10 percent of all pregnancies. The exact cause of PPROM is unknown; many authorities believe it is caused by a uterine infection. Other less common but still possible causes include trauma, cervical insufficiency, multiple pregnancies, amniocentesis, too much amniotic fluid (polyhydramnios), abruptio placenta, genetic abnormality, poor hygiene, smoking, and inadequate nutrition.

If your membranes rupture prematurely, you may feel a sudden gush, a steady leak, or a trickle of fluid from your vagina. Slow leaks also occur, in which a small amount of liquid leaks from the vagina and is sometimes confused with urine. If this happens to you, you should immediately go to the hospital, because once the sac has been broken, there is a greater risk of infection. If your membranes rupture, labor almost always begins within twenty-four hours. If labor does not occur within twenty-four hours and there are no strong, rhythmic contractions, then labor will be induced to prevent infection both of the membranes and in the newborn. Some physicians may choose to wait longer than twenty-four hours.

Treatment depends on your stage of pregnancy. For the most part, the management of PPROM is highly controversial and often a matter of preference. Some women will be placed on bed rest (see Chapter 8). Some physicians may take a wait-and-see approach, especially if the woman is less than thirty-six-weeks pregnant.

Post-Term or Prolonged Pregnancy

Post-term or prolonged pregnancies are those that continue past your expected due date (EDD), or date of delivery, or past forty-two weeks. Most pregnancies are maintained for thirty-eight to forty-two weeks. However, from 8 to 11 percent of all pregnancies continue longer. Sometimes the woman's due date is incorrectly calculated because she does not remember the first day of her last menstrual period. In this case, the fetus's age must be determined by ultrasound.

Despite these indicators, you should understand that your delivery may occur anytime between two weeks before and two weeks after your EDD.

Even so, some women are at greater risk for carrying a post-term pregnancy, such as those pregnant for the first time, those over the age of thirty-five, and those with a previous prolonged pregnancy.

In many cases, carrying the baby a bit longer will have minimal consequences. However, in some cases, it can be associated with placental tears, lack of oxygen supply to the fetus, a large baby, growth restriction, meconium in the amniotic fluid (which indicates distress), or death. The most difficult part of prolonged pregnancies is the emotional aspect. Some women feel as if their pregnancy will never end and they will never get to hold their precious little bundle. It is normal for post-term mothers to feel frustrated and to feel as if they have lost control over their pregnancy.

Ultrasounds, oxytocin challenge tests, nonstress tests, tests of amniotic fluid (for amount and quality), and fetal breathing movement tests will be done to ensure fetal well-being. If the fetus is normal and your cervix is ripe, your physician may choose to induce labor. If your cervix is not soft or you have passed two weeks of your EDD, labor will probably be induced. In some instances, the cervix may be primed with prostin gel.

If you are past forty weeks, you should be particularly aware of fetal movements and phone your physician immediately if you notice any change (see Chapter 7). The risk of postterm or prolonged pregnancy is postmaturity, which is a more serious condition in which the baby's health declines as a result of the delayed birth. The placenta may shrink and the amount of amniotic fluid decrease. When this happens, the baby becomes inadequately nourished and will show signs of distress. A cesarean delivery may be necessary.

Cancer in Pregnancy

According to the Mayo Clinic, about one in a thousand pregnancies is complicated by cancer, but, in general, the incidence of cancer does not increase in pregnancy. The most common types of cancers that occur in women of childbearing age include breast cancer, cervical cancer, ovarian cancer, and melanoma, which is a type of skin cancer.

In most cases, if you were diagnosed with cancer prior to your pregnancy and began treatment, your practitioner will suggest that you postpone your pregnancy until after treatments are completed.

Most of the decisions about the management of cancer during pregnancy depend on the type of cancer, the timing of the pregnancy, and your prognosis. If you have a history of cancer or are newly diagnosed during pregnancy, you will be monitored by your obstetrician as well as a cancer specialist (oncologist).

If you are diagnosed with cancer in the third trimester, chances are your physician will let you deliver your baby normally, and then cancer treatment will begin after your baby is born.

If you are diagnosed in the first or second trimester, your obstetrician should meet with your cancer specialist to decide on a plan, keeping you and your baby's best interests in mind. It is a good idea for you to also be in the meeting, because there might need to be a discussion about terminating the pregnancy.

The usual treatment for cancer is surgery and/or chemotherapy and/-or radiation. Some cancers, such as breast cancer, might require surgery, and although it may be emotionally stressful undergoing surgery during pregnancy, it is perfectly safe. General anesthesia is typically well-tolerated by the unborn baby. Certain types of chemotherapy treatments may also be tolerated by the baby. Some cancer medications, such as methotrexate, cannot be used during pregnancy. If radiation therapy is necessary, it should be discussed in detail with your high-risk obstetrician.

Many of the decisions about the treatment of cancer in pregnancy depend on what the mother and/or couple wants, the type of cancer, and when it is diagnosed. Often, the decision is made to deliver the baby early so that the mother's cancer can be treated in a timely manner. In general, the baby remains unaffected by the cancer. Studies have shown that melanoma is the only type of cancer that can cross the placenta and affect the baby.

Women may wonder how the pregnancy can affect the cancer. Some cancers can change in the presence of the hormonal changes associated with pregnancy. For example, with breast cancer, which is a type of hormonally responsive cancer, there is the potential that pregnancy can exacerbate the cancer, and an early delivery may be recommended, but in most situations, this is not the case.

Medications Used In High-Risk Pregnancies

There are some medications that the high-risk mother may take for the treatment of certain pregnancy-related problems (see Table 5.1). Although there may be side effects associated with some of these medications, they are usually prescribed because the benefits for the baby far outweigh the risks. Have faith in your physician: It makes a difficult pregnancy much easier. If you do not have faith, it is important to obtain more information or consider changing physicians.

Table 5.1: Some Medications Used in High-Risk Pregnancies

Medication	Use
Aldomet	Hypertension
Betamethasone	Fetal-lung maturity
Ergotrate sulfate	Uterine stimulant
Indomethacin	Labor suppressant
Magnesium sulfate	Labor suppressant, preeclampsia
Nifedipine	Labor suppressant
Pitocin	Uterine stimulant
Prostaglandins	Uterine stimulant
Prostaglandin inhibitors	Labor suppressant
Rh immune globulin	Rh incompatibility prevention
Ritodrine hydrochloride	Labor suppressant
Syntocinon	Labor stimulation

Labor Suppressants

These medications are prescribed for premature labor prior to the thirty-fourth week. Taking them will give your baby more time to grow and mature inside your uterus. Labor suppressants are rarely administered if your membranes have ruptured prematurely, and if they are given, they are usually given in conjunction with antibiotic therapy. Some common types of labor suppressants include beta-adrenergic receptor stimulants such as ritodrine (Yutopar), terbutaline sulfate (Brethine), indocin (Indomethacin), and magnesium sulfate.

Beta-Adrenergic Medications: Ritodrine was first approved by the FDA in the 1980s. Today, it remains the only drug that is FDA-approved for the treatment of preterm labor. However, ritodrine is no longer available in North America because it has been shown to be dangerous to the pregnant woman.

Ritodrine is the medication that I took on bed rest during my second and third pregnancies. I suppose I am lucky to have not had any of the dangerous side effects. I took the medication in 1989 for the birth of my third child. My side effects were minimal, and less bothersome than those associated with Vasodilan, which I took during my first pregnancy. When on ritodrine, I had occasional palpations. Although I never experienced any other symptoms, I remember some friends sharing complaints of nausea, sweating, and headaches.

Terbutaline sulfate is a beta-adrenergic medication, similar to ritodrine. In the United States, it is available and used to suppress preterm labor by relaxing the uterine muscles. Some women have reported side effects such as nausea, sweating, palpitations, and headaches. These may be related to the dosage and may not occur with small or moderate doses of this medication. In general, these side effects are considered to be safe for the developing fetus. Some practitioners claim that these side effects may increase the baby's heart rate and cause a decrease in blood pressure and blood sugar. Following delivery, these babies are carefully watched. Terbutaline is usually given by injection, but you may be sent home with the oral form of the medication.

Magnesium Sulfate: This medication was first used nearly fifty years ago for severe preeclampsia to prevent seizures, and only recently has it been utilized for treating preterm labor. It is given only in the hospital by injection. As with most medications, there are side effects, including nervousness, breathing difficulties, flushing, warmth, altered heart rate, and changes in muscle reflexes. The most serious side effect is pulmonary edema (water in the lungs), seen in about 2 percent of women. However, some believe that this medication has fewer side effects than others, and it is therefore the medication of choice in high-risk pregnancy. In addition, it is relatively safe for the baby—side effects are rare. Following delivery, babies may be monitored for lower calcium levels and decreased muscle tone.

Nifedipine: This medication was first used to treat those with an irregular heartbeat and is now used to decrease uterine contractions. It works by interfering with the action of calcium, which plays a major role in muscle contractions. Women who cannot tolerate terbutaline are often prescribed nifedipine. Side effects can include dizziness, headache, and lowered blood pressure. Some providers might recommend that before swallowing nifedipine, the woman chews the capsule to break it up.

Indomethacin: This medication is a prostaglandin inhibitor and is used prior to thirty-two weeks. It has been found to be very effective in stopping preterm labor, with only rare side effects to the mother. However, long-term use of this medication may result in a decrease in amniotic fluid and/or possible heart, lung, digestive, or kidney problems for the baby. Usually this medication should not be taken more than forty-eight hours at a time. For these reasons, most practitioners consider indomethacin to be a second-line medication.

Special Concerns: Because most of these medications cause an elevated heart rate, it is a good idea to take your pulse at the same time each day to ensure that your dosage is properly adjusted. Most health-care providers expect your pulse to be between 90 and 100 beats per minute, but you should notify your caregiver if it rises over 120. You should report any complaints of chest pain or shortness of breath. Also, you should notify your provider of any feelings of nervousness, agitation, and/or tremors. These signs may indicate your dosage needs to be adjusted.

Journaling Corner

Is there something your provider has told you that concerns or upsets you?

Are you in any support groups or meeting with other mothers? If yes, describe.

How does your partner feel about your pregnancy?

How has your life changed since you have been pregnant?

How do you feel about your body right now?

Write about some happy moments.

6

Genetics and Birth Defects

It's gonna be a long hard drag,
but we'll make it. — Janis Joplin

According to the March of Dimes Foundation, a birth defect is "an abnormality of structure, function, or body chemistry, whether genetically determined or the result of environmental interference before birth. It may be present at or before birth, or appear later in life." In 1985, more than two hundred and fifty thousand infants in the United States had birth defects resulting in physical or mental damage. Today, birth defects affect more than one hundred and fifty thousand babies, or one in five babies annually, and birth defects remain the leading cause of infant death. Approximately 3 percent of infants have malformations and 1 percent have multiple malformations. Some are more serious than others, but, needless to say, defects are not easily accepted by parents. Many months of imagining the "perfect baby" are suddenly shattered.

A study by D. A. Beckman and R. L. Brent concluded that 15 to 25 percent of birth defects are caused by genetic diseases or chromosomal abnormalities. Approximately 8 to 10 percent are the result of environmental factors, such as maternal infections, exposure to chemicals or medications, and diseases. The remaining 65 percent of birth defects are caused by unknown reasons or may be due to many factors.

A teratogen is an agent that may cause a birth defect. Some examples of teratogens include chemicals, medications, infections, and diseases. The actual effect of the teratogen will depend on a number of variables, including the fetus's vulnerability, when you are exposed, the nature of the teratogen, the dosage, and your general health. The most vulnerable period for the fetus is during the first two months, when the basic organ systems of the body are being formed.

Some Possible Teratogens

- alcohol
- tobacco
- venereal diseases: syphilis
- caffeine
- infections: cytomegalovirus, rubella, toxoplasmosis
- medications: Accutane, anticonvulsants, Coumadin, DES (diethyl-stilbestrol), illicit drugs (cocaine), methotrexate, oral hypoglycemics, retinoids (vitamin A), thalidomide
- environmental and occupational hazards: DDT, lead pollution, poor nutrition, X rays

To discuss each teratogen in detail is beyond the scope of this book. Therefore, only the most common ones will be discussed. A detailed discussion of infections and sexually transmitted diseases can be found in Chapter 5. The effects of poor nutrition are discussed in Chapter 2.

There are many possible causes of birth defects, and often the problems are due to genetic factors, environmental hazards encountered during pregnancy, a combination of both, or untraceable errors in development. The following sections will discuss affected babies in terms of the genetic, environmental, and multifactorial causative factors. A basic overview of genetics will help you understand the genetically acquired diseases discussed in this chapter.

A human being originates from the union of two gametes: the ovum and the sperm. These cells contain half of the inherited characteristics (genes) of each parent. Genes are arranged on rodlike structures called chromosomes that bear each person's genetic material. Chromosomes occur in pairs and are present in almost every cell of the body.

At conception, there is a union of twenty-three of your chromosomes and twenty-three of your partner's (or one of each pair), giving your baby a total of forty-six chromosomes in every normal cell. Twenty-two pairs of these chromosomes are called autosomes and are identical in males and females. The twenty-third pair, however, are referred to as "the sex-determining chromosomes." Females have two X chromosomes and males have one X and one Y. These sex chromosomes determine not only sex but also certain diseases that may affect either males or females.

Genes are the basis of heredity, and they may be thought of as the storehouse of information that determines how your baby develops. The combined set of your and your partner's genes, as they interact with environmental factors, form the picture of your child's characteristics, including his or her physical appearance, health status, and life span. In a sense, genes join the past and the present to the future.

Genes can either be dominant or recessive. Dominant genes show their effect, even if there is only one copy of that gene in the pair. For a person to have a recessive disease or characteristic, the person must have the gene on both chromosomes of the pair.

Who Is at Risk?

During one of your earliest prenatal visits, you will be asked if there is any family history of genetic problems. All physical or mental problems among family members should be mentioned, including miscarriage, stillbirth, and early infant death. If there is a history of an inherited problem, you may be referred to a genetic counselor or specialist for further investigation. More recent studies have shown that the mother's age is the priority risk factor for genetic problems, particularly in the case of Down syndrome. Women over the age of thirty-five on their expected due date are at the greatest risk of having a child with genetic problems, such as Down syndrome.

Risk situations include:

- couples with a genetic condition themselves
- women who have had a stillbirth or a live birth with a genetic condition
- couples who have a family history of a genetic abnormality
- women who are suspected or known carriers of sex-linked disorders (e.g., hemophilia, muscular dystrophy)
- women who have phenylketonuria (PKU)
- couples who are blood-related
- women who have had two or more miscarriages

It is amazing how much must go right in order to bring a healthy child into the world! It is also surprising that more errors do not occur during the reproductive process. However, spontaneous losses, such as in the case of the blighted ovum discussed earlier, do occur.

Genetic disorders fall into three major categories: chromosomal, single-gene, and multifactorial. Approximately 7.5 percent of all congenital malformations are due to single-gene defects; 6 percent are due to chromosomal problems; 28.5 percent are multifactorial; and nearly 60 percent are due to what experts call unknown factors.

Chromosomal Defects

In general, chromosome defects are caused by errors in cell division that may be the result of either too much or too little genetic material. Unlike single-gene defects, which may reoccur with subsequent pregnancies (see the discussion on the next page), chromosomal defects affect only one specific pregnancy. Some chromosomal defects may be hereditary, and this possibility needs to be explored with each individual family. Approximately one infant in every 150 to 200 is born with a chromosomal abnormality. Down syndrome and Turner syndrome are two examples; the former is the most common chromosomal disorder in live-born infants.

Down Syndrome

Down syndrome (mongolism, or trisomy 21) is the most discussed sex chromosome abnormality, *not* because it is the most common, but because it is the one that is most likely to produce a viable child who tends to vary in his or her capabilities and who most often lives well into their thirties or forties, and sometimes much longer.

Down syndrome is characterized by different degrees of mental retardation and multiple physical defects. The average child with Down syndrome has an IQ of about 24, but some may have an IQ as high as 70, which is considered mildly retarded. An encouraging and stimulating environment helps these children develop to their fullest potential.

Half of these children will have heart problems, and some will have problems involving the bowel, blood, or other body systems. It is important to remember that 50 percent of these children will have no structural abnormalities. Their most outstanding physical features include upward-slanted eyes, small ears, and a protruding tongue because of an undersized mouth.

The incidence of Down syndrome, as indicated in Table 6.1, depends on maternal age. It is most often caused by the presence of an extra number 21 chromosome.

Table 6.1: The Incidence of Down Syndrome

Mother's Age	Risk of Down Syndrome
25	1 in 1,250
30	1 in 952
35	1 in 378
40	1 in 106

If you are over the age of thirty-five, your physician may suggest either an amniocentesis or chorionic villus sampling to verify the number of fetal chromosomes (see Chapter 7). It is important to know, however, that the screening tests for Down syndrome are just as reliable for women under the age of thirty-five as they are for those over the age of thirty-five.

Turner Syndrome

Turner Syndrome is a less common chromosome abnormality, occurring in about one in twenty-five hundred babies where one X chromosome is abnormal or absent. The condition affects only females, and there may be few symptoms in the newborn period. In some cases, however, the baby may have puffy hands and feet, a webbed neck, and cardiac problems. Later in childhood, the female child may have short stature, late breast development, and lack of menstrual periods because of small ovaries. These girls need to take hormonal supplements throughout puberty. Unfortunately, they are almost always sterile, but they can otherwise lead a normal, productive, and full life. Intellectually, they do not have any significant mental problems.

Single-Gene Defects

Single-gene defects occur when a change or a mutation involves one or both of a single pair of genes. Dominant means that the abnormal gene will dominate over the "normal" one. A dominant condition is one in which only one member of the pair of genes needs to be altered in order for the condition to be expressed. The condition may be passed from generation to generation, with the risk of inheriting the gene being 50 percent (see Figure 6.1 on the next page). For example, if one parent has high cholesterol with a predisposition to heart disease, there is a 50 percent chance that the offspring will have heart disease.

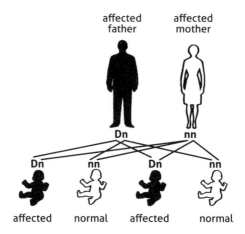

Figure 6.1: How dominant inheritance works: One affected parent has a single faulty gene (**D**) which *dominates* its normal counterpart (**n**). Each child's chances of inheriting either the **D** or **n** from the affected parent are 50%. (courtesy of March of Dimes Foundation)

A recessive gene is expressed only when present in two copies or if the other copy is missing. Recessive genes are masked in the presence of dominant genes.

Most genetic abnormalities are seen at birth, except for Huntington's chorea. In this disorder, only the father is affected and will show symptoms of the disease only when he approaches his thirties or forties.

The term *penetrance* is often used in genetics to describe the proportion of individuals carrying a particular variation of a gene that also expresses a particular trait (phenotype). In other words, if you inherit a particular disease from both of your parents, you might be better or worse off than your parents. Your body may manifest the disease differently and there is no way to predict how that will be. For example, a mother may have a mild form of sickle-cell disease (a recessive gene) but gives birth to a child who has it much worse.

Some rare dominant disorders are listed below. Detailed discussions are beyond the scope of this book.

- achondroplasia (dwarfism)
- high blood cholesterol levels
- polydactyly (extra fingers or toes)

- osteogenesis imperfecta (very brittle bones)
- von Willebrand disease (poor blood clotting)
- Huntington's chorea (progressive neurological deterioration)

A recessive gene problem manifests only when both members of the gene pair are abnormal. Usually both parents have one copy of the abnormal gene, and yet are healthy themselves. A child who receives an autosomal recessive gene from both parents shows its trait. For example, having blue eyes is a recessive trait. Recessive genes are rare, and so the chance of marrying a carrier of the same genetic disease is unlikely if you marry outside of your own family. We are all carriers for some recessive conditions; our children have problems only if our partner is also a carrier and they inherit two copies of the harmful gene. When both parents are carriers, the risk with each pregnancy is 25 percent (see Figure 6.2).

Researchers have found that ethnicity is important with recessive disorders. For example, sickle-cell anemia is more common among African-American women; cystic fibrosis is more common in Caucasians, and Tay-Sachs disease is more common in Ashkenazi Jews. If you are of

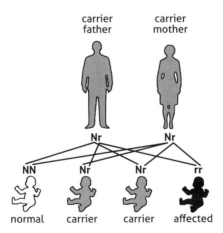

Figure 6.2: How recessive inheritance works: Both parents usually unaffected, carry a normal gene (**N**) that takes precedence over its faulty recessive counterpart (**r**). The odds for children are: 1) a 25% risk of inheriting a "double dose" of **r** genes, which may cause a serious birth defect; 2) a 25% chance of inheriting two **N**s, thus being unaffected; and 3) a 50% chance of being a carrier as both parents are.
(courtesy of March of Dimes Foundation)

a certain ethnic group, you might undergo special tests during your prenatal period. If you are negative for the disease, no further testing will be
done. However, if you are positive for the gene defect, further testing will
be performed, usually on the baby's father, and if necessary, on the fetus.
Only if you and your partner have the gene does your baby have a one-in-
four chance of also getting the disease.

Some examples of recessive disorders are:

- phenylketonuria (PKU)
- sickle-cell anemia
- beta-thalassemia (blood disorder)
- cystic fibrosis (affecting secretions in the lungs and pancreas)
- galactosemia (inability to metabolize milk)
- Tay-Sachs disease (fatal neurological disease)

The most common recessive disorders are discussed below.

Cystic Fibrosis

Cystic fibrosis is a metabolic disorder that affects the mucous glands of
the body and results in thick secretions. The bodily systems that are affected include the lungs and the pancreas. It is an inherited recessive disorder affecting about one in two thousand newborn Caucasian children
and about one in twenty-five people carry this abnormality in one of
their genes. According to the Cystic Fibrosis Foundation, about thirty
thousand children and adults have cystic fibrosis in the United States.
The carrier rate in the general population of a single abnormal gene is
one in twenty-five.

The American College of Obstetricians and Gynecologists (ACOG)
recommends screening all couples for cystic fibrosis carrier status. This
screening involves a blood test for the mother. It only needs to be done
once in a person's life, since your genes do not change over time. If a
woman is negative, then no further testing is needed.

Cystic fibrosis is transmitted to a child when he or she inherits an abnormal gene from both parents and therefore has two abnormal genes
and no normal ones. The parents are typically normal, although they do
carry the recessive gene and one or both of them can have the disease. If

both parents are carriers, there is a 50 percent chance that the child will just be a carrier, a 25 percent chance that the child will be unaffected, and a 25 percent chance that the child will have cystic fibrosis.

Cystic fibrosis is often recognized early in life. The infant may have a chronic cough, foul-smelling stools, difficulties metabolizing sugar, and heat intolerance. Chronic lung infections are common due to the thick lung secretions, which serve as a nourishing medium for bacterial growth. Cystic fibrosis is diagnosed with a sweat test, which measures the amount of salt in the sweat.

There is no cure for cystic fibrosis, and it is usually managed at home. The standard treatment is to deal with the symptoms as they arise. The child is often given antibiotics to liquefy the characteristic thick secretions, and is given aggressive physical therapy to keep the lungs free of secretions.

Sickle-Cell Disease

Sickle-cell disease is an inherited blood disorder characterized by red blood cells that when stressed assume an abnormal rigid shape. This unusual shape restricts them from movement in the bloodstream and therefore deprives the surrounding tissues of oxygen.

The disease can cause anemia, pain, frequent infections, and damage to vital organs. It is usually diagnosed in infancy with a simple screening test called hemoglobin electrophoresis. There is no cure for sickle-cell disease; however, medications are used to treat the pain and to prevent further problems.

There is a difference between having sickle-cell disease and the sickle-cell trait. To have sickle-cell disease, the child must have two abnormal genes, one from each parent. If the child has only one abnormal gene, he or she is healthy but is a carrier and can pass this abnormality to their offspring. Being a carrier offers protection against malaria, which is probably why this gene is still common among those of African ethnicity.

Phenylketonuria (PKU)

Phenylketonuria is a rare recessive condition that affects one in approximately twenty-five thousand births in the United States. All newborns are routinely tested for PKU within a few days of birth. A small amount of blood is taken from the baby's heel to see if there are abnormal amounts of phenylalanine. If the baby is premature or is born at home, arrangements are made for his or her screening.

PKU is most frequently seen in those of Northern European and Native American ancestry. PKU is characterized by the child's inability to process or metabolize the amino acid phenylalanine. One consequence of this inability is the excessive production of phenylketones, which are excreted in the urine. The disruption of phenylalanine metabolism can prevent the child's brain from developing properly and can lead to severe mental deficiencies, behavior disturbances, and sometimes seizures.

If you have PKU and were treated as a child, your own child may be at risk during pregnancy. It is important for you to maintain a strict diet before and during pregnancy because high levels of phenylalanine may cause a miscarriage or increase the risk of having a child with PKU symptoms.

Infants born with PKU appear normal for the first few months. Treatment, which must be initiated within the first few weeks of life, is with a special diet providing low amounts phenylalanine. The diet can help prevent brain damage and must be continued at least until adolescence.

Infants who are untreated begin to lose interest in their surroundings by the age of three to five months. By the time they reach their first birthday, they show progressive mental retardation accompanied by physical symptoms such as dry skin, foul-smelling urine, skin odor, and very fair hair.

Tay-Sachs Disease

This disease is an autosomal recessive disorder resulting in progressive deterioration of the neurological system. The disorder is most common among those of Ashkenazi Jewish ancestry. The symptoms include the child's loss of interest in his or her environment, poor head control, and loss of muscle tone, all of which may appear between three and six months of age. When the child is eighteen months old, he or she may become deaf and blind and display uncoordinated muscle movements. By the time they are three to five years old, these children usually die of a respiratory infection. Tay-Sachs can be detected by a routine blood sample taken from a pregnant woman, but the test is not done unless specifically requested. When both parents are carriers, prenatal diagnosis is available by amniocentesis and/or chorionic villus sampling, and if the fetus is affected, the couple may decide whether to continue or terminate the pregnancy. There is no cure for this tragic disease, and the treatment is merely to support the child and to treat the symptoms as they arise.

Sex-Linked Disorders

Sex-linked defects are traits carried on the X or Y chromosome. Because the Y chromosome is largely rudimentary (i.e., it has very few genes), most examples of sex-linked diseases are X-linked disorders. In X-linked recessive diseases, only the males are affected and the females are carriers of the disease (see Figure 6.3). There are many X-linked disorders. The traits may be either dominant or recessive; the latter are more common. In X-linked recessive disorders, a woman may be a carrier of the disease or defect that is manifested only in her male children. If you are a carrier of an X-linked disorder, the risk for a male or female to inherit the abnormal gene is 50 percent. Some examples of X-linked recessive disorders are:

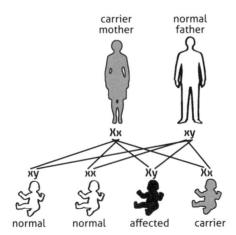

Figure 6.3: How X-linked inheritance works: In the most common form, the female sex chromosomes of an unaffected mother carry one faulty gene (**X**) and one normal one (**x**). The father has normal male x and y chromosome complement. The odds for each *male* child are 50/50: 1) a 50% risk of inheriting the faulty **X** and the disorder and 2) a 50% chance of inheriting normal x and y chromosomes. For each *female* child, the odds are: 1) a 50% risk of inheriting one faulty **X**, to be a carrier like mother; and 2) a 50% chance of inheriting no faulty gene.

(courtesy of March of Dimes Foundation)

- agammaglobulinemia (lack of immunity to certain infections)
- color blindness
- Duchenne muscular dystrophy
- hemophilia (bleeder's disease)

Multifactorial Disorders

Many inherited problems are caused by a complex interaction of genetic and environmental factors that are called multifactorial disorders. The incidence of some of these disorders is low, as is the chance of them recurring in subsequent children. Some examples of multifactorial disorders include the following:

- cleft lip/cleft palate
- congenital hip dislocation
- congenital scoliosis
- some urinary tract malformations
- hydrocephalus (water on the brain)
- some congenital heart defects/diseases
- Hirschsprung disease (congenital large colon)
- pyloric stenosis (narrowed/obstructed opening from stomach to small intestines)
- club foot
- mental retardation
- some diabetes mellitus
- spina bifida (open spine)

Mutations

Certain environmental factors may cause a chemical change in the gene, resulting in mutations. Mutations occur spontaneously in the population. Mutations can be caused by certain types of radiation, such as X rays (see Chapter 2).

Fetal Surgery

Fetal surgery is reserved for life-threatening fetal abnormalities where it might be too late to operate after the baby is born. For some, fetal surgery is a possible alternative to abortion or to the birth of a special needs child.

Fetal surgery in humans began in the 1960s with intrauterine red blood cell transfusions for those with Rh disease. Prior to the advent of this procedure, the fetus would have died of complications such as anemia and swelling (edema). Since ultrasound was introduced in the 1970s, it has been used to diagnose certain problems that can benefit from surgery after twenty-four weeks of pregnancy. Fetal surgery has been used since the early 1980s to treat fetal blockages. This has been done by inserting a catheter or tube through the mother's uterus to facilitate drainage of excess fluids. Today, most types of fetal surgery involve the use of a catheter passed into the mother's abdomen.

Basically, there are two types of fetal surgery. The first is open fetal surgery. In 1981, Dr. Michael Harrison, at the University of California at San Francisco, did the first open fetal surgery to treat a severe fetal blockage in the urinary tract (hydronephrosis). In this type of surgery, an incision is made in the mother's abdomen in the same way as in a cesarean delivery. The fetus is partially removed from the uterus so that the problem can be exposed and then repaired. The fetus is then returned to the uterus. There is a risk of preterm labor, and the surgeon will be ready to perform an emergency cesarean delivery.

The second type of fetal surgery is more commonly performed today. It is performed through a fetoscope and compared with open fetal surgery, it is minimally invasive. The technique uses a small surgical opening in the mother's abdomen and then the use of a fiber optic telescope to correct the fetal problem. There is less of a risk of preterm labor.

Fetal surgery should be done prior to the twenty-fourth week because this is when the baby becomes viable and the surgery could precipitate preterm delivery. However, there are significant maternal risks that should be considered. To date, studies have not shown that fetal surgery makes a huge difference in the outcome for the fetuses. However, there are four major fetal problem areas where fetal surgery might be considered: congenital hydronephrosis, congenital diaphragmatic hernia, sacrococcygeal teratoma, and neural tube defects.

Congenital Hydronephrosis

Congenital hydronephrosis, or urinary tract obstruction, prevents the kidneys from developing normally, thus causing a blockage in the urine flow. It usually develops early in pregnancy and affects the ureters and urethra. In severe cases, the mother has less amniotic fluid because the fetus is not excreting the normal amount of urine. The fetus's lungs are also poorly developed because they are dependent on fluid for their growth and development. If detected early in pregnancy, those with severe forms of the disease would be good candidates for surgery.

This type of surgery is performed during an ultrasound. A small catheter is placed into the fetal bladder to temporarily drain the urine into the amniotic fluid and to bypass any obstruction. The tube is left in place until after delivery, at which point the surgery is performed to correct the blockage. The fetal mortality rate from this procedure is about 4 percent, and the survival rate following birth is close to 50 percent. If left untreated, the mortality rate from the disease itself is much higher.

Congenital Diaphragmatic Hernia

In this birth defect, the fetus's diaphragm fails to develop properly, leaving a hole. This makes it difficult for the baby to breathe. The other organs, such as the stomach, small intestines, and other organs slip into the fetus's chest, crowding the lungs and interfering with proper development. As a result, at birth, the baby's lungs are so small that he or she cannot breathe.

The incidence of diaphragmatic hernia is about one in every twenty-two thousand births. About 50 percent of these fetuses die, often in the delivery room. Prior to surgical intervention for the fetus, the standard treatment had been to wait for birth, attach the newborn to a respirator, and then operate on the hernia as soon as possible.

With the assistance of ultrasound, diaphragmatic hernias are detected during routine ultrasounds at about eighteen weeks. However, only about 10 percent of fetuses are suitable for this type of surgery. The surgery was first performed in 1990 by Dr. Michael Harrison on a mother who was twenty-four weeks pregnant. A small incision was made in the uterus, and then the fetus's left arm was lifted aside, the baby's chest was opened, and the abdominal organs were pushed into their proper places. The fetus's diaphragm was then closed with a patch of Gore-Tex (the waterproof material used in ski jackets). The operation took less than one hour, and seven weeks later baby Blake was born. Many of Dr. Harrison's patients did quite well, although there was one trial study published in 1998 indicating that this procedure did not improve the baby's survival, as compared to babies who were repaired after birth.

Sacrococcygeal Teratoma

Sacrococcygeal teratoma is the most common type of congenital tumor that affects newborns. The tumor is located at the base of the baby's coccyx (tailbone). These tumors can sometimes grow quite large but are usually benign. They are often detected through routine prenatal ultrasound. If the tumor is larger than 10 centimeters, the baby may have to be born by cesarean delivery. Most babies survive and do quite well following surgery in the early newborn period. Sacrococcygeal teratoma occurs in about one out of every forty-eight thousand births; 80 percent of babies with this condition are females.

The Fetus as Patient: Now that practitioners have found ways to see and treat the unborn child, they are faced with complex decisions. Today, both mother and child are considered patients during pregnancy. Medical advances may help fetuses survive who, under "normal" circumstances, would not have had the gift of life.

Ethical, legal, and economic questions will continue to be raised as long as medical technology advances at such an unrelenting pace. Questions are being posed about the rights of both the mother and the fetus. A procedure will be advocated if it is beneficial to mother as well as to child. If either the mother or the baby is put into danger as a result of the procedure, it will probably not be performed.

Ethical questions arise when the mother waives her right to have fetal surgery. Is it her right to decide? Who makes the decision? Can we make analogies with the choice to have a cesarean or an abortion? In a 1987 article in *Current Problems in Obstetrics, Gynecology, and Fertility*, Dr. Sherman Elias and Professor George Annas state that society should honor a mother's refusal of intervention, since we assume that the mother has the fetus's best interests in mind. In the journal *Nursing Clinics of North America* (1989), author J. G. Twomey argues that court resolutions of such situations should be reserved for situations in which the mother and father disagree or the mother's competence or judgment is in question. The author goes on to say that adequate prenatal care helps to reduce the very problems that may force the mother to contemplate fetal surgery.

There are also certain dilemmas from an economic standpoint. The cost of surgical intervention is high, but so is the medical care required for a child with severe defects. Caring for the chronically disabled is very costly, especially if it is necessary to keep these children institutionalized.

Although surgical intervention can help many, a certain risk is always present and must be weighed against the benefits. Careful assessment of the fetus by a skilled team is essential before the decision is made to recommend fetal surgery. The fact that a procedure can be performed does not always mean that it should be performed.

Although professionals may believe intervention is necessary, you, the parent, have the right to decide what you think is best for your unborn child, based on all the information that you have gathered. The best decision is an educated one. Whatever you decide for your unborn child, you can be thankful that today you have the option to choose sophisticated interventions, a choice parents of previous generations never had.

Genetic Counseling

Many couples seek genetic counseling long before trying to conceive a child. The most frequent candidates for genetic counseling are women over the age of thirty-five; however, just because you are an older mother, it does not necessarily mean that you will need genetic counseling. It is critical that you receive good counseling if you have a family history of genetic disorders. Typically, the genetic counselor has special training in hereditary diseases and in birth defects in general, and he or she may be a physician or a trained health professional.

The genetic counselor will need to know about any hereditary diseases in your family, the causes of death of family members, and any previous stillbirths or miscarriages. It is important that you bring forward as much information as possible. Talk to your family members to gain a complete picture of your family history. If you already have an affected child, he or she needs to be investigated.

If there is unexplained mental retardation in your family, you should tell your provider. He or she may want to screen for something called fragile X or Martin-Bell syndrome. This genetic syndrome results in a spectrum (from none to severe) of characteristic physical, intellectual, emotional, and behavioral features. It is associated with the extensive repetition of a gene on the X chromosome resulting in the failure to produce a certain protein (FMR-1), which is essential for neurological development in the fetus.

The two most important components of genetic counseling are the pedigree charts (family tree) and the mother's ethnicity. Certain ethnic groups are more prone to certain genetic problems. If your physician inquires about your ethnic background, chances are he or she merely wants to gather information to guide your prenatal care to ensure you have a healthy baby. Table 6.2 below lists some diseases associated with particular ethnic groups:

Table 6.2: Some Diseases Associated with Particular Ethnic Groups

Ethnic Group	Possible Disease
Ashkenazi Jews	Niemann-Pick disease (Type A), Canavan disease, Gaucher disease (Type 1), Tay-Sachs disease
Caucasians	Cystic fibrosis
Mediterraneans	Thalassemia
African-Americans	Sickle-cell disease

To help the counselor understand your potential risks, he or she may recommend various diagnostic tests, including blood and skin tests. If you are already pregnant, you may be advised to have certain prenatal diagnostic tests, such as amniocentesis and ultrasound, to detect fetal defects. If you are planning to use in vitro fertilization (IVF), a preimplantation genetic diagnosis (PGD) may be offered (see Chapter 1).

Your counselor will discuss what has been ascertained from all the gathered information. Your family history will be drawn in the form of a pedigree chart that illustrates your family tree and any diseases of its members (see the example in Figure 6.4 on the next page). The risks, if any, to yourself and/or your offspring will be discussed with you in detail. This information, along with your counselor's guidance, should help you to make an informed reproductive decision. Couples face difficult issues and questions when genetic disease is confirmed or is a possibility. All of these factors are considered during the counseling sessions.

One mother had the following to say about her decision:

"I had to make the most difficult and painful decision of my life, which was to terminate my pregnancy. I was fourteen weeks pregnant. My husband and I made our decision based on statistics and risk. At eleven weeks, I had a severely abnormal nuchal translucency test (almost 7 mm), so they suggested a CVS test. The tests were normal. I had numerous normal ultrasounds, but the doctors all said it was probably too early to detect problems.

"We met with a genetic specialist who reviewed the list of possible disorders and diseases associated with a high nuchal and normal CVS. We were told that there was about a 60 to 70 percent chance that either I would miscarry or that some disorder would be found. During three weeks before our decision, we talked to every expert we could find and had every possible test, and we finally decided to terminate the pregnancy. The nightmare continued. I bled for weeks almost nonstop, and my doctor did a couple of ultrasounds and then referred me to a specialist. The specialist also wasn't sure, and referred me for an MRI. My doctor called that night to tell me I had placenta accreta, which is when the placenta has implanted in the muscle of the uterus. It's a very dangerous condition during delivery and usually leads to hysterectomy. The following week I was referred to a gynecological oncologist for treatment with methotrexate.

"After some months, we conceived again. Initially everything looked fine, but my doctor wanted to follow me carefully. I had a number of blood tests and ultrasounds, which showed an ectopic

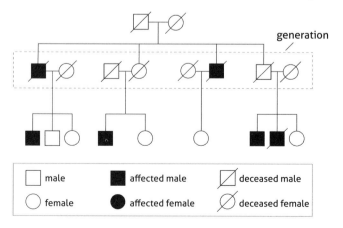

Figure 6.4: A sample pedigree chart

pregnancy. I was numb. We were concerned that there was a lot of scar tissue from my C-section and/or the D&C, so I had a hystero-salpingogram, which was normal. Finally, several months later, we conceived again. I loved being pregnant, but after having gone through what I did, I had a lot of anxiety about whether this baby would be normal.

"I now have a beautiful four-year-old son, and he has a six-month-old brother, who I'm so thankful for. I think it actually took me a couple of months after he was born to really feel attached to him, because of the stress from the previous two years."

Your Emotions

Learning that your child is affected by a chronic illness or disability is probably one of the most painful and stigmatizing experiences in your life. As one mother of a hemophiliac said, "No matter how it is presented, the fact of serious chronic illness is always difficult to accept."

One single mother observed:

"At first, I was in total despair. It somehow seemed to me that I couldn't do anything right. First, I had failed as a wife and now as a parent. But in the long, dark night that followed the disclosure of the news, I had a real change of heart. As an only child, I had been very much protected and I realized this was not standing me in good stead in life. I now realize that I was at a real crossroads. I could have either continued being a weak person, now with a perfect excuse of a very sick child, or I could grow up that minute—take charge of a new baby and my own life—and do something about my son and get moving. I did grow up that night and it is a decision I never regretted."

Early in your pregnancy, you and your partner began to imagine what your child would be like. This image was carried throughout your pregnancy, up to the birth of your child. After learning of your child's disability, it is normal for you to feel inadequate and helpless. It is normal to fear the reaction of loved ones, including grandparents, who may have long awaited the birth of this child. These feelings may be magnified if you have had infertility problems.

It is normal to feel your faith shaken. You may ask yourself questions like "Why did this happen to me?" "What kind of world is it in which such pain can be inflicted on people?" "Is there any meaning to our suffering?" One woman who cared for a daughter with hydrocephalus until she died at six years of age states:

> "She was our only child and we did everything for her, including feeding, dressing, and bathing, because of her physical and mental handicap. She could not walk or sit or even talk to us. We accepted that she would never be normal and that we would do everything in our power to make her life as comfortable as possible. That was the decision we made."

In Rayna Rapp's article in *Ms.*, "The Ethics of Choice," she writes about learning through amniocentesis that her fetus had Down syndrome. She discusses decisions women must make when they find they are carrying a handicapped fetus:

> "Making the medical arrangements, going back for counseling, the pretests, and finally, the abortion, was the most difficult period in my adult life. I was then twenty-one weeks pregnant, and had been proudly carrying my expanding belly. Telling everyone—friends, family, students, colleagues, neighbors—seemed an endless nightmare. But it also allowed us to rely on their love and support during this terrible time.... Our community was invaluable, reminding us that our lives were rich and filled with love despite the loss."

Whatever decision you make regarding your baby-to-be, these will be difficult times for you. If you decide to have an abortion, it is normal to take a while to get over your loss. You may continue to wonder if you made the right decision or you may feel comfortable knowing that you were correct. If you decide to care for the child yourself, you should be prepared for the unavoidable strain the handicap will place on you and your family. You should also be prepared for society's reaction to your special-needs child. It is common for society to set you apart and make you feel different. It will be your own creative efforts that will make the difference in combating the loneliness often felt by handicapped people and their families.

Journaling Corner

What genetic issue are you most concerned about?

Are there any genetic issues in your family? If yes, describe.

Are you seeing a specialist? How do you feel about him or her?

Do you understand all the risks of your situation?

Who provides you with the most support during your pregnancy?

What have you read lately?

Write about things you need to keep in mind right now.

7 Tests, Tests, Tests

A mother's joy begins when new life is stirring inside...when a tiny heartbeat is heard for the very first time and a playful kick reminds her that she is never alone. — AUTHOR UNKNOWN

Tests during pregnancy are inevitable. They answer many questions and help provide a sense of security about what is going on. Medical testing today is a bit more sophisticated than it was years ago. Women today know a lot more details about their pregnancies, such as what to expect and their possible risks.

Whether you are contemplating pregnancy or are already pregnant, you will be asked numerous questions about your past and present health the first time you meet with your physician. You may be asked questions about your mother's history, since many female characteristics are inherited. Some other questions you might be asked include the following:

- When was your first menstrual period?
- What is the duration of your period?
- How heavy is the flow?
- How long is your cycle?
- Have you ever been pregnant before?
- Have you ever had an abortion? A miscarriage?
- Do you have any health problems?
- Are you taking any medications?
- Have you ever had urinary or vaginal infections?

All of this information provides a baseline history that will subsequently help to plan your prenatal care. For example, if you have a family history of genetic disorders, such as hemophilia, Down syndrome, or birth defects, your physician may recommend certain genetic-screening tests. If you have had uterine fibroids (benign tumors on the wall of the uterus), an ultrasound may be recommended to detect their presence, size, and growth rate. Tests may be done at various stages of your pregnancy to assist the physician in detecting any high-risk problems before they arise.

There are two categories of tests given during pregnancy: screening tests and diagnostic tests. A screening test is performed to determine if you have a particular disease. These tests assist the physician in deciding if you belong in a low- or high-risk category. If you fall into a high-risk category, your physician will suggest further tests, called diagnostic tests. A diagnostic test is performed to confirm or refute the presence of a particular disease. If a diagnostic test is positive, it means you have the disease. If you know that you might be at risk for a particular disease and want to forgo the screening test and go directly to a diagnostic test, make sure to mention this to your provider.

Ultrasound Tests

An ultrasound is a painless and safe method of scanning your abdomen with high-frequency sound waves to assess your baby's growth and development. These sound waves have a frequency of approximately twenty thousand vibrations per second. During your ultrasound, a transducer will be placed on your abdomen (see Figure 7.1). This emits high-frequency sound waves that pass into the body and are reflected back to the transducer, which also serves as the receiver. The variation in rate and intensity of the sound waves is interpreted electronically to form a picture of the medium through which they pass. In this case, the medium is your abdomen.

There are three parts of the baby that are measured on the ultrasound:

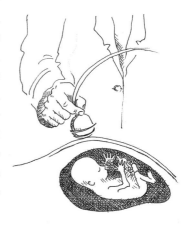

Figure 7.1:
Ultrasound testing

the head circumference, abdominal circumference, and femur length. These numbers are then put into an equation in the computer that estimates the fetal weight. Of these three measurements, the abdominal circumference is the most important because it is indicative of the baby's weight/proportions. Similar to adults, when fetuses gain weight, they gain it in their abdomens. Sometimes the baby's weight as indicated by an ultrasound is not precise or accurate. In fact, it has a margin of error of approximately 15 percent. The actual weight of the fetus in pounds/-grams will not be determined until the twenty-fourth week. Prior to this time, the fetus weight and estimation of the fetal size is calculated using measurements of the head and long bones of the leg.

Uses of Ultrasound Testing

Many women get an ultrasound very early in the pregnancy to obtain an accurate due date, especially if they are not sure of the first day of their last period or if they have irregular periods. A woman with vaginal bleeding in the first trimester may also get an ultrasound to make sure everything is okay and that she is not having a miscarriage or an ectopic pregnancy.

The next ultrasound is usually performed between seventeen and twenty weeks to survey the baby's anatomy. Certain abnormal findings on ultrasound are linked to particular known disorders (see Chapter 7).

Every pregnancy is different, so the number of ultrasounds a woman receives will depend on her particular risk. If you are being monitored by a high-risk obstetrical center, there is a good chance that you will receive more ultrasounds to ensure that everything is okay.

Below is a list of some high-risk situations in which ultrasound is routinely performed, and more specific reasons are shown in Table 7.1.

Maternal Problems	Fetal Problems
• diabetes	• multiple pregnancies
• hypertension	• placental problems
• thyroid disease	• two-vessel umbilical cord
• obesity	• poor fetal growth
• autoimmune disorders	• cervical insufficiency
	• abnormal amniotic fluid volume

Table 7.1: Why Ultrasounds Are Performed

Use	Reasons
Estimate fetal age	Time cesareans or induction of labor
Evaluate fetal growth	Ensure good growth
Determine vaginal bleeding	Determine source
Determine fetal position	When difficult to palpate
Determine multiple pregnancy	Monitor pregnancy
During amniocentesis	Ensure correct needle placement
Suspected hydatidiform mole	Confirm diagnosis
Suspected cervical insufficiency	Measure the cervical length
Following cervical cerclage	Aid in timing and correct placement of suture for cervical insufficiency
Suspected ectopic pregnancy	Confirm diagnosis
During special procedures	Amniocentesis, intrauterine transfusion, IVF, embryo transfer, fetoscopy, CVS
Suspected fetal death	Confirm diagnosis and initiate treatment
Suspected uterine problem	Monitor fetal growth
Ovarian-follicle growth	Determine treatment for infertility
Suspected excessive or insufficientamniotic fluid	Confirm diagnosis and identify cause
History of previous congenital abnormality	Preventive measure
When turning a breech presentation	Facilitate safety of procedure
Suspected abruptio placenta	Confirm diagnosis so treatment may be recommended
Screen for abnormalities	Routine screening to check growth and development
Prolonged pregnancy	Assess fetal health

Other Applications: Vaginal ultrasounds may be performed to assess fetal heart rhythms and to be sure that the fetal sac is in the uterine cavity and that you are not having an ectopic pregnancy. Until the thirtieth week of pregnancy, the cervical length may also be known through ultrasound. An ultrasound may be performed to detect less common abnormalities such as hydatidiform mole. Ultrasound is also used for guidance during an amniocentesis.

Most providers will not order an ultrasound to determine your baby's gender; however, if you are having an ultrasound for another reason and you want to know the sex of your child (which is best seen after sixteen weeks), you should feel free to ask. On the other hand, if you do not want to know, then it is important you tell the person before beginning the scan, so as to prevent the technician from blurting the news out by accident! Although gender determination by ultrasound is quite accurate, you should know that it is not 100 percent predictive.

Ultrasounds may also be used in the case of prolonged or postterm pregnancy because they can help identify potential complications before they arise.

What to Expect

Ultrasound may be performed either in your physician's office or in the hospital. You will be instructed to drink about six glasses of water about one hour prior to the test. Early in pregnancy, the image of your uterus shows up more clearly on the ultrasound when you have a full bladder. You will probably notice that you will be more uncomfortable during your second ultrasound than your first because of your larger size. Waiting for the administration of the test will probably be more of a problem than the actual ultrasound itself. The discomfort does not last long, and you can urinate as soon as the test is completed.

During your ultrasound, you will lie on your back on an examination table. You will be asked to bare your abdomen, and either a gel or an oily substance, serving to improve ultrasound-wave transmission, will be rubbed onto your abdomen. A transducer that is hooked up to a computer screen will be placed on your abdomen, and by looking at the image produced by the transducer, the technician or physician will be able to observe your baby's status. You can also ask to see your baby and its position. An ultrasound takes approximately fifteen minutes, depending on the pace of the technician administering the test.

If an ultrasound is being done before the twelfth week, doctors will often perform a vaginal ultrasound. The use of a vaginal transducer does not require a full bladder. This procedure can be somewhat uncomfortable; however, it does provide a better image of the baby.

Special Concerns

Ultrasounds have been used since the 1960s and are completely safe and noninvasive. As in many diagnostics of this type, the results are only as accurate as the person interpreting the data. Ultrasound has opened new horizons in obstetrics, where the well-being of the fetus is always of primary importance. Today, many potential problems are avoided by early detection.

There are two relatively new types of ultrasounds that are sometimes performed on the pregnant woman: the 3D ultrasound and the 4D ultrasound. The 3D ultrasounds are performed to provide a more detailed look at the fetus. They take longer to perform, but they provide a realistic image of how your baby looks as it grows inside of you. Seeing such realistic images of your baby can be very emotional, particularly if you spot your baby smiling or waving. Although it might enhance your own and your partner's pregnancy experience, it can also be upsetting, because sometimes the images might be distorted and can make your baby look deformed when it is not. Sometimes this type of ultrasound is useful if your baby has something like a cleft palate and seeing the image might prepare you for what your baby will look like.

The 4D ultrasound is similar to the 3D; however, in this version the image is seen along with the baby's movements inside of you.

First Trimester Risk Assessment

This relatively new and noninvasive evaluation can assess the mother's risk of having an abnormal baby. The test combines an ultrasound evaluation of the fetus for specific chromosomal abnormalities, such as Down syndrome, along with a maternal blood screening.

The blood portion of the test measures the levels of the hormones hCG and PAPP-A (pregnancy-associated placental protein-A). The fetal ultrasound measures the nuchal translucency (NT), which is a measurement of the thickness of the skin at the back of the baby's neck. (This is not a structural defect, but it has been shown as a possible indication for Down syndrome.) The results of the blood tests and ultrasound measurements, in conjunction with the maternal age, help to determine the risk of having a baby with trisomy 21, or Down syndrome.

Typically, this test will be done between your eleventh and thirteenth week. It is used to help decide if you should have further testing, such as chorionic villus sampling and/or second trimester amniocentesis. It is usually at this point that the physician may recommend you and your partner meet with a genetic counselor.

A study published in the November 2005 issue of the *New England Journal of Medicine* ascertained that this test is the most accurate, noninvasive screening test available.

Expanded AFP Screening
(Triple Marker and Quadruple Marker Screen)

You may be asked if you want to have this optional test. Using a blood sample, the triple marker screening test checks for three substances: alpha-fetoprotein (AFP), human chorionic gonadotropin (hCG), and unconjugated estriol (UE) in the mother's blood.

The hormones hCG and UE are produced by the fetus and the placenta. AFP results provide information regarding the risk of abdominal wall defects, Down syndrome, and trisomy 18 (Edwards syndrome). Abdominal wall defects occur when a fetus has an abnormal opening on the abdomen allowing the intestines and other organs to form outside of the body. This is deformity can be corrected surgically after birth.

The AFP portion of the test also checks for neural tube defects. Early in pregnancy, this protein is produced by the fetal liver and secreted in the area where the spinal canal, spinal cord, and brain are developing. By the end of the first trimester, when the spinal canal is closed, this protein is present in smaller amounts in the amniotic fluid. If there is an excess of this protein, it may indicate that the baby has serious disorders, such as spina bifida (open spine) or anencephaly (absence of brain).

The quadruple marker test is basically the same as the triple marker test, except it also measures an additional marker in the maternal blood, called inhibin A. More recent studies have shown that it is much more effective in determining fetal abnormalities because it tests for one more marker in the maternal blood.

What to Expect

Because the amounts of the tested substances in the mother's blood change throughout pregnancy, this test is reliable only if performed between the fifteenth and twentieth weeks.

A normal test result provides reassurance that there is little chance of your baby having any problems. However, if the test shows your baby might have a problem, this is a good time for a genetic counselor to be contacted to discuss the possibility of an advanced ultrasound or amniocentesis. If an ultrasound does not provide an explanation for the initial test result, an amniocentesis will be performed to confirm the diagnosis.

Special Concerns

The screening program described here is a simple, safe, and relatively reliable group of tests. The only disadvantage is that it may provide false positive results. False positive results may also be due to a poor dating of the pregnancy. High levels of the tested hormones may be associated with a miscarriage, intrauterine growth restriction, or a multiple pregnancy. Most women who have positive results give birth to healthy babies.

According to California's Department of Health Services, among those who have had the expanded AFP blood test and follow-up tests in California:

- 97 percent of the cases of anencephaly are found
- 80 percent of the cases of open spina bifida are found
- 85 percent of the cases of abdominal wall defects are found
- 50 percent or more of the cases of trisomy 18 are found
- 40 to 66 percent of the cases of Down syndrome are found among women aged thirty-five and younger

All pregnant women should be offered the triple or quadruple marker test and the AFP test, but it is strongly recommended for women in the following categories:

- those with a family history of birth defects
- those over the age of thirty-five
- those with a personal or family history of genetic defects
- those who used possible harmful medications during pregnancy
- those with diabetes and who use insulin

Amniocentesis

Amniocentesis is a procedure in which a sample of amniotic fluid is taken from the uterus by inserting a needle through the woman's abdomen into the amniotic sac. It is almost always performed using an ultrasound to ensure that the needle is well-positioned. The amniotic fluid, which holds the baby's chromosomal content, is then sent to the laboratory for analysis. Amniocentesis is usually performed between the fifteenth and eighteenth week of pregnancy, and results usually take between two and three weeks. Early amniocentesis is no longer recommended because there are more risks if it is performed too early.

Uses

Amniocentesis has many applications. Its most frequent use is for women over the age of thirty-five. Other reasons for amniocentesis include genetic evaluation, checking for metabolic disorders, blood incompatibilities, infection, or neural tube defects, and assessment of fetal lung maturity as the time of birth approaches.

Advanced Maternal Age: The purpose of amniocentesis for an older woman is to ensure that there are no signs of genetic abnormalities (see Chapters 5 and 14). Because the procedure is performed earlier in pregnancy, it gives the couple a chance to make the decision to abort an abnormal fetus.

History of Genetic Problems: If there is a history of genetic problems in your family, if you are taking medication for seizures, or if you are an insulin-dependent diabetic, you should be referred for genetic counseling. Counseling will also be recommended if you have had a child with a genetic or chromosomal disorder, such as Down syndrome, or if either you or your partner carries a recessive trait for a disease.

The cells collected in the amniocentesis sampling can identify the sex of your child. This is particularly important information in certain sex-linked disorders, such as hemophilia, in which females carry the factor and males manifest the symptoms of the disease.

Metabolic and Hematologic Disorders: If your physician suspects a metabolic or hematologic disorder such as beta-thalassemia or sickle-cell anemia, an amniocentesis may be advised. Beta-thalassemia is a rare metabolic disease, seen most often in Mediterranean regions, that results in severe anemia in the newborn child. In certain population groups, there may be increased incidence of Tay-Sachs disease (see Chapter 6). This error of metabolism is characterized by severe neurological problems in the fetus.

During routine prenatal blood testing, high-risk women are screened as carriers of these diseases. If both partners are found to be carriers, an amniocentesis is performed to confirm the diagnosis or to ensure the baby's health.

Blood Incompatibilities: If this is your second pregnancy and you have had blood incompatibilities with your first child and have formed antibodies, then an amniocentesis may be performed to ensure that your antibodies are not harming your baby-to-be. Your amniotic fluid will be analyzed for bilirubin, a yellowish pigment that is formed as a result of broken-down red blood cells. If the resulting anemia is harming your unborn child, an intrauterine blood transfusion may be given. When an amniocentesis is performed for this reason, it is usually repeated every two to three weeks.

Lung Maturity: Amniocentesis helps determine the lecithin/sphingomyelin (L/S) ratio, a ratio that is indicative of fetal lung maturity—in other words, the fetus's ability to sustain life on its own. This older test is usually performed after the thirty-fourth week of gestation. The test is performed to predict the probability of respiratory distress syndrome (RDS), which is a common problem among premature babies or babies born with immature lungs (see Chapter 12).

If the test indicates that your baby's lungs are adequately matured, delivery is usually not a problem. However, if the test indicates immature lungs, you may receive an injection of steroid hormone (betamethasone), which helps to facilitate the baby's lung maturation.

Generally, an L/S ratio greater than or equal to 2:1 indicates that your baby's lungs are mature and that there is a minimal risk of respiratory distress following birth. The results of this particular test will be available within two to three hours.

A new test called phosphatidyl glycerol (PG) is sometimes used instead of the L/S ratio. It uses the amniotic fluid and takes a little more time to perform.

What to Expect

Amniocentesis for genetic screening is usually performed around the fifteenth to sixteenth week of pregnancy. It may be performed either in your physician's office or, more commonly, in genetic centers. You will be told to empty your bladder. Your skin will be cleansed with a special antiseptic solution to prevent infection. During the test, you will lie on your back on the examination table with a sterile cloth placed on your abdomen. The cloth will have a hole in it, through which the needle will pass and enter into your womb. Some women say the injection feels like an insect sting and only lasts a moment.

Guided by the image on the ultrasound screen, the physician will insert the needle into the amniotic sac to obtain a sample of the fluid. The needle insertion sometimes causes uterine contractions. These are usually not serious. After the fluid sample is removed, a small bandage is applied. After the test, your baby's heart rate will be checked to make sure that the procedure was well tolerated. If you are lucky, you may be able to see your baby-to-be move on the ultrasound screen. For most expectant mothers, this is very reassuring and exciting. The actual test takes ten to fifteen minutes; however, you may be asked to remain in the room for about thirty minutes to make sure that both you and your baby are well.

By the time you go home, you should feel fine. If you notice any of the following signs or symptoms, be sure to notify your physician: unusually frequent uterine contractions, abdominal pain, decreased fetal activity, fever, vaginal drainage, or vaginal bleeding. Do not be alarmed by any bruises on your abdomen following the test—they will soon disappear.

Special Concerns

The main concern of an amniocentesis is the risk of miscarriage, which occurs in about one in four hundred procedures. Some women will experience other side effects, such as cramping, soreness, spotting, vaginal fluid leakage, or premature rupture of the membranes. The decision to have an amniocentesis involves balancing the pros and the cons. The most difficult aspect of having an amniocentesis is having to wait at least two to three weeks for the results.

Fluorescence in Situ Hybridization (FISH)

FISH is a relatively new and commonly used test. The results can identify whether the fetus's chromosomes are normal or abnormal. The test is very accurate if it detects an abnormality. If it identifies trisomy 21 (Down syndrome), for example, the child definitely has the syndrome. However, studies have shown that the FISH test does have a 10 to 15 percent false-negative rate.

FISH is performed by collecting fetal cells from the amniotic fluid, fixing them on a slide, and then staining them with antibodies against specific chromosomes. Each antibody is labeled with a different color. A normal cell should have two copies of each autosome—a nonsex chromosome (13, 18, and 21) and two sex chromosomes (XX for female and XY for male).

Because the test is done using fresh cells and not cultured cells, the results are usually received within twenty-four to forty-eight hours, which is a huge advantage over some other tests.

Chorionic Villus Sampling (CVS)

The chorion is the outermost embryonic membrane, which develops about two weeks after fertilization. It eventually becomes the placenta. An analysis of this tissue early in pregnancy can detect chromosomal abnormalities. Chorionic villus sampling should ideally be performed between ten and fourteen weeks of gestation.

Uses

The uses of CVS are similar to those of amniocentesis. Certain fetal-blood disorders, such as hemophilia and beta-thalassemia, are also detected in the first trimester by CVS. The decision about which procedure to use depends on the country, the institution, and the physician.

Depending on the results, the decision to terminate the pregnancy can be made at this time. Although it is no longer used for this reason, CVS was first used in China in 1975 to determine the sex of the child. Since 1982 it has been used in the Soviet Union to determine sex-related genetic disorders and continues to be used extensively in other parts of the world.

What to Expect

The test may be performed either through the vagina or the abdomen. Today, the abdominal approach is more common because it has a lower risk of causing miscarriage. First, your baby will be located with an ultrasound. Next, a special needle will be inserted through your abdomen and a small sample of tissue will be removed from the placenta. These sample cells hold your baby's genetic composition and are sent to the laboratory for analysis.

Similar to having an ultrasound, it is important for you to have a full bladder. You may feel a small amount of discomfort as the needle enters your abdomen, and it is normal to spot or bleed slightly after the test. However, you should report any unusual vaginal leakage or increase in the amount of bleeding.

Special Concerns

While CVS identifies the same defects as amniocentesis, it has some advantages. First, it may be performed much earlier in pregnancy and the results are usually available within one week. This takes a huge stress off the waiting time. In addition, if a fetal abnormality is detected, it will not be too late for a first trimester abortion.

At the present time, this procedure is performed only at major medical centers in the United States and may not be available to all women. The main risk is miscarriage, which is slightly higher than for amniocentesis. Studies have shown that the risk of miscarriage from CVS ranges from one in two hundred to one in three hundred women.

Percutaneous Umbilical Cord Sampling (PUBS)

This technique, also called funipuncture, involves taking fetal blood samples from the umbilical cord. It is performed in a similar way to amniocentesis.

Uses

This technique may be used after the eighteenth week to determine the fetus's condition and to identify inherited disorders. The main advantage of this test, like CVS, is that the results are received within one week.

The procedure can also be used to perform an intrauterine blood transfusion. Women who are Rh-negative will need an injection of anti-D antibody after this test, in case any fetal cells are disturbed, which could increase the risk of the development of antibodies against the fetus's blood.

What to Expect

The preparation for this procedure is similar to that for amniocentesis; however, the main difference is that the needle is left in place for a longer period than during amniocentesis.

The umbilical cord is located with the ultrasound. Then a special needle is inserted through your skin into your uterus and then into your umbilical cord. The ultrasound transducer will move along your abdomen, aiding the physician in finding the umbilical vein. If the fetus is very active, a mild sedative may be given so the umbilical cord remains still long enough for the procedure to be performed.

Special Concerns

In many ways, PUBS has gone one step beyond amniocentesis because it examines the fetal blood rather than just the amniotic fluid. Today, this procedure is considered both diagnostic and therapeutic. For example, if the fetus has a problem due to a blood incompatibility with the mother, it may be given a transfusion while in the uterus. Years ago, these babies would have had to be delivered prematurely. The risk of miscarriage as a result of this procedure is about five percent.

Fetoscopy

Fetoscopy is a relatively new procedure, available only in a select number of specialized obstetrical-care centers. The instrument used to perform the test, called a fetoscope, is a telescope or narrow tube about the diameter of a large needle, with a light at the end of it. The fetoscope is inserted through the abdomen in order to view the fetus.

Uses

The most common usage of fetoscopy is for laser therapy for twin to twin transfusion syndrome (TTTS). In this situation, both babies share a placenta and blood supply, but they do not share it equally. In other words, one baby is taking blood from the other. During this procedure, the technician uses a fetoscope to identify where the shunts in the placenta are going from one baby to the other. With the use of a laser, these shunts are destroyed.

Blood samples can be taken at the same time to detect inherited abnormalities, such as sickle-cell anemia, hemophilia, and beta-thalassemia. The results are usually received within five days, which is a quarter of the time it takes for the results of amniocentesis to be processed.

After a possible birth defect is detected via fetoscopy, a physician may choose to do surgery on the fetus using the fetoscope. In some instances, photographs of the fetus may be taken with a special camera located at the end of the fetoscope.

What to Expect

A fetoscopy is usually performed in the hospital between the seventeenth and twenty-second week, and it does not involve an overnight stay. Similar to an amniocentesis, an ultrasound is done before the test. You will have an intravenous drip that may contain a medication to help you relax. Prior to the procedure you will be given a local anesthetic near the site of your incision, which will only be about ⅛ of an inch. A tiny tube is inserted alongside the fetoscope to obtain the blood sample.

Special Concerns

A fetoscopy is a delicate and costly procedure that must be done under highly supervised and specialized conditions. It is the only test that actually comes into direct contact with the fetus, and this obviously has its risks. The risks to the mother include rupture of membranes, preterm birth, bleeding, and infection. With a 5 to 70 percent chance of miscarriage, most practitioners consider PUBS to be preferable; however, others believe that fetoscopy is worth the risk because of its high accuracy rate.

Fetal Fibronectin (fFN)

Fetal fibronectin is a glycoprotein that glues or binds the fetal membranes to the underlying uterine lining. Between twenty-two and twenty-five weeks this glue should not be detected in vaginal secretions, unless there is a premature separation or disruption between the membranes and the uterine lining.

Uses

This test measures the level of fFN in your vaginal discharge between twenty-two and thirty-five weeks of gestation. Used to identify women at high-risk for preterm delivery, this is not a routine test. It is typically performed in women who are having contractions or showing signs of premature labor. If you have a history of stillbirths or multiple pregnancies, your provider may also choose to perform this test even if you do not have any symptoms. If your levels of fFN are high, you have an increased chance of delivery.

Negative test results (low levels of fFN) are reassuring and indicative that there is a 95 percent chance that you will not deliver within the next seven days. The test is reliable for one to two weeks after it is performed. If the test is positive (high level of fFN), it means that you have a higher risk of delivering prematurely. Your provider may want to monitor you more closely, decrease your activity level, or consider giving you steroid injections to help mature your baby's lungs. It is important to know that three out of four women who have a positive fFN test still deliver at term.

What to Expect
A cotton swab will be used to obtain a sample of discharge from inside your vagina near the lower part of your cervix. The results are usually available within a few hours, depending on the facility and who performs the test.

Special Concerns
Due to the recent approval of this test, many insurance companies and physicians may not be aware of its existence. Ask your physician or health-care provider for more information.

Fetal-Movement Counts

This is probably one of the oldest and most reliable tests of fetal well-being and also a reassuring sign of a healthy pregnancy. The best time to count fetal movement is after the twenty-eighth week. This test is usually performed in high-risk women after thirty-two weeks.

Uses
Fetal-movement records are especially important if you are having a difficult or problem pregnancy. Your physician will probably make a special note of the reports you provide at each visit. If you say that the movements

are less frequent or less intense, further investigations may be undertaken to ensure fetal well-being. A "movement diary" may be recommended from the sixth month onward. Often, babies who are in distress as a result of nutrient or oxygen deficiency in the last trimester of pregnancy tend to slow down their movements or may not move at all.

What to Expect

This is the only test that you, as the mother, supervise. It is done at home with a paper and pencil. On the top of your page write the days of the week, and on the left side, write the time of day. (See the example in Figure 7.2.)

There are a few different ways to do a fetal-movement count, but the most effective one is to see how long it takes for your baby to kick ten times. An even older method is to jot down the number of kicks in twelve hours (you should feel at least ten kicks). Whichever method your practitioner recommends, it is suggested that you per-form this exercise twice a day—once after breakfast and once after dinner.

	SUN	MON	TUES	WED	THUR	FRI	SAT
9 00		✓					✓
9 30	✓						
10 00			✓		✓		
10 30			✓			✓	
11 00	✓			✓			✓
11 30		✓					
12 00				✓			
12 30						✓	
13 00			✓				
13 30							

Figure 7.2: A sample fetal-kick chart

To do the count, lie on your left side and place your hands on your belly. It is a good excuse to put your feet up, something pregnant women probably do not get enough time to do!

Some centers might suggest counting the movements in a twelve-hour period, just in case your baby is having a quiet day. Sometimes in the later part of pregnancy, you may feel a fluttering sensation, which is the baby having a hiccup. Researchers are unsure why babies hiccup, but it is a common phenomenon and seems to be perfectly normal.

Special Concerns

Most physicians will ask you at your prenatal visits about the nature of your baby's movements. You should take this question seriously and try to take note of your baby's activity.

Your baby's movement may depend on his or her position in your uterus. Also, the number of kicks felt varies from one person to another. Some babies seem to be moving all the time, while others are less active. One woman said that with her first pregnancy, she had far fewer kicks than with her second. In general, if you feel three movements in one hour, this is indicative of a healthy baby.

The chart will provide a baseline for your practitioner. If a change is detected from one chart to the next, it might necessitate further testing, such as a nonstress test.

There are many benefits to the fetal-movement test. Studies have shown that this test has a major impact on fetal outcome. Also, the test is not expensive and it is highly reliable, simple, and safe to perform. One disadvantage is that some women tend to panic unnecessarily if they believe that movements are not occurring frequently enough. Remember that babies have patterns of being awake and asleep, just like you do. Some may sleep for long periods of time and may have gentle movements.

Typically, babies are more active at night. Unless you notice a deviation from your baby's normal pattern, it is not necessary to become alarmed. Call your physician or midwife if you have any questions—you owe it to yourself to put your mind at ease.

Monitoring Devices

Today, most women delivering in urban North American hospitals will be exposed to some type of monitoring device. Most hospitals will have you monitored electronically as soon as you are admitted to the maternity unit. There are various types of devices, all with a similar objective of assessing either fetal well-being or uterine contractions. Monitoring can be done both before and during labor.

Typically, there are two types of electronic monitoring devices: external fetal monitors and internal fetal monitors. Both devices send information to a machine that records a tracing of the fetus's heart rate and uterine contractions on graph paper.

The external fetal monitor is used in both low- and high-risk cases to determine the fetus's status and/or to determine how the baby is or will handle the stress of labor. The external electronic fetal monitor is also used in both the fetal nonstress and stress tests. This monitor consists of two small ultrasonic devices strapped around the abdomen; one of them records fetal movements and the other records the muscle tightness of the abdomen or the uterine contractions.

The internal fetal monitor is an option only if your membranes are ruptured and delivery is expected within a few hours. This monitor consists of an electrode (a small clip), inserted vaginally, that attaches to the scalp of the fetus to measure its heart rate. A tube or catheter can be placed in the uterus to measure the strength of the uterine contractions. Although the external fetal monitor is used more often, the internal fetal monitor is more sensitive and can provide important information for a high-risk mother during labor.

The internal monitoring device is used if external monitoring is not providing the desired results, or if there are any questions about fetal well-being.

Both electronic monitoring devices are often used for continuous monitoring during hospitalization, either for high-risk situations, such as premature rupture of membranes, or during your actual labor. If your condition is stable and the fetal heart rate is stable, your monitor may be removed for a while so that you can get up and move around.

Nonstress Test (NST)

The nonstress test (NST) assesses your baby's well-being by observing the baby's heart rate in relation to its movements. The best time to perform this test is after thirty-two weeks. Before this time, the fetal brain is too immature for any changes to be seen in the fetal heart rate. This noninvasive test is performed without medications or anesthesia. It is called a *nonstress test* because no additional stressors are placed on the baby and the uterus, other than the pregnancy itself.

The test involves monitoring the fetal heart rate with a special fetal electronic monitoring device (Doppler) that is located on a belt placed on your abdomen. The monitor is then connected to a machine that resembles a cardiograph machine and provides a printout of the fetal heart rate.

Uses: The nonstress test is usually performed in high-risk situations and in more specific situations, such as:

• Your baby is less active than usual.

• You are having a multiple pregnancy.

- Your baby has been diagnosed with intrauterine growth restriction.

- You have diabetes or high blood pressure.

- You are in a high-risk category for stillbirth.

- You are having premature contractions.

- You are bleeding in the third trimester.

- You are having a prolonged pregnancy.

What to Expect: The nonstress test is performed in the hospital. The nurse will ask you to go to the bathroom and then to lie in bed on your left side. You will be hooked up to two monitors connected to your abdomen. One is an ultrasound Doppler transducer that monitors the baby's movements and heartbeat through sound waves and the other is a tocodynamometer that measures your uterine contractions.

The technician will ask you to push a button each time you feel your baby move, and these movements will also be recorded. At the same time, your baby's heart rate will be graphed on a chart. Babies are usually less active when they are sleeping, so sometimes it takes longer to perform the test. In general, this test usually takes from ten minutes to one hour.

Some women find that these devices restrict their activity because they may need to stay in a certain position to get the best results. Slight movements will show up on the graph, but if they are intermittent, they should not affect the results.

This test is fairly straightforward and safe, and it is not painful or uncomfortable. After the monitor is applied, you will be observed for about twenty minutes or until two to five fetal movements or contractions are felt. If none have occurred, you will be observed for another twenty minutes. If movements are still not felt, you may be given a snack containing glucose, which often results in an active response. At some point, your examiner may choose to stimulate your baby by manipulating your abdomen or ringing a bell to see if there is a response, since fetuses are known to hear sounds from within the uterus. One woman shares this experience:

> "After waiting for what seemed like forever—but was actually only
> an hour—the nurses decided to excite my baby. I laughed when

they walked into my room and dangled a bell over my tummy. I was about six months pregnant, and I think it was the first time I thought of my child as real. It was amazing how quickly my baby responded with kicks. It was within moments of hearing the bell. Of course, I sighed with relief and was sent home because all was well."

Your practitioner will want to know if your baby is testing reactive or nonreactive. Reactive, which is normal, means that the heart rate speeds up when the baby moves. It is normal for there to be two accelerations, each lasting fifteen seconds or more over a twenty-minute period.

Special Concerns: The most difficult aspect of this test is waiting for fetal movement so that the recording can be completed. The best thing to do if the test lasts longer than anticipated is to be patient and to bring along your partner or a friend, or to bring a book or a magazine with you. Babies born within seven days of a reactive NST are usually in good health.

As mentioned earlier, some babies move more than others and some are more sluggish than others. This is not always indicative of a problem. Some specialists might recommend you have a light snack before the test to try to get the baby moving during the test.

The electronic monitor is accurate in assessing well-being; however, it does restrict your activity, and after each major movement the tocotransducers may have to be readjusted on your abdomen.

Contraction Stress Test (CST)

This test, which is seldom done today, has also been called the oxytocin challenge test. It has been performed in high-risk situations to determine how the fetus reacts during uterine contractions. During careful monitoring, oxytocin, a hormone that stimulates uterine contractions, is given intravenously. The amount of oxytocin injected is increased until there are about three contractions in ten minutes (similar to labor). The test takes fifteen to twenty minutes.

Uses: This test helps to determine if the baby can handle the labor process and is used for the same reasons as the nonstress test. It is usually performed after thirty-four weeks.

What to Expect: This test also uses ultrasound, and it is performed in the hospital in a similar way as the nonstress test. You will be told not to eat for at least four to eight hours prior to the test, and just before the test you will be reminded to empty your bladder. You will be given a medication to induce contractions. The practitioners will then monitor your baby's fetal heart rate and your number of contractions. To complete the test, you must have three contractions in ten minutes. Because your baby may have quiet moments, this test often takes a few hours to complete.

Some women claim that this test can be uncomfortable, but it is certainly not as uncomfortable as labor. A negative test indicates that the fetus is in good health; a positive test is indicative that delivery is necessary. The exact management depends on how far advanced you are in your pregnancy.

Special Concerns: This test is usually performed if a nonstress test provides unclear results. The ratio of nonstress tests to stress tests being performed is about a hundred to one.

Sometimes nipple stimulation is performed to stimulate the release of oxytocin from the mother; however, most practitioners agree that it is very difficult to control the contractions this way and in fact, the contractions may become too strong.

Biophysical Profile (BPP)

A biophysical profile (BPP) is a very accurate test that measures the overall fetal well-being, using a scoring system. It can be performed as early as twenty-six weeks, but it is usually done in the last trimester. The profile examines five parameters: fetal heart rate, amount of amniotic fluid, fetal movement, fetal tone, and fetal breathing pattern. The test is now performed for both term and preterm babies.

Uses

This test is frequently performed in high-risk pregnancies. Basically, it relies on an ultrasound and nonstress test to create a profile that provides information such as the amount of amniotic fluid, fetal tone, fetal heart rate, fetal movement, fetal tone, and fetal breathing patterns (see Table 7.2 on the next page).

Table 7.2: Biophysical Profile

Biophysical Attribute	Normal	Abnormal
Breathing	One breathing episode within 30 minutes	No breathing episodes within 30 minutes
Movement	Two or more movements within 30 minutes	Fewer than two movements within 30 minutes
Muscle Tone	One or more episodes of active extension/flexion of limbs, etc. (i.e., opening and closing a hand).	Slow extension/flexion of limbs, partially open fetal hand, etc.
Heart Rate	Two or more episodes of reactive heart rate acceleration within 20 minutes	One or more episodes of unreactive heart rate acceleration
Amniotic Fluid	One or more adequate pockets of fluid	Either no pockets or inadequate pockets of fluid

(Courtesy of American Pregnancy Association, 2006)

What to Expect

Each characteristic is measured on a scale of 0 to 2, with a total of 10 points. If your score is 10 points, it means that your baby is doing perfectly well. Depending on your score, your health-care provider will decide on the next step. Typically, if your test gives you a score that is more than eight and you are past your due date, you might need to have the test repeated once or twice a week. If your BPP is low, the tests will be repeated and you will be monitored closely. If your score is low, it does not necessarily mean that your baby is in distress; it might just mean that you will have to be monitored more closely during the later part of your pregnancy.

There is a small risk of false-positive results with this profile.

Specific Blood Tests

There are a number of blood tests that might be performed later in pregnancy and these include the glucose screen, the glucose tolerance test, and the group B streptococcus (GBS) test.

The Glucose Challenge Test (Glucose Screen)

The glucose challenge test (GCT), or glucose screen test (also known as the glucose-loading test or one-hour glucose test), is a nonfasting test usually performed at about twenty-four to twenty-eight weeks. It tests for gestational diabetes. You will be given a drink containing 50 gm of glucose. One hour later, your blood will be drawn and tested. It is considered abnormal if your blood-sugar level is more than 130. If it is higher than 130, a glucose tolerance test will be performed. Having this test does not mean that you have gestational diabetes, but it will simply confirm your diagnosis of gestational diabetes. It takes about twenty-four hours to obtain the test results.

Glucose Tolerance Test (GTT)

The glucose tolerance test (GTT) is usually performed after an elevated glucose challenge test. Prior to having this test, you must fast for at least eight hours. The primary goal is to diagnose gestational diabetes, a high-risk condition during pregnancy.

The test is a four-step process:

1. You are fasting.
2. Your blood is drawn.
3. You drink a sweet drink (containing 100 grams of glucose).
4. Your blood is drawn every hour for three hours after the drink is finished. You are not allowed to eat during this time. Some women get queasy or nauseated when drinking the glucose mixture because of its high sugar content.

Group B Streptococcus (GBS)

The Centers for Disease Control and Prevention suggests that every pregnant woman between her thirty-fifth and thirty-sixth week be screened for this organism. The test is performed by taking a swab from the mother's vagina and rectum. This swab will detect any potentially harmful bacteria in these areas. Twenty percent of all women of childbearing age harbor these bacteria, and although it is harmless to adults, it can be transmitted to the newborn during delivery.

If babies have skin contact with the bacteria, they can become quite sick, and although this is rare, it does affect about one in a thousand newborns. If the results of the swab are negative, nothing is done. If the results are positive, during labor you will receive intravenous penicillin.

This antibiotic will destroy the bacteria so that the baby cannot get infected. If you are allergic to penicillin, another antibiotic will be given. Ideally, the antibiotic is administered four hours before delivery.

The Ethics of Prenatal Testing

The goal of prenatal testing is to detect any problems early, so that they can be diagnosed and treated. For years, women went through their entire pregnancy without knowing any details about their baby-to-be. Those who delivered special-needs babies after nine months of imagining a perfect baby found the shock to be terribly painful. It seems that there is less psychological damage to the mother if she knows early in her pregnancy that she may have a baby with disabilities.

Despite the advantages, the entire area of prenatal diagnosis remains controversial, since there are a number of ethical questions that arise. First, are all these tests necessary, and who decides if they are? The physician? The woman? Or the community as a whole, through the establishment of universal criteria? Second, what happens if the tests indicate a problem with the fetus? Who decides what to do and what happens if there are differing opinions? The issue of abortion emerges.

Difficulties also may occur if you have different beliefs from your physician and/or your partner. It is important for you to make your wishes known and understood. Remember that it is your body and your baby-to-be. If you are over thirty-five years of age and your physician does not recommend an amniocentesis, it is your right to ask for one. If you feel that your physician has ordered too many ultrasounds, you should discuss this concern with him or her.

Advocates of amniocentesis believe that since the advent of regular prenatal testing there are fewer babies born with serious handicaps. They argue that the woman now has a choice whether she wants to continue her pregnancy or to abort if tests have shown there to be the possibility of a special-needs child. The opponents of excessive testing argue that the world has gotten along well for countless generations without all of this testing and that because many of these tests are new, their long-term effects have yet to be determined.

For some women, it may be difficult to decide whether to have prenatal diagnostic tests. Others undergo testing without thinking twice when they consider that the health of their baby is at stake. The best advice is to be as informed as possible so you can make educated decisions. It is important that you speak to your practitioner about how he or she will use the results obtained from the test. If the results will not be used in a way to help both the mother and the child, it might be unnecessary to perform them in the first place.

Be sure that you understand the reasons for your test and its possible advantages, disadvantages, and risks. Knowledge means confidence, and confidence helps you make the correct decision. If you want additional information, make sure to ask your provider where to obtain it.

Journaling Corner

What was your reaction when you saw your baby on ultrasound for the first time?

If this is not your first child, compare the testing in this pregnancy to your previous ones.

Write about your expectations and fears about becoming a mother. How do you feel about becoming a mother?

Does your physician explain the tests and the results in a way that you can understand?

Have you had any surprises you want to write about?

Bed Rest

Having a baby is like taking
your bottom lip and pulling
it over your head. —Carol Burnett

About one in five women are prescribed some sort of bed rest during their pregnancy. In some cases, bed rest may be suggested as a preliminary treatment until the source of your problem is identified. It may also be used as an extended final treatment to prevent premature labor after other treatments have been unsuccessful. *Bed rest* is a general term used when limited activity is advised for your fetus's well-being. There are many types of bed rest and they each mean different things to different practitioners. It is important that you understand exactly what yours means. Bed rest is often accomplished at home, but in some instances hospitalization may be necessary.

Below are the most common types of bed rest prescribed, but be aware that, depending on your condition, your practitioner might custom-design your protocol.

Types of Bed Rest

Bed rest is a common recommendation during high-risk pregnancies. Although the idea of bed rest remains controversial amongst practitioners, it is still widely recommended for a variety of reasons. Women may be placed on brief or extended periods of bed rest. Your bed-rest experience will be highly individualized and will depend upon the reason for your bed rest and the type of bed rest that is prescribed for you. Below is a list of the most commonly suggested types of bed rest.

Scheduled Bed Rest: This type of bed rest is usually prescribed during the third trimester to avoid the more intense types of bed rest. It is commonly suggested for older moms or those bearing multiple pregnancies. You may be told to rest for a certain amount of time each day, to shorten your work day, or to limit exertions such as climbing stairs, walking, or standing for extended periods of time each day.

Modified or Partial Bed Rest: This type of bed rest means spending part of the day in bed or lying down and resting. The range of hours your provider prescribes for you to be in bed may vary from a couple of hours to a large part of the day. Most often women prescribed this type of bed rest are prohibited from working, driving, climbing stairs, house cleaning, sexual intercourse, exercise, and any type of lifting. Often, you will be able to sit at a desk and work for a short period of time, but your time will generally be divided between lying down and sitting, depending on your practitioner's guidelines.

Strict Bed Rest: This type of bed rest is exactly what it sounds like! It means that you must be in bed all day, and if you are lucky, you will be granted bathroom and shower privileges. Some practitioners may recommend using a bedpan. In some cases, you may be allowed to sit and eat, while at other times you will be required to recline all day long. If you have stairs in your home, you will probably have to decide where to spend your time. Some practitioners might allow you to make the round-trip once a day. During my pregnancy, I was allowed this privilege and I chose to go downstairs for lunch because I found it broke up my day, plus I could go to the door to greet the mailman, which in a funny way was the highlight of my day. Your provider may also recommend "pelvic rest." This means that you should not use tampons, douche, or have intercourse.

What to Ask Your Doctor about Bed Rest

- Is it okay to drive?
- How much walking is safe?
- Can I get up to use the bathroom?
- Can I take a bath or shower?
- Can I get up to prepare quick meals or to do light chores?
- What position should I maintain while in bed?
- Can I go to work or work from home?
- How much and what kind of sexual activity is okay?
- What activities or exercises do you suggest?

Complete or Hospital Bed Rest: This is the most serious type of bed rest and it means that your pregnancy is so high-risk that you will require twenty-four–hour monitoring. You will have to use a bedpan, and your hygienic care will also be attended in bed by the hospital staff. Women prescribed this type of bed rest have usually gone into preterm labor and need an intravenous infusion of medications to slow down their contractions. Women with a bleeding placenta previa may also be prescribed this type of bed rest. In some instances, the hospital staff may elevate your feet higher than your head (Trendelenburg position) to minimize the stress on both your cervix and your baby.

The following are some common situations in which bed rest may be prescribed for you.

Bleeding

Bleeding during the second or third trimester is usually due to a problem with the placenta, such as cervical erosion, placenta previa, and abruptio placenta. Bed rest may be recommended to minimize the bleeding, and sometimes a stay in the hospital is advised until the bleeding subsides. A relaxing and calming environment augments the effects of bed rest. Studies have shown that increased activity, and even sensory stimulation, may actually increase bleeding. Sometimes the best place to rest is in the hospital.

Heart Disease

Women with a history of cardiac disease may be advised to minimize their activity and/or maintain bed rest, especially in the latter three months of pregnancy, when the strain on the heart is the greatest. If you have heart disease, it will be worth investing in well-fitting support hosiery, which help massage your legs and improve blood flow from the legs back to the heart. Many women claim that this hosiery is very comfortable and makes them feel stronger when on their feet. During the winter months, this hosiery provides warmth. Today, support hosiery comes in attractive colors and styles.

Hypertension and Preeclampsia

Hypertension and preeclampsia are two diagnoses that are often added to other problems associated with high-risk pregnancy. They are also two situations where bed rest may be considered as adjunct therapy to other recommendations. In this case, bed rest decreases blood pressure, ankle swelling, and protein in the urine. It also increases oxygen and nutrient supply to your baby. Again, the left side–lying position may help to lower blood pressure, because it decreases pressure on the inferior vena cava—the large blood vessel in the back that brings blood back to the heart for oxygenation—and improves blood circulation and urine output.

Pregnant women often feel more tired and find themselves benefiting from a few nap periods each day. Women who are at high-risk for developing elevated blood pressure during pregnancy really benefit from this extra rest. It is a good idea to have eight to twelve hours of sleep with two nap periods during the day. This may be difficult to manage, especially if you have younger children at home, but you should do your best. It may be a good time for your children to learn that there are some things they can do for themselves.

For mild preeclampsia, either bed rest or limited activity is usually advised. In some cases, your physician may choose to admit you to the hospital for close observation. Sometimes women actually request hospitalization, especially if there are other children at home and it is difficult to get adequate rest in the home environment. In most cases, resting is enough to reduce elevated blood pressure.

Intrauterine Growth Restriction (IUGR)

When your baby's growth lags behind what it should be for his or her age, your physician might recommend bed rest. This may involve a reduction in your activity and when in bed, lying on your side. A baby that is small for his or her age is usually associated with a small placenta. Bed rest may increase the blood flow to the placenta, thus helping the baby to grow properly and increase the chance of having a normal delivery.

Multiple Pregnancy

Bed rest for the mother facing a multiple pregnancy is a common recommendation, although when it should start and finish is a personal decision made by the practitioner and the woman. The left side–lying position is recommended. Some believe that short naps in the morning and afternoon are sufficient, while others might advise modified bed rest to prevent premature labor. Some studies show that bed rest should begin prior to the critical period of twenty-seven weeks and continue until thirty-four weeks. Often, bed rest is discontinued when tests show that the fetal lungs are mature enough to sustain life on their own.

Premature or Preterm Labor

You should call your provider if you have any of the signs of preterm labor (see Table 8.1). He or she might tell you to rest for an hour and then call back. You might also be told to drink a few glasses of fluids and in some instances you might be told to come into the office.

Table 8.1: Signs of Preterm Labor

Symptom	Feels Like
Abdominal contractions	A tightening fist every 10 minutes or more
Vaginal discharge	Clear or bloody discharge
Cramping	Menstrual period
Low back pain	Dull aching
Pelvic pressure	Baby moving downward

If your physician establishes that you are in premature labor, bed rest will probably be prescribed, particularly if it is prior to your thirty-fourth week of pregnancy. You will probably be advised to lie on your left side, as lying on your back tends to increase uterine contractions and reduce blood flow to the placenta. Those of you who have been pregnant before know about pregnancy-related back problems; lying on your side may help you to avoid this complication. The side-lying position may decrease the chances of the cervix dilating and effacing. If you are on bed rest for premature labor, your treatment will probably also include medications to decrease contractions.

Preterm Premature Rupture of Membranes (PPROM)

When the membranes rupture prematurely, there is a gush or dribble of fluid from your vagina. This condition demands careful attention. If this happens to you, the first recommendation is to maintain complete bed rest in order to prevent excessive drainage of amniotic fluid. After about twelve to twenty-four hours, your physician may allow you to walk to the bathroom rather than using a bedpan. Most women who have premature rupture of the membranes are hospitalized until delivery; however, if you are sent home, you may be instructed to stay quiet and to avoid engaging in too much activity. You should clarify this recommendation with your physician, but do yourself and your baby a favor—take it easy!

After the membranes have ruptured, it is very important to avoid any chance of infection; therefore, intercourse is not recommended. You should only take showers and not baths, and monitor your temperature in the morning and evening. If you find that it is over 104°F, notify your physician as soon as possible. With these safety measures, chances are that you will successfully carry your baby without problems.

Threatened Miscarriage

If your pregnancy is threatened, you will most likely experience some bleeding, and if your physician believes that you are at risk of miscarrying, bed rest may be prescribed. If you have a blighted ovum (see Chapter 9), you will miscarry whether or not you are on bed rest. The loss will be due to a malformed embryo and not to the level of your activity. If the embryo is viable, it is hoped that bed rest will optimize its internal environment and minimize your uterine contractions. The length of bed rest depends on you as an individual, your physician, and how you feel. Bed rest is sometimes recommended until the bleeding has subsided. Others may recommend bed rest until the end of the first trimester. Remember that your participation in the decision is very important, and you should discuss any of your concerns or questions with your practitioner.

Women with a history of cervical insufficiency may be advised to go on bed rest following the surgical placement of a small suture on the cervix (cervical cerclage), in order to avoid any strain on the cervix and the temporary suture. If you are on bed rest for this reason, your physician may prescribe medications to avoid contractions and to decrease the risk of premature labor. These medications are discussed later in this chapter.

Coping with Bed Rest

Bed rest is not fun at the best of times, nor is it an absolute cure for any high-risk problem. Even though the idea of bed rest might initially sound welcoming and seem to present you with time to catch up on your reading, after a while you will find it to be an exhausting experience. Because you are not using your muscles, you may tire more easily or might become sore in some areas of your body. Also, because you have significantly reduced your activity level, you are at great risk of developing blood clots in your legs. Depending on your level of bed rest, it might be a good idea to wear compression stockings to keep your circulation moving as much as possible while you are immobile.

In addition to being fearful for your baby's life and the outcome of pregnancy, one of the most difficult aspects of going on bed rest is giving up control of managing the home and family. Sometimes it is aggravating to watch other people do tasks differently from how you would do them. The healthiest thing to do is to let go and pass on the responsibility, reminding yourself that the situation is a temporary one.

Many women are filled with guilt, resentment, and anger about having to put everything aside and put their lives on hold for a few months. You might feel as though your emotions are constantly in flux, and often this is connected to feelings of helplessness and being pulled out of your normal routine.

The emotional adjustment to bed rest may be very difficult, especially if you have always led an active life, working full-time at home or at a career. Becoming dependent when you are used to being independent is never easy, and you may find that the smaller things in life, like phone calls and visits, will become the highlights of your day!

Other Children: If you have other children at home, it may be difficult for them to understand your inactivity. When I was on bed rest with my second pregnancy, my two-year-old, who enjoyed being held, could not understand why I was no longer able to lift her. She was deeply hurt, feeling that I did not love her anymore, and she had great difficulty coping. She used various types of attention-seeking behaviors to test my love for her. I made a point of sitting on the floor with her and hugging her. This meant a lot to her—as most parents will agree, there can never be enough hugging.

Another woman with an older child shares her sentiments:

> "Joan was seven years old when I was told I would have to be on bed rest with my second child. Somehow it wasn't much of a problem,

because she was already well-established in school and the school bus picked her up and dropped her off each day. As a matter of fact, I think she liked having me on bed rest because it was probably the only time, both before and after the pregnancy, that she knew where to find me. I was simply always in bed and there when she needed me."

A good book for kids between the ages of four and eight is *Mommy Has to Stay in Bed*, by Annette Rivlin-Gutman.

Support Systems: Your partner will also feel burdened with more responsibilities and may feel intense pressure at times. Many women sense feelings of resentment from their partners. It is normal for him to occasionally lose patience with you. Try to be patient and loving and keep the communication channels open.

My husband was very strong during my pregnancies, offering ongoing love and respect. Understandably, there were days when the tension got to him because for him it was also a time when he was beginning a new business and so he had pressure from all sides. I often wondered if I would have been as intensely patient and loving as he was.

Adequate support systems are important during this time. If you are able, you should seek home-care help to assist both you and your family. People who will clean and do the shopping are invaluable. A list of students who can run errands may be helpful if you live in a school community. Remember that even though you are on bed rest, you can continue to manage your household.

Keeping Busy: Keeping busy is often difficult for the bedridden mother-to-be. Try to contact other mothers who have been on bed rest and ask how they spent their time. This will boost your confidence and provide you with guidance. Inquire about home manicures, massages, hairstyling, and other pampering and relaxing activities. This is a good time to catch up on reading, knitting, sewing, writing, and other activities that you used to say you never had time for. Also, some women can do light upper-body work with weights; however, it is a good idea to first check with your health-care provider.

Mental Health and Bed Rest: There are many things you can do to maintain a good state of mind during your bed-rest experience. The first recommendation is that each morning you still get dressed, because this makes you feel "less sick." I did this and it did wonders for me. In addition, mental rest is as important as physical rest for the high-risk mother. One way to support your mental balance is by listening to calming music, which will have a positive effect on both you and your baby. Your environment should be relaxing, with quiet diversional activities. And remember you are in bed not because you are sick but because you are maintaining your health and awaiting the birth of your child.

It is helpful for some women to practice stress relief activities such as meditation and visualizing. Not only does this help you cope, but visualization exercises can connect women with their new baby. According to Dr. Joel Evans in his book, *The Whole Pregnancy Handbook* (2005), one way to start is to dedicate five to fifteen minutes each day to visualizing your healthy baby surrounded by water and warm light, safely tucked into your womb. He goes on to explain that you could imagine the placenta and umbilical cord, the physical connection between the two of you and the pulsing cord connecting you. This entire image should fill you with love and joy and bring lots of positive energy into your life.

If you find bed rest emotionally overwhelming, you might want to mention it to your practitioner, as he or she might be able to recommend a mental-health professional for you to talk to. You also might want to connect with support groups in your area or a group specializing in your type of difficult pregnancy complication. (See Appendixes B and C.) Below are some exercises you may be able to do while on bed rest. However, it is important that you first check with your provider before engaging in any of these exercises.

Passive Exercises for Bed Rest

Modest activity during bed rest can help to minimize stiffness, improve circulation, and promote relaxation. Before taking part in any exercise regime, be sure to check with your health-care provider. If he or she agrees, try incorporating passive exercises into your daily routine. Typically, these are done with another person's assistance. You can, however, do some of the exercises described below on your own, such as abdominal breathing and Kegel exercises, but you should ask your partner or another adult to help you with the others.

Kegel Exercises: Lie on your back or sit up. Tighten your pelvic floor muscles (as if stopping your urine). Hold for three counts, then relax.

Abdominal Breathing: Lie on your back with two pillows behind your shoulders and with your knees bent. Breathe in deeply, letting your abdominal wall rise. Exhale slowly through your mouth as you tighten your stomach muscles.

Bridging: Lie on your back with two pillows behind your shoulders and with your knees bent. Raise your hips off the bed while keeping your shoulders down.

Leg Sliding: Lie on your back with two pillows behind your shoulders and with your knees bent. Slide your legs out, slowly straightening your knees against the bed. Slowly pull both knees back up.

Modified Leg Raises: Lie on your back with two pillows under your head and bend one knee. Bend the other knee up toward your chest, then straighten your leg by kicking upward toward the ceiling, and then lower your leg to the bed. Repeat with the other leg.

Abduction: Lie on your back with two pillows underneath your head and bend your knees. Let your knees come apart, and then squeeze them back together.

Ankle Circles: Lift your ankles up and down. Rest your right ankle on your left knee and rotate the ankle circularly in both directions. Repeat with the left ankle on the right knee.

Arm Lifts: Exhale deeply through your nose as you lift one arm up to the side over your head. The sides of your chest should expand. Exhale as you bring your arm down. Repeat with the opposite arm.

Some Things to Do for a Mom on Bed Rest

- Bring her a pint of ice cream.
- Fluff up her pillows.
- Lend her books about childrearing.
- Change the sheets on her bed.
- Call her on the phone…often.

Some Things to Do for a Mom on Bed Rest (cont'd.)

- Send her a card for no reason
- Bring her a flower from your garden.
- Bring her old magazines.
- Do her laundry or fold clothes while you visit.
- Bring her some scented lotion or shower gel.
- Give her a pedicure and paint her toenails.
- Bring her some chap stick and breath mints.
- Visit her at home or in the hospital (but make it short).
- Buy her the latest book on the best-seller list.
- Take her a bottle of flavored sparkling water.
- Bring her take-out food from her favorite restaurant.
- Shave her legs and rub on heavy cream.
- Remind her of the wonderful thing that she is doing.

(Courtesy of Sidelines National Support Network)

Recovering from Bed Rest

How to cope with the aftereffects of the bed rest experience following the birth of your baby depends to a large extent on the nature of your bed rest and what physical condition you were in prior to going on bed rest. As a result of your inactivity, many of your muscle groups will be weakened and they will need time to rebuild themselves. The rest of your body also needs time to heal. You might notice changes in your strength and energy. It is important to be patient and give yourself time to recover. Your physical recovery might be slow and sometimes physical therapy or an exercise program may be prescribed to help you get back into your routine. It is critical not to get overtired and to maintain a healthy attitude.

Journaling Corner

How do you feel about the bed-rest experience?

How are you keeping busy?

How does your family handle your being on bed rest?

How has your appetite and activity level changed while on bed rest?

Are you taking any special medications, like something to prevent early labor?

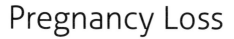

Pregnancy Loss

*I believe that imagination is stronger than knowledge—
myth is more potent than history—dreams are more
powerful than facts—hope always triumphs over
experience—laughter is the cure for grief—love is
stronger than death.* — ROBERT FULGHUM

The five most common types of loss during pregnancy and
immediately afterward include abortion, miscarriage, stillbirth, neonatal
death, and sudden infant death syndrome (SIDS).

Elective Abortion

An elective abortion is an option for an unwanted pregnancy, and it is
also a decision some couples make when a fetal abnormality has been
detected. Women who might opt for an elective abortion include those
who have a medical problem; those who have contracted rubella (German measles) early in pregnancy; those exposed to environmental hazards such as radiation, toxic chemicals, or certain medications; and those
carrying a baby with a genetic disorder or structural abnormality.

The Decision

Most of the tests that indicate a fetus has an abnormality are performed
during the fourth month, and in many cases this is after a woman has begun to feel her baby move. It may be difficult to make the decision to terminate a pregnancy once this sign of life has been felt. Deciding the fate
of a fetus is a huge responsibility.

Couples choose prenatal tests for a variety of reasons. Some choose
them for reassurance (about 98 percent of the results are normal), while
others choose them if they suspect a fetal problem. Some couples choose
not to have the tests because they have no intention of having an abortion, even if a severe abnormality were detected. Other couples are quite
sure that they would be unable to devote their lives to raising a child with

severe disabilities. Others use the knowledge gained from these tests to help them prepare for a child who may require specialized care. Those who are less sure of what they would do in such a situation are the ones who find the decision-making process most difficult of all.

If a test detects a fetal abnormality, your physician will meet with you, accompanied by a genetic counselor. All of the options should be discussed. Remember that these professionals will not make your decision for you, but they may offer you perspectives that will hopefully help you come to your own terms with the situation.

Your options might include repairing a fetal anomaly. If this option is not possible or if you decide you do not want to go that route, the details about terminating your pregnancy will be discussed. The type of elective abortion depends on the stage of your pregnancy.

Options

There are two ways to terminate a pregnancy, both of which are typically performed prior to the twentieth week of gestation. They are a D&C, or a D&E, and often their difference is purely semantic. Often times, the term D&C refers to a procedure performed on the nonpregnant woman or for those early in pregnancy if the cervix is already dilated or the fetus is not viable. A D&E is a term typically referring to an elective termination done during pregnancy.

Less Than Fourteen Weeks: If your pregnancy is less than fourteen weeks, you will typically have a simple D&E (dilation and evacuation) under either local or general anesthesia. This procedure involves dilation, suction, and evacuation of the uterine contents. If this has not already been performed, your physician should discuss the option of having chromosomal testing. An alternative for women less than seven weeks pregnant is to take the oral abortion pill (RU-486), which is also known as mifepristone. It is 95 percent effective in initiating abortion without the need for a D&E. In about 5 percent of women, a D&E might be necessary because of excessive bleeding.

Fourteen to Eighteen Weeks: If your pregnancy is between fourteen and eighteen weeks, a D&E will also be performed, but the preparation for the procedure is slightly different than that discussed above. A day before the procedure, you will be admitted into the hospital to have one or more laminaria sticks (seaweed rods) inserted into your cervical opening. Over the course of the next twenty-four hours, these expand to three to four times their original size and gently dilate your cervix. This makes the procedure to evacuate the fetus safer and less complicated. The use of the seaweed rods also eliminates future problems, such as injury to the cervix and cervical insufficiency in future pregnancies. On the day of your procedure, you may also be given an oral medication called misoprostol (prostaglandin E1). This helps to prepare the cervix and also helps to minimize the risks from the procedure.

Eighteen to Twenty-Four Weeks: If your pregnancy is between eighteen and twenty-four weeks, the suggested type of termination varies. Some practitioners recommend that your labor be induced with misoprostol, so that you may deliver the baby vaginally. Other providers may suggest a late D&E. This latter procedure requires more diligence and experience to perform.

In either case, you will receive laminaria sticks one to two days prior to the procedure to help open the cervix. Most providers will encourage you to have an amniocentesis with an injection of potassium chloride to stop the fetal heart prior to having the laminaria sticks inserted. Doing this ensures that the baby is not born alive and makes the procedure much less stressful for the couple, physician, and nursing staff. On the day of the procedure, you will also be given an oral dose of misoprostol.

Your provider will also discuss the option of genetic testing and a possible autopsy to confirm the fetus's anomalies. Burial options should also be discussed.

More Than Twenty-Four Weeks: In most states, it is not legal for you to have an abortion after twenty-four weeks. If you live in a state where it is illegal and you decide this is the route you want to take, you might consider traveling to a state where abortion could be performed legally under special circumstances.

What to Expect

The details of your procedure should be explained in detail, and you will be asked to sign a consent form. You will then be given a bimanual exam during which your practitioner can feel the size of your uterus and determine the stage of your pregnancy. Then a speculum will be inserted into your vagina. You may feel some pressure, but this should not hurt. Your vagina will be cleaned to prevent infection and a local anesthetic will be injected into the cervix. Since the cervix has only a few nerve endings, you may only feel a pinch. An instrument will be inserted to keep the cervix steady, and the cervical opening will be gradually stretched. You may feel some mild cramping, similar to menstrual cramps. A strawlike tube, or cannula, is inserted through the cervix and connected to a bottle, which is connected to a vacuum pump. A gentle suction will remove the pregnancy tissue. The aspiration takes only a few minutes, depending on the stage of your pregnancy. You may feel some cramping, which should subside shortly after the cannula is removed.

Before you leave the hospital or surgical center, you may feel weak, tired, and nauseated for a while. Your provider will give you instructions on what symptoms to watch out for, such as increased bleeding or abdominal cramping.

Having an abortion does not decrease the chance of having a healthy baby in the future. Some studies have indicated that repeated abortions may slightly increase the chances of miscarriage and premature birth because repeated dilations of the cervix may, in some women, weaken the cervix.

Your Emotions

Positive, negative, and mixed emotions are all common following an elective abortion. For some, the procedure may provide relief of an unwanted pregnancy. You and your partner will probably feel that it is the right decision for you at this time. Knowing this, however, does not give immunity from the emotional impact of your experience. Feelings of guilt are common and may be reinforced by the discomfort you feel after the actual procedure. You may wonder once again if you made the right decision, what the child may have looked like, and the effect the child might have had on your life. These questions must remain unanswered, but the most difficult and the most important question has been answered and you should have the confidence to agree that it was the right decision.

Recovering from an abortion is not easy. As Rayna Rapp said in a *Ms.* article entitled "The Ethics of Choice":

> "Recovering from the abortion took a long time. Friends, family, co-workers, and students did everything they could to ease me through the experience. Even so, I yearned to talk with someone who'd 'been there.' Over the next few months, I used my personal and medical networks to locate and talk with a handful of other women who'd opted for selective abortions. In each case, I was the first person they ever met with a similar experience. The isolation of this decision and its consequences is intense. Only when women (and concerned men) speak of the experience of selective abortion as tragic but chosen fetal death can we as a community offer support, sort out the ethics, and give the compassionate attention that such a loss entails."

Miscarriage

A miscarriage is sometimes called a "spontaneous abortion," and it occurs when a pregnancy ends naturally prior to the twentieth week of gestation. An "early" miscarriage occurs prior to twelve weeks, while a "late" miscarriage occurs between the twelfth and twentieth week. Nearly 20 to 25 percent of all pregnancies result in miscarriage, most often during the first three months of pregnancy, making it the most common type of pregnancy loss. Many miscarriages are not even recognized because they happen so early.

Many women also prefer not to talk about their miscarriage because of its personal nature and the accompanying feelings of failure and loss. For them, this can be a lonely time. Other women say that they never realized how many women have miscarriages until they started speaking to others about it. As one woman says:

> "After I miscarried, it seemed as if everyone I spoke to either had experienced a miscarriage or knew someone who had. It was unbelievable. It certainly helped me feel less alone, knowing that other women knew what I was going through. It didn't take the pain away, but it certainly facilitated the grieving process."

Without question, miscarriage has a strong emotional and physical impact on a woman. How she copes with this tragedy will depend on how she has coped with other traumas in her life. Even for the strongest person, the loss of a baby is psychologically and emotionally very difficult. Both partners feel the impact deeply. Those who have never experienced a miscarriage often do not see it as the death of a baby, and they may regard it as a rather common occurrence. Thus, the grief a couple feels is often downplayed by others who do not understand what they are going through.

There are many causes of miscarriage. The exact cause is usually difficult to establish unless you have a structural abnormality in the reproductive system that is well documented through tests, such as the hysterosalpingogram, or have had an infection that was not adequately treated.

What Happens?

Not all women have warnings before their miscarriage. The earliest sign is vaginal bleeding, ranging from a heavy flow to a few drops every few hours, during the first three months of pregnancy. The spotting is initially dark, as progesterone and estrogen levels decrease, causing the endometrium to slough. The blood color may then turn to pink or bright red, as the blood vessels open and the products of conception begin to separate. One woman remarks:

> "It was the most unusual thing. We were sitting down to have a quiet supper one evening, when I was exactly three months pregnant. Suddenly I experienced abdominal cramping as if I had suffered some form of food poisoning. I immediately went to the bathroom and was lucky I did, because right there I began losing what seemed like an enormous amount of blood. I sat on the toilet and could feel the fetal products leaving me, forever. We went right to the hospital and I had a D&C. It all happened so quickly."

Another woman recalls the following experience:

> "I denied everything that was happening to me. I spotted on and off during the first three months. I vividly remember one day at work when I spotted more than usual. I called my obstetrician and he advised me to go home immediately. He suggested that it may or may not be serious but advised bed rest until the bleeding stopped. It took about three days for the bleeding to stop, and since the third

day landed on a Friday, I decided to also spend the weekend in bed—just to ensure that all was well.

"Everything was fine for the weekend and I returned to work on Monday. I saw my obstetrician on Tuesday for a checkup and all was well. Thursday night I was having intense abdominal cramps accompanied by heavy bleeding and went immediately to the emergency room. I lost my baby in the hospital. It was the most traumatic experience in my life."

Cramping and vaginal bleeding during pregnancy sometimes indicate that a miscarriage is occurring, and whenever possible you should save all tissue and products that you pass. If it is during your physician's office hours, bring them there, if not, bring them to your local hospital's emergency room. When the physician sees you, you will probably have an examination with a speculum to try to determine the source of your bleeding. You may also have an ultrasound. If you do miscarry, your breasts may also begin to feel less tender and less full. After the miscarriage has occurred, some physicians recommend certain blood tests or even an endometrial biopsy. The blood sample will be analyzed for various hormonal levels, which may provide a clue as to the cause of your miscarriage.

Types of Miscarriages

There are several types of miscarriages, some of which require more medical attention than others.

Threatened Miscarriage

A threatened miscarriage refers to any bleeding or spotting in early pregnancy, which may or may not be associated with cramping or back discomfort, indicating that a miscarriage may occur. If you are having a threatened miscarriage, you might bleed while your cervix remains closed and the pregnancy is still healthy inside your uterus. The physician cannot predict if your pregnancy will survive or if it will end. Your physician will tell you to either come to his or her office or to go to the hospital. At that time, your blood will be drawn to establish your blood type. If you are Rh-negative, anti-D immunoglobulin (Rh[D]) will be given.

Waiting to see if your pregnancy will survive will be an uneasy time, because you do not know whether to plan for your baby or not. Everything seems to be up in the air. Your physician will probably recommend restricted activity, bed rest, avoidance of douching and tampons, and abstinence from intercourse for anywhere from a few days to two weeks after bleeding begins.

Inevitable Miscarriage

A threatened miscarriage is similar to an inevitable miscarriage, except that in the latter instance the cervix is open, and therefore a miscarriage is inevitable. Symptoms include bleeding and pain that may be cramp-like at the beginning and then become more intense. Your physician will probably recommend bed rest for forty-eight hours. If bleeding continues and/or fever develops, a D&C will most likely be performed.

Here is one woman's experience with her inevitable miscarriage:

"I vividly remember just having finished the first trimester. It was my second pregnancy, and for me the first three months is always the worst time. I am one of those people who gets extremely nauseated and feels faint half of the time. I saw my obstetrician at about twelve weeks and she was unable to find a fetal heart rate. She recommended having an ultrasound, but I felt it was too early to start with tests. The following week I started bleeding and visited my obstetrician again, and that's when we decided to do an ultrasound. I was shocked—the report showed that there was no fetus. As hard as it was, I went home, only to return a few weeks later to have a D&C."

Complete Miscarriage/Spontaneous Abortion

A complete miscarriage means that you miscarry, your cervix closes, and you return to your normal lifestyle. The products of conception may pass on their own or be reabsorbed into your body. In other words, the miscarriage occurred by itself and there is nothing that needs to be done. These types of miscarriages generally occur before the twelfth week of pregnancy. You should arrange for a follow-up appointment with your physician, which should include blood work and an ultrasound to make sure that you had a complete miscarriage.

Missed Miscarriage/Abortion

A missed miscarriage is an unpleasant circumstance in which the first few weeks of pregnancy progress normally, and then the fetus dies and remains in the uterus. Some women may have intermittent vaginal bleeding or a brownish discharge.

Other symptoms include an obvious decline in uterine growth and a lack of fetal development. Your breasts also return to their normal size. Eventually, the fetus aborts. If it does not, you may develop serious blood abnormalities and a D&C may be necessary. It is best to have a D&C as soon as it is established that the fetus has died. The longer you wait, the greater your chances of getting a uterine infection or a condition called disseminated intravascular coagulation (DIC), a serious bleeding problem. It is also better for you to terminate your relationship with your fetus, because it can be very draining, psychologically, to carry a dead fetus.

If you had a missed miscarriage that occurred early enough in pregnancy, you might be offered a medication called misoprostol, given orally, vaginally, or rectally. Misoprostol brings on an abortion so that a D&C will not be necessary.

Recurrent Miscarriages

If you have had recurrent miscarriages or three or more unexplained miscarriages in the first trimester, your physician may call you a "habitual aborter." This may indicate a hidden problem of either fetal, genetic, or maternal origin. About 70 to 80 percent of these women will go on to have normal subsequent pregnancies, even without practitioner intervention. Some possible causes of recurrent miscarriages include structural abnormalities of the uterus (i.e., cervical insufficiency), genetic problems in either parent, maternal health problems (i.e., thyroid), antiphospholipid disorder (autoimmune problem where antibodies attack healthy cells), and hormonal imbalances. The idea that an imbalance of hormones causes recurrent miscarriage remains controversial.

If you have had more than one miscarriage after sixteen weeks of pregnancy, your physician will probably suspect cervical insufficiency. If a chromosomal disorder is suspected, you and your partner may need to be evaluated genetically. If a hormonal imbalance seems to be your problem, your physician may recommend hormonal suppositories, such as progesterone, which are usually started at the time of ovulation and continue until the twelfth to fourteenth week of gestation (other physicians may begin it as soon as you have a positive pregnancy test). Some may choose to give progesterone or hCG injections at the first sign of bleeding and once more two weeks later.

Causes of Miscarriage

There are several causes for miscarriage; and some of the best-understood ones are discussed below.

Chromosomal Abnormalities

About 85 percent of miscarriages are due to a genetic disorder in the makeup of the egg that causes the fetus to develop improperly. When this occurs, the embryo disintegrates or is absorbed by the surrounding tissue early in pregnancy. The empty gestational sac is then expelled with the other products of pregnancy (amniotic sac, placenta, and amniotic fluid).

Over 60 percent of early pregnancy losses are a result of the products of the embryo having an extra chromosome or an extra set of chromosomes. The development of an embryo with abnormal chromosomes is most often an accident of that particular pregnancy, but in a small proportion of these instances the condition is inherited.

This cause of miscarriage is diagnosed by analyzing the embryonic tissue that the woman passed or what was extracted during a D&C.

Structural Abnormalities in the Female Reproductive System

Structural abnormalities in the female reproductive system are seen in about one in seven hundred women. Having a congenital abnormality does not mean that you cannot bear children, but it may increase your chances of having a miscarriage or a preterm delivery. Malformations may have occurred during your own fetal development that have gone unnoticed until you try to have a baby. The malformations may be detected before your pregnancy, but they are usually discovered only when investigative tests are performed after multiple miscarriages. If your physician suspects a malformation in your reproductive system, he or she may order a hysterosalpingogram (HSG). This test involves injecting a dye into the uterus through the vagina so that your reproductive system is highlighted when an X ray is taken. The dye outlines the uterine cavity and fallopian tubes so that abnormalities can be easily seen by the specialist.

Anatomical malformations that may trigger a miscarriage include a septate uterus/bicornuate uterus, a congenital abnormality where the uterus is partitioned in two, with one cervix; a double uterus with two cervixes; cervical insufficiency; and uterine fibroids. If you have cervical insufficiency, you may experience a painless miscarriage between the sixteenth and twentieth weeks of your pregnancy. A woman with a septate uterus will have a miscarriage associated with discomfort. (These conditions are discussed in detail below.) Yet another structural cause of miscarriage is Asherman's syndrome, characterized by scar tissue inside the uterus resulting from overly vigorous D&Cs or from an infection following an abortion.

Bacterial and Viral Infections

Infections such as rubella or German measles, active herpes simplex, chlamydia, and cytomegalovirus may affect fetal development and result in miscarriage. At the beginning of your pregnancy, you will probably have a test for rubella. However, if you are not immune to German measles and are considering pregnancy, it is a good idea to get vaccinated and then wait one to three months before trying to conceive.

Pregnant women are prone to vaginal infections. If you are pregnant and have a vaginal infection, it is important to have it treated promptly, because the effects on the fetus are still unknown. Treatments with suppositories and creams are usually successful. Signs of vaginal infection include genital itching, unusual vaginal odor or discharge, and discomfort or a burning feeling during urination.

Maternal Diseases

Diabetes, hypertension, thyroid imbalance, sickle-cell anemia, and autoimmune disorders, if not adequately controlled, may result in the loss of a fetus. These conditions will be discussed in further detail in the latter part of this chapter.

Women with systemic lupus erythematosus, an autoimmune disease, have an increased incidence of miscarriage, especially if the disease is not in remission. Some women's bodies may respond to the new fetus as a foreign object and reject it. One woman who had six miscarriages before it was learned that she had lupus says:

> "I'm glad we decided to start having a family soon after we got married, because only after six miscarriages and one stillbirth did doctors realize what was wrong with me. Autopsies showed that my placenta was completely disintegrated. Finally, my obstetrician prescribed prednisone early in pregnancy to prevent my placenta from disintegrating. It was a long time coming, but it was worth every minute, as I am enjoying my five-year-old daughter so much."

Hormonal Imbalances

Hormonal imbalances may be another cause of miscarriage, although some authorities admit that there is a great deal of uncertainty about the relationship between hormonal imbalances and miscarriages. Some sources believe that inadequate progesterone production, also known as corpus luteum deficiency, may result in early miscarriage. The corpus luteum is the empty follicle in the ovary that has released the egg. If conception occurs, it serves as a temporary endocrine gland that secretes progesterone, the hormone that thickens the lining of the uterus in preparation for the egg's implantation and prevents menstruation. When progesterone levels are too low, the egg has difficulty implanting itself in the uterine wall or the pregnancy is not maintained until the developing placenta makes its own hormones.

In some instances, spotting in the early stages of pregnancy may indicate a hormonal deficiency during the implantation period. If a blood test indicates that your progesterone levels are low, your specialist may give you progesterone suppositories, vaginal cream, or injections, either for the duration of your luteal phase or in two injections spaced two weeks apart. The injections, often given in the gluteal (buttock) muscles, may be painful because of their oil base. The causes of a decreased progesterone level have not yet been established.

Some authorities believe that adrenal gland problems and a decrease in the secretion of thyroid hormones may also cause miscarriages. Routine blood tests performed early in the pregnancy and yearly physical examinations help in identifying hormonal imbalances.

Amniocentesis and Chorionic Villus Sampling (CVS)

Although the benefits of these tests often outweigh the risks, in rare instances they can cause miscarriage. Performing amniocentesis and CVS early in the pregnancy is thought to carry a slightly higher risk; however, results tend to fluctuate from health-care center to health-care center. Couples should consult their caregiver before making the decision to incorporate these procedures as part of the mother's prenatal testing.

Antiphospholipid Antibody Syndrome

Recurrent miscarriage may also be caused by the presence of certain antibodies made against phospholipids, which are the building blocks of all cell membranes. A simple blood test may be performed to catch the problem early. Treatment includes aspirin and heparin. In rare cases, steroids may be recommended.

The Emotional Impact of Miscarriage

Once a woman has had a miscarriage there is a 15 to 20 percent chance that she will miscarry again. Miscarriages are difficult emotionally, especially if you have been trying to have a baby for a long time. Some women who have had a miscarriage say that they find it hard seeing other babies without bursting into tears. Adjusting to the loss often takes time and a great deal of support.

The most important aspect of adjusting to a miscarriage is understanding that it was not your fault and was not due to anything you might have done. Miscarriage is an event that affects both the woman and her partner—though the actual impact is almost always different for each, which often results in additional stress. This is because the bonding that occurs with the unborn baby is different for men than it is for women.

Although having a miscarriage is scary, it is rarely life-threatening today, and the most difficult part is the aftermath. When a woman's body heals and she goes home without her baby, she is often overwhelmed by grief and sadness. It may seem to her like everything is coming to an end. In addition to the emotional impact of losing a baby, her hormones are also returning to their pre-pregnant state and depression may accompany this adjustment.

After a miscarriage, you may experience emotions such as anger and disappointment at having lost the baby, and guilt about whether you caused it. These feelings are normal and are part of accepting your loss. You may become angry with yourself and with those around you. This anger is marked by questions such as "Why me?" If you have had more than one miscarriage, you may begin to wonder why pregnancy is so easy for some and so difficult for you. One obstetrician says that although most of his patients have "accepted it as a fact of life," many feel "It was my fault. I should have taken better care of myself." Sometimes the guilt is magnified by other people's comments. One woman remarks:

> "I'll never forget my sister's comments when she phoned me at home following the miscarriage. Her exact words were, 'Maybe they made a mistake; maybe it really wasn't a miscarriage.' I couldn't believe what she was telling me. She was denying that anything happened to me, and here I was absolutely devastated. Nobody would let me grieve. Nobody seemed to understand that I was experiencing an enormous amount of emotional pain."

Another woman shares her experience:

> "I remember trying to open up to an orderly who was looking after me in the hospital. I always related better to men. I broke down in tears when we spoke. The next thing I knew, he was asking me if I was religious because I was so upset. I was so insulted."

Feelings of guilt may be very strong in some women and may last for many years after the miscarriage. If you have any guilt feelings, it is best to verbalize them with your loved ones rather than keeping them pent up inside you. Another alternative is to seek professional one-on-one counseling to discuss what you are going through.

Some couples find it easy to speak about their loss; while others find it difficult. Support groups can be encouraging for those who feel comfortable in group situations. If you want to share what you have been through and are more comfortable in a one-on-one situation, ask about the services offered by your hospital, such as those provided by social workers.

Everyone reacts differently to loss. Some women say that each time they see an infant, they burst into tears. You may find yourself avoiding visits to or contact with women who have babies. You may find that you break down each time you hear a baby cry. You may be filled with unrelenting pent-up emotions—emotions that you never thought existed inside of you.

One woman comments:

> "Others who have never had a miscarriage really don't understand what a woman goes through. I remember people questioning my grief the following week. My own sister couldn't understand why I was still so emotionally upset. Most people expect women to just shake off the event—however, in reality, this is impossible."

Socializing following a miscarriage may be difficult, especially during the immediate mourning period. It may be best to integrate yourself gradually with those around you, starting with those who are closest to you and then expanding to people who are less familiar to you.

It is normal for your grief to take you by surprise. You may think you have rid yourself of the grief, only to find yourself unexpectedly breaking down and even crying for some time after the loss. This hypersensitivity varies from one person to another and may last days, weeks, months, or years. This mourning period is considered healthy, and it helps to heal the wounds of the loss.

As one woman who had three miscarriages states:

> "It's amazing how we hear only what we want to hear. I remember blocking out all the negative situations or problems during my childbirth-education classes. They told us all about miscarriage, stillbirth, and even neonatal death. It is as if I don't remember a thing about what they said. After I miscarried, I tried to mobilize the information I learned at these classes and my mind went completely blank."

Essentially, the loss you and your partner feel is the loss of a child you never knew. It is particularly difficult if you have been trying for a long time to become pregnant. In their book *Coping with Miscarriage*, Christine Palinski and Hank Pfizer say that the fear takes two forms: agony over the chances for subsequent pregnancies to succeed and the fear that the physician would say that something even more terrible (perhaps life-threatening) than miscarriage was occurring.

Deciding when to become pregnant again is often a frightening and difficult choice for the couple. Some say that the right time to become pregnant is when you feel ready—that is, when you and your partner have acknowledged that the miscarriage was not your fault and was beyond your control. This often means that the mourning period is essentially completed.

While 70 to 90 percent of women who miscarry eventually become pregnant again, there is a 15 to 20 percent chance of having a subsequent miscarriage. If your previous pregnancy was the result of months of temperature charts and infertility workups, the thought of reliving that laborious process may not be very tempting.

You waited so long for that pregnancy—and now you are back to square one. You may become impatient with yourself and with your partner, but it is important for both of you to be sensitive to each other, tolerant, and accepting. You should wait three months before trying to get pregnant again. The key is not to worry about the chance of having a miscarriage. As one obstetrician put it, "You cannot live your life in fear."

Coping with Miscarriage

- Be patient with yourself.
- Spend time with those close to you.
- Speak with other women who have miscarried.
- Join miscarriage support groups or get private counseling.
- Communicate openly and honestly with your partner.
- Cry if you feel like crying.
- Remember 15% of all pregnancies end in miscarriage; you are not alone.
- Wait at least three months after a miscarriage before trying to become pregnant again.

In addition to miscarriage, there are other types of losses in pregnancy. If you have had a high-risk pregnancy, you have probably thought about the possibility of the death of your child. These fears are perfectly normal. It is healthiest in the long run to discuss them with your partner, a friend, a relative, or your childbirth educator. Some women may detach themselves from the loss of their child, and this may result in unresolved grief. These denied feelings will likely and unexpectedly surface later.

No matter how prepared you are, when your baby dies, you will experience a wide range of emotions, including shock, despair, and frustration. This is especially true if getting pregnant was difficult and/or if this pregnancy and previous ones were complicated. You will want to hold on to that baby's life and you may find yourself denying the loss.

A baby may die at any point during pregnancy or immediately afterward. Researchers believe that the effects of loss are in direct proportion to the closeness of the relationship prior to death.

Stillbirth

A stillbirth, also known as an intrauterine fetal death, is the birth of a fetus that has died at any time after twenty weeks of pregnancy. In 50 percent of cases, there is no known cause of the stillbirth; however, studies have shown some possible causes including rare, unexplained blood clots forming in the umbilical cord, preventing oxygen from getting to the baby, or the placenta prematurely separating from the baby, cutting off its oxygen. About 5 to 10 percent of all stillbirths are due to chromosomal abnormalities or congenital deformities. If you have a history of stillbirths and early miscarriages, your physician may recommend genetic screening to rule out any genetic problem in either you or your partner. Certain maternal high-risk medical conditions may also be potential causes of stillbirth. For example, those with diabetes mellitus, high blood pressure, or preeclampsia may be more predisposed to stillbirth because there is poor blood flow and nutrition to the fetus. In general, the cause of stillbirth in diabetics is less well understood. Other causes include IUGR, post-term pregnancy, advanced maternal age, and umbilical cord accidents.

In other cases, the woman and fetus may be perfectly healthy when stillbirth occurs. One woman comments:

"We were really taken by surprise because my pregnancy was progressing so well. On Monday my obstetrician heard the baby's heartbeat, and on Saturday I was told my baby had died inside of me three days earlier. The autopsy seemed to show that everything was normal, and the baby—we named him Pascal, was perfectly formed. My obstetrician was reluctant to give me a cause of the stillbirth, but after I pressed him, he said that I may have had a virus or something that caused the baby to die."

Many couples are dissatisfied with the explanations given by health-care professionals, but, in many cases, professionals do not have all the answers. The most useful test is an autopsy performed on the baby to determine if there were any major abnormalities. Many couples do not want it, but it is an option. You must give a consent for the medical staff to perform this procedure. Genetic testing is also performed to look for chromosomal problems. The placenta is always sent to a pathologist (a specialist who studies the cause of disease by examining human tissues) for examination, and they will be looking for such things as infection or blood clots.

In addition to examining the fetus, the specialists will want to determine if the mother's health could have caused a stillbirth. A blood test will be taken to see if she is diabetic, because this could be a factor resulting in stillbirth. In addition, the mother might have another blood test called a Kleihauer-Betke (KB) test that detects if there are large numbers of fetal red blood cells in the mother's circulation. If there are, this means that the baby might have had a large hemorrhage that caused it to die.

What to Expect

If this unfortunate event happens to you, you may no longer feel the fetus moving. One woman shares her experience:

> "The week before my baby died, I had a feeling that something was not right. By the sixth month of pregnancy, I was quite familiar with my baby's habits. I knew that the baby moved a great deal after I ate, but it had not done so for about one week. I also remarked that when I lay in bed on my side, it felt like my baby was very heavy on the side I was lying on, almost like dead weight, and certainly much heavier than she had been the week before. That's when I decided to go to the hospital."

Report any unusual occurrences to your physician. He or she will listen to your baby's heart rate with a fetoscope, and an ultrasound will be performed to assess your baby's well-being. The incidence of stillbirth is lower today, thanks to technological advances. Fetal monitors help detect the need for immediate interventions, such as a cesarean, when the baby's oxygen supply is diminished.

If your baby has died (there is no heartbeat), you will be given the difficult choice of either being induced or waiting until labor begins on its own, which may take up to two weeks. If you choose induction, prostaglandins will be used. If you choose to wait for labor to begin naturally, the waiting may seem long, although some claim that it can give you and your partner time to work through your grief. When given the choice, most women choose to be induced within one to two days.

When you are told your baby has died, you may be in shock; it is normal to deny everything you hear. You may not remember all of the details of what you are told. It is important to ask again later to ensure that you are adequately informed and prepared. No question is a stupid question, especially when it is your body and your baby that are concerned.

Your Emotions

It is normal to have feelings of anger and emptiness following a still-birth. For so many months, you and your partner have organized your life around your child-to-be. The bonding that occurred will leave you with a sense of disorganization. You may be inclined to brood over what you might have done to save the child. There is no reason to feel guilty or to try to bear the blame for this mishap. There is nothing you could have done to change the situation. Chances are that you did all you could do, and that was to seek professional attention.

Mourning the loss of an unborn child is different from mourning the death of someone who has already lived. When we mourn for a deceased person, we have actual memories to hold on to and to think about. With an unborn child, there are only the dreams and fantasies that have occupied your mind from the beginning of the pregnancy. It is important to express these dreams and to talk about your pregnancy. Talking may help you come to grips with your situation and assist you in getting back into your life.

Some mothers find that being able to hold their baby, even for a few minutes, helps them to acknowledge the loss. Taking a picture of the baby, taking footprints, saving the hospital bracelet, and giving the baby a name are also recommended. Some hospitals take routine photos and keep them on file, should the mother want to have them in the future. Seeing your baby right away may be difficult, but as time goes by you may regret not having that small yet sacred memory.

If you do decide to hold your baby, you should be aware that your baby may be different from your dreams and fantasies. Your baby will be cool to the touch and will be pale in color. Its skin may be peeling, and its head size may be smaller than expected. For some women, the thought of holding their dead baby is something they are unable to fathom. This is fine, too.

Today, most hospital staff will try not to admit you to a maternity unit if you have lost a baby. It is difficult to be surrounded by women carrying their newborn bundles as you stroll the corridor empty-handed. This makes the grieving process much more difficult. If you find yourself on a unit with pregnant women or crying babies, either ask to be transferred to another unit or to be discharged home. It is your prerogative.

One woman who had a stillbirth comments:

> "The year following the death of my baby was the hardest year of my life. Nobody seemed to understand what I was going through. They didn't understand that my baby was a real person to me and that I was very sad when it died. I felt very isolated and depressed. I found that friends were avoiding me. I remember one incident where I saw a childhood friend on the street who knew I lost my baby, and she turned around and walked the other way when she saw me. I understand that at times people don't know what to say—but this made it particularly hard on me at a time when I really needed love."

Today, some hospital centers will prepare a memory box that includes the baby's footprint, photograph, what would have been their hospital bracelet, and the little cap given to all newborns. This is a lovely gesture and if your hospital does not offer this service, you should ask them for any keepsakes so that you can prepare your own memory box.

Newborn Death

Neonatal death is a death within the first four weeks after birth. The birth of a premature baby is most often associated with neonatal death because the baby's systems are too immature to allow it to sustain life on its own.

The baby's lungs may be unable to provide the needed oxygen, and its immune system may not have developed enough to fight infections. Severe congenital problems may also cause neonatal death because the nature of the abnormality is incompatible with life. These include problems associated with the heart, brain, kidneys, lungs, and/or endocrine system. Other possible reasons for neonatal death include those babies with Rh disease, those in fetal distress, those with chromosome abnormalities, and those with a combination of these factors.

After enduring labor or cesarean birth, the couple has already formed a bonding relationship with the new baby. The child may have had health problems that the couple has had to learn to accept. There may have already been some thoughts about the loss of the child. As the child goes through the crisis period, the parents experience a sense of uncertainty as they are torn between becoming more attached to the child and slowly distancing themselves in preparation for possible death. One husband explains:

> "One of the hardest aspects of having our daughter in the premature nursery was the fact that although she was surrounded by excellent quality care, she was also surrounded by death. There were so many infants so much sicker than she was—the sounds of emergency alarm systems beeping intermittently made me feel very ill at ease. We had already lost a baby from miscarriage, and I couldn't bear losing another, especially one that I was already able to touch and hold."

In some cases, the couple is aware of the possibility of death immediately following birth. The newborn may be in the high-risk unit being monitored very carefully. Twins are often at risk, and parents surviving the loss of one twin may have great difficulties coping. In most instances, when a couple experiences the death of a twin, it is very difficult to grieve over the loss while rejoicing at the birth of the other baby. It is normal for the parents to have conflicting emotions as they try to retain enough strength and positive energy to give to the surviving child. Speaking with other parents who are in or were in similar situations can be very helpful. If you are comfortable in group situations, you should seek out a support group in your area. Or you may prefer the help of counselors specially trained in working with couples who have lost a baby or child.

In other cases, the death of a newborn is entirely unexpected. One woman explains:

> "Two years ago, our baby was born four weeks early and was doing extremely well. Although she was in the premature nursery, she was one of the healthiest newborns there. I was nursing her and she didn't have any tubes and wasn't hooked up to any machines. After having already had two miscarriages, I was sure that I was going to take this baby home. Well, I never did. Four days before I was to take her home, she developed what was to be a fatal staphylococcus infection. To this day, the shock I feel is overpowering."

Sudden Infant Death Syndrome (SIDS)

Sudden infant death syndrome, sometimes called crib, or cot, death, is the unexpected death of an apparently healthy infant. In the United States, SIDS is responsible for approximately seven thousand to eight thousand deaths each year. In Canada, approximately one thousand infants die from this syndrome each year. It is the leading cause of death in children one month to one year old. SIDS is not predictable or preventable, nor is it anyone's fault. It may happen to breast-fed or bottle-fed babies.

How It Happens

When and why SIDS happens remains an ongoing question for both parents and professionals. Typically, an infant is put to bed for the night or for its usual daytime nap with no suspicion of anything out of the ordinary. After some time, the child is found dead. Parents and caretakers have remarked that the baby does not seem to struggle, nor are there any crying or unusual sounds prior to death. The event is devastating.

Researchers agree that the highest incidence of SIDS occurs between the ages of two and four months, with a peak at twelve weeks. The child often has a cold or other minor illness. It occurs most commonly in the winter months, although it may occur during any season.

The American Academy of Pediatrics has initiated what it calls the "back to sleep plan," which means when babies are put down to sleep, they should only be placed on their back to reduce the risk of SIDS. Since

1992, the year this recommendation was made, the rate of SIDS has dropped by 38 percent in the United States.

One father recounts his experience:

> "We lost our second child, Maddie, to SIDS when she was four months old. That was sixteen years ago, and today the one thing that echoes in my mind are the words of the Colorado SIDS program director sitting in our living room telling my wife and me how we were going to grieve differently. Everything else remains a blur of pain. I am not sure we could have survived without the love and support of a huge community of relatives, friends, coworkers, and strangers.
>
> "We have both learned that the saying, 'Time heals,' is true. Over time, the pain comes less frequently, but it will forever be present. When I start thinking about Maddie, I still cry. The intensity of the emotions of losing her will be with me forever.
>
> "We continue to honor Maddie's short life by living ours, and trying to be helpful to others and to appreciate everything we have. During the years after Maddie's death, my wife, Karen, endured four miscarriages. Six years later we received a very special gift—the birth of our only son, Jesse. I believe that everything happens for a reason, and if Maddie hadn't died, we probably never would have had Jesse and for this I am thankful. This week Jesse will have his bar mitzvah, and every day with him has been a blessing."

Causes of SIDS

Some infants are considered to be at high-risk for SIDS, and professionals recommend that these infants have baby monitors in their room that ring when breathing ceases. Some professionals believe that the problems begin during prenatal development. An abnormal or underdeveloped respiratory system may prevent these infants from responding to carbon-dioxide levels in the blood that serve as the signal to breathe. As a result, they have periods of apnea (nonbreathing) even when they are awake.

Remember, most of the babies who fall into one or more of these categories thrive and do very well. If your baby falls into any of these categories, it does not mean that he or she will have the symptoms most commonly associated with SIDS, but that the risk is greater than for the general population.

Babies at Increased Risk for SIDS

- premature babies
- twins and triplets
- children of adolescent mothers
- children of low-income families
- Native Americans and African Americans
- children of mothers who did not receive adequate prenatal care
- low-birth-weight babies
- children of smokers
- children of methadone addicts

Many theories about the causes of SIDS have been proposed, including an allergy to cow's milk, viral infections, spinal hemorrhages, calcium/magnesium deficiency, excessive sodium (salt) in the blood, carbon dioxide pooling in the blood, heart/lung defects, house-mite allergy, stress, and lack of lung surfactant—a substance produced in the fetal lung necessary for lung maturity. Its purpose is to control the surface tension in the lungs.

Coping with SIDS

Coping with the loss of a child to SIDS is very difficult because the situation is completely out of your control, and it may take a long time to resolve your feelings of helplessness. It is normal to feel guilty and angry, especially when it is difficult to identify the cause of your child's death. It is not uncommon for marriages to weaken after such an incident, or for fathers to immerse themselves in their work as their way of coping with the stress of losing a child. You may find that your partner is less communicative during this time and, like yourself, needs extra love and understanding.

Explaining what happened to other siblings may be a trying task, depending on their ages. Younger children may not comprehend what has happened but may be sensitive to your moods and feelings of depression. They may need more love and affection and may use attention-seeking behaviors to get it. It may help if you can clarify or interpret your child's perception of what has happened. It is common for adults to deny that children are sad. Experiencing a loss can be a learning experience for a child—he or she can learn that the sadness is eventually resolved.

With younger children, try to be as simple as possible with your explanation. Mention that the baby died suddenly and unexpectedly, and that the baby seemed well and healthy when it died. They should be told that the death was nobody's fault. Older children may be told the facts about SIDS discussed above. Remember that children have different ways of coping with grief. They may become naughty, have nightmares, revert to bedwetting, or have other problems at school or at home.

Family, friends, and neighbors need to understand as much as they can about SIDS. The popular misconceptions may make you uncomfortable when speaking with these people. Uninformed persons may believe that the baby was abused or neglected, or suffocated in its bedding. These misconceptions and the negative attitudes associated with them make coping difficult. You may feel that you have nobody to talk to and that nobody understands what you are going through. If this is the case, you should seek professional help from someone who has experience with couples like yourself. It is important that significant others understand that SIDS is not preventable, nor is it anyone's fault.

Future Pregnancies

The loss of a child to SIDS should not prevent you from becoming pregnant again. It is usually recommended that the mother not become pregnant until she has had an opportunity to deal with the loss of her baby. Having one SIDS baby does not necessarily lead to having another SIDS baby. Your pediatrician may carefully monitor your baby after birth for any clues of respiratory difficulties. For the first year of your baby's life, it may be recommended that you use a monitor in your baby's room. Rather than being afraid, you should be confident in knowing that you are doing everything in your power to ensure that it does not happen again.

The Grieving Process

Accepting your baby's death does not occur overnight, but rather over weeks or months. It may take some women up to a year to begin recovering from the deep pain of this tragedy. You may be surprised at yourself for being so grief-stricken. What you are feeling is perfectly normal. Grieving is an important part of the resolving process, and of accepting your loss so you can move on with your life.

No two people react in the same way to the stress of the death of a loved one. The way you cope may be similar to the way you have coped with other stresses. Sharing your feelings with others who have experienced loss can help you cope during this difficult period. The Compassionate Friends is a group with over five hundred chapters throughout the United States and over thirty in Canada, plus chapters in other countries, and its goal is to support and provide friendship and education for bereaved parents. One representative comments:

> "Sharing and telling our stories over and over again is what the healing process is all about. We also learn that we are not going crazy and most of our feelings and the things we do or do not do after the death of our children are really normal. Others tell us what it was like for them, too. We read books, listen to tapes, and listen to others who have succeeded in resolving many of the problems and concerns of bereaved parents."

The loss of a child is a loss unlike any other. It is the loss of something you have created. It is the loss of a loved one whom you hardly knew, but knew very well. It is the loss of a special and intense bond that was created over a very short period of time. In a sense, when you lose a baby, you lose part of yourself.

When you lose a baby, there is deep disappointment, a loss of hope and of plans for the future. Accepting this change in your dreams and goals is not something that is accomplished overnight. Your dreams are destroyed as you realize that the baby you grew to love is no longer there.

One woman said that she was thankful to those who let her grieve:

> "I'll never forget the emotional support I got from my closest friend. You really learn a great deal about people during these difficult times. It was especially surprising because she had never lost a baby, but she really knew me well. She was the only one who remembered the date of my child's death and one year later to the date sent me a card. It was nice to see that someone else also remembered my loss. Sometimes it's what people call 'the little things' that really count."

Feelings of despair are common among those who lose a baby. These feelings are especially common in those who have had infertility problems or high-risk pregnancies. Where before all their energy and time centered around the new baby, now their life suddenly feels meaningless and empty. Susan Borg and Judith Lasker, in their book *When Pregnancy Fails*, state that feelings of despair may increase if the baby's sex was the one the parents had wished for. For example, if a family had three girls and wanted a boy and the boy died during delivery, the despair will be much more profound.

Everyone is affected differently following the loss of a loved one. The following are some of the most common reactions:

Physical Signs of Grieving

- difficulty sleeping
- bad dreams
- loss of appetite
- loss of energy
- restlessness
- muscle aches and pains
- palpitations
- stomachaches
- diarrhea, constipation

Emotional Signs of Grieving

- crying
- apathy
- irritability
- feelings of going crazy
- confusion
- indecision
- uncontrollable sadness

Few people experience all these symptoms. You may have some, or none at all. But remember that they are normal expressions of the stress that you are going through.

Some women have identified grief as feeling as if they were locked in a dark closet without the key. You may feel that life is passing you by and you are just a spectator, unable to become involved. You may need someone, a dear friend or a professional, to help you get out of that closet. It is normal to have your ups and downs as you begin healing from your loss. You may take your problems out on others—this, too, is normal. It is a good idea to vent your concerns. Speaking with those who care is very important. One woman comments:

> "Keep in the company of those who make you feel happy and good about yourself rather than those who tend to bring you down. It is important that you get on with your life while at the same time understanding that you should give yourself the necessary time to mourn."

The grieving parent cannot look to family and friends for understanding if they have not experienced the death of a child themselves. They will go back to their regular routines soon after the funeral, and we cannot count on them for the support we so need. Six months after the death, they expect us to be back to normal, and this is totally unrealistic. It is common for people to say, "Get on with your life and forget it." We do not want to forget our child. I feel that "to forget" means we could not have loved very much. We shall never "get over" the death, but we will learn to live with our grief, and the pain somehow becomes bearable.

Significant Others

For most women, the pregnancy experience is not a lonely one, but rather one they share with their loved ones, partners, family, and friends. When there is a pregnancy loss, loved ones also experience grief. In addition, the relationship between the pregnant woman and her loved ones may itself be affected.

Fathers

Your partner will not be exempt from the grief-stricken reaction. You may think your grief is deeper because you were closer to the child, but chances are that he is hurting and is sheltering you from his pain. It is common for men to bond with the baby either later in pregnancy or after delivery, and therefore they tend to mourn the loss of a child differently than a woman. He may sublimate his pain by working long hours. If he was talkative before, he may become more quiet. It is not uncommon for the partner to block out the loss at first, and when the mother has begun to accept the loss a few months down the road, he may be starting to hurt.

You may be busy trying to resolve your own grief, and if you have other children, your energy may also need to be extended to them. Often the husband's needs are either neglected or overlooked. Although they too have experienced loss, men are still expected to continue making major decisions and to remain strong for their wives. Marriage failure and divorce are common following the death of a child. Studies have shown that divorce occurs in over 50 percent of those couples sustaining perinatal death, serious newborn abnormalities, and/or mental retardation. In many cases, the partners are unable to support one another because they are both having difficulty navigating through their own journey of grief. It is common for one partner to place blame on the other to cover up for their personal sense of failure. One woman comments:

> "Losing our child was the most traumatic time in both our lives. Although we had known the child for such a short period of time, we felt a terrific void in our life. If it wasn't for local support groups for bereaved parents, I don't know what might have happened to either of us, or our relationship, for that matter."

Partners or husbands often feel helpless, as if they are "onlookers" during the pregnancy. When death occurs, they may feel even more alienated. It is important that both partners make an effort to give strength to one another. Couples should try to talk about the baby and about what their aspirations were.

Siblings

Siblings will grieve in their own way. Some may act out inappropriately. The child senses the parents' tension and reacts to these feelings. It may be their first loss, and often they are unsure how to act, what to say, and how to grieve. If they are old enough, it is important to give them accurate and honest information about what has happened. Children also need to be told that they were not responsible for the loss and that feelings of guilt are unnecessary. Try not to alienate them. Try to involve them in as many activities as possible. If they are older, there is no reason they cannot be a part of family discussions.

Children in their early childhood may have a more difficult time dealing with the death because they do not understand why it happened. They also have difficulty understanding that events such as death are final. These children are usually governed by their own experiences and tend to believe that everything in their world is alive, including inanimate objects. They may be very fearful about what has occurred. They may also blame themselves for the death because they might have said something about not wanting to have a sibling. If they are under the age of five, they may fear being abandoned following the death of a sibling. Younger children may also surprise you with their reaction to the loss. As one woman says:

"Josh was two when his brother died. Although their relationship was short-lived, he seemed to be as grief-stricken as we were. His rapport with the baby began when I was pregnant, and how he enjoyed feeling and seeing the baby move inside of me. When the baby was born, he was very protective and loving to his younger brother. Now, two years after his death, he continues to ask questions about how and why his brother died. I find this amazing for a four-year-old. We decided to plant two trees in our backyard—one for each boy. Josh was very proud to help me do this. He tells everyone who the second tree was for—'That was for my baby brother who died a long time ago,' he says."

It is common for children to feel that wishing will bring the baby back, and it is important to explain to them that this will not happen. Tell them that most people live to be older before they die, but sometimes little babies and kids die because they are sick. Answer all of their questions as simply as possible, without overwhelming them.

Those in their late childhood or in the preadolescence time will understand death as a permanent event. They might be very curious and interested about the process of dying.

No matter what age the children are, the sense of loss will be felt by everyone in the family. Sometimes siblings develop symptoms of anxiety, depression, aggression, and/or difficulty sleeping. Sometimes parents are submerged deeply in their own grief and do not spend the time attending to the emotional needs of their children. It is a good idea to call on the support of family or support groups listed in Appendixes B and C. Typically, it takes a couple at least one to two months to work through their grief, but it may take the siblings longer—sometimes up to six months.

Friends

Sometimes friends want to be supportive, but often during times of grief, they do not know what to do or say. If they have not experienced the loss of a child, they might make insensitive or inappropriate comments. Even though they are well-intended, they can be hurtful and in some cases, they might belittle the experience of a pregnancy loss.

If you know someone who has lost a baby, here are some helpful and soothing words:

- I am sorry.
- What can I do to help?
- Cry when you need to cry.
- Can I bring you dinner?
- I am here for you if you want to talk.
- Be patient with yourself and take time to heal.
- Can I take the baby's sibling on an outing?
- Don't feel guilty if you laughed today.
- What errands can I do for you?
- Tell me more about your pregnancy and baby.
- When you are ready, I will help you sort through the baby's items.

It is also a good idea to refer the women to support groups in your community and if you do not know where to turn, use the resources and associations mentioned in Appendixes B and C at the end of this book. The national organizations can lead you to local groups.

Future Pregnancies

Experiencing the loss of a baby should not prevent you from becoming pregnant again. Some women speak of another pregnancy even while they are in the hospital, with a sense of urgency to become pregnant again, while others fear the thought. However, it is important that you recover both physically and psychologically first. Many professionals recommend waiting anywhere from six months to one year before becoming pregnant again.

If you are over the age of thirty, you are probably battling time constraints and know that if you want to have several children it is not a good idea to wait too long. Some women find it easier to have a child very soon after they lose a baby, while others are too afraid that the same thing will happen again. One woman who had one child and then a stillbirth said that she needed a break and was going to go back to school for a couple of years before deciding if she was going to have a second child.

It is normal to have fears and concerns with your subsequent pregnancy, but it is important not to let these emotions overwhelm you, because they could be detrimental to both you and your child-to-be. You may feel nervous and unsure of your situation. You may magnify each symptom and event, and fear that any and every symptom will result in the death of another baby. Remember, do not be hard on yourself or on others.

For the high-risk mother, having another baby is often a relief. It is common to have feelings of elation and appreciation for everything that goes right. Many women compare the new baby with the deceased one because the memories live on. But remember, this baby is a new one in its own right, with an identity of its own.

In some cases, another pregnancy may not be feasible because of your age or the complications of the earlier loss. Perhaps adoption is your only option. The waiting is sometimes lengthy, but raising your child will be well worth the wait!

Today, there are a number of helpful books that will assist you in coping with the loss of a baby. One reference that is highly recommended is Dr. Michael Berman's book, *Parenthood Lost: Healing the Pain After Miscarriage, Stillbirth, and Infant Death*. Appendixes B and C list associations and websites that can also offer you solace during these difficult times.

Journaling Corner

Writing down your thoughts and feelings about your experience is a good way to come to terms with your loss. The writing journey helps you dig deeper into yourself so that healing will happen. Daily journaling not only records your feelings but it saves all the precious memories you have of your baby. Writing these down will help you through your grief journey.

It is a good idea to buy a journal that you can carry with you so that whenever the mood strikes, or if you start feeling sad, you can sit down and write.

You can use your journal daily, but you may also want to say good-bye to your baby in a creative way. You can do this either in the form of a letter or a poem.

- Write a letter to your baby relating all the feelings in your heart.

- Write a poem to your baby to say good-bye. Start the poem with your own title, or use one of these. Remember that your poem does not have to rhyme.

  — Good-bye, My Baby

  — To My Baby

  — What I Remember

  — I Will Always Love You

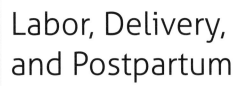

Labor, Delivery, and Postpartum

Life is a flame that is always burning itself out, but it catches fire again every time a child is born. — George Bernard Shaw

Just because you survived a high-risk pregnancy, that does not necessarily mean that you will also have a high-risk labor and delivery. The good news is that you have made it to this chapter! Certain women are more prone to having a high-risk labor and delivery. They might include women who have experienced the following:

- gestational diabetes
- multiple pregnancies
- preeclampsia or hypertension
- uterine fibroids
- too much or too little amniotic fluid
- large babies

Others in this category may include those with a

- breech presentation
- fetal genetic abnormality
- vaginal birth after cesarean (VBAC)
- fetus with intrauterine growth restriction (IUGR)

Whether you had a high-risk pregnancy or not, there is no way to predict when your baby will be born. It may arrive prematurely, at term or post term. In each situation, it is a good idea to be prepared for your baby's arrival. Here is a suggested checklist of how to prepare during the latter part of your pregnancy:

- Pay your bills.

- Wash all the baby clothes.

- Buy the baby a crib.

- Send out the necessary e-mails or correspondences.

- Preregister at the hospital so the staff is ready to receive you.

- Set aside a day of pampering—get a hair cut or coloring, have a massage, or get a natural manicure and pedicure (unless this is not recommended by your physician).

- Prepare your baby's room with all the necessities, such as diapers, baby wipes, T-shirts, and sleepers.

- Pack your suitcase (two nightgowns, robe, socks, slippers, lotion, toiletries, camera, address book, photos of other children, reading material, lip balm, a notebook, tennis ball, baby bag with receiving blanket).

- Have your suitcase and the car seat parked near the front door.

Labor Defined

Labor is a physiological process by which the fetus or fetuses are expelled from the uterus into the outside world. This process is facilitated by uterine contractions that eventually result in cervical effacement and dilation. These events begin even before your membranes rupture. Spontaneous rupture of the membranes before contractions is seen in only about 8 percent of all pregnancies.

Your physician will suspect you are in labor if you have regular painful uterine contractions, your cervix is beginning to efface (thin) and dilate (open), and you have a bloody discharge (show). At this time, you will get a complete physical examination, which will include having all your vital signs taken. Your provider will also want to make note of your baby's position and presentation inside of you. This is done by palpating your abdomen or with ultrasound viewing. Sometimes fetal monitoring devices will be used to assess your baby's well-being. At the same time, you will be asked to report the frequency, duration, and intensity of your uterine contractions.

While you are in labor, your practitioner will regularly check your cervix for dilation and effacement. He or she will also check the position and placement of your baby's head. This should really be done at indicated intervals because too many exams can increase the risk of infection to the amniotic fluid. If an examination is deemed absolutely necessary, make sure that in the urgency of the moment your practitioner uses a sterile lubricant and sterile gloves.

Signs of Labor

- dilation (opening) of the cervix
- effacement (thinning) of the cervix
- breaking of the water
- diarrhea or nausea (sometimes)
- regular uterine contractions lasting thirty to seventy-five seconds, every five to ten minutes

Stages of Labor

You will likely think of labor as one long, continuous process when you go through it; however, health-care professionals divide the labor process into three stages: first, second, and third.

First Stage or Early Labor

During the first stage, your uterine contractions cause your cervix to open and thin, two signs that your body is preparing for your baby's arrival. Sometimes the early contractions are quite painless and many women do not even realize that labor has begun.

You will probably be admitted into your hospital's labor and delivery unit and an intravenous drip will be started. A fetal monitor will be used to assess your baby's well-being. At this time, your practitioner will ask you about pain medication and whether you want an epidural later on in labor.

The first stage of labor continues until your cervix is completely dilated to 10 centimeters. Typically, this is a large enough opening to allow your baby's head to pass through the birth canal. This is the longest stage of labor and can last up to twenty hours.

During this stage, your baby will drop into your pelvic canal and your water may break. If your labor progresses slowly and your water has not broken, your provider may artificially rupture your membranes to augment labor. When labor does begin, many women experience backache, an upset stomach, and sometimes diarrhea. It is a good idea to empty your bladder every hour during this stage.

Many women feel elated during this stage because they sense the impending birth of their baby. Sometimes a little walking during the first stage of labor may decrease your discomfort, and hopefully this will be encouraged by your providers. You should keep in mind that this activity will not affect the length of time you are in labor, or whether or not you will need to be augmented or given Pitocin to speed up labor. During this phase, your labor coach or doula will be very helpful to you, and she will probably remind you not to start pushing until your cervix is completely dilated, because this can cause complications.

This first stage is further divided into two phases: the latent phase and the active phase.

The Latent Phase: The latent or early phase is the time between the onset of labor and the cervix dilating to 3 centimeters. This phase is the longest phase of labor and can last from a few hours to a few days. This stage might require a huge amount of patience on your part.

The Active Phase: The active phase begins when your cervix begins to rapidly dilate from 3 to 10 centimeters. This is the time when your contractions become stronger and you will have to work very hard. Each contraction usually lasts about forty-five seconds and may occur three to four minutes apart. During this phase, you will have more bloody show and muscle aches in your back and legs. Some women experience nausea and vomiting. Remember to stay well-hydrated during this phase.

Women who elect to have epidurals will usually receive them during this phase. If your cervix has dilated past 7 centimeters, it may be too late for the epidural to be effective, and it therefore will not be given.

Second Stage of Labor

The second stage of labor starts when your cervix is completely dilated and lasts until the moment your baby passes through your pelvic area and is born. After the baby's head is out (crowning), your provider will tell you to stop pushing. You may be advised to pant instead of push. This minimizes your chance of having skin tears.

For those women having their first baby, this stage normally lasts for about two hours without regional anesthesia, and about three hours with regional anesthesia. Women who have had previous deliveries will usually push for a maximum of one hour without regional anesthesia and two hours with regional anesthesia.

During this stage, your provider will likely assess your baby's heart rate about every fifteen minutes and also after each uterine contraction, just to make sure that your baby is not in distress.

Here is a comment from one father in the delivery room:

"My wife's second stage of labor was quite dramatic. The baby's heart rate started decreasing and the doctors suspected the cord was around her neck. Two doctors were on either side of her and they began rotating the baby's position. I was nervous because I noticed the doctor was sweating and then someone announced, 'Okay, everybody push hard.'

"There was about thirty seconds of silence. It seemed like forever. It was awful. Finally, our little baby girl was born, but she was all blue and not moving at all. They immediately suctioned her and gave her oxygen. It was an extremely urgent situation. My wife looked at me and she was absolutely expressionless. I could not console her because I didn't know what the outcome would be.

"Then all of a sudden, our baby let out a sound. The air in the room was very heavy. The doctor apologized but finally said she was a healthy baby girl weighing 8¼ pounds. I had no idea that she would be so big, because my wife is so tiny.

"I am so glad I went to the childbirth classes and had a doula, because I would have been much more frightened had I not known what was going on."

Your Baby Is Born: When your baby is completely out of your body, he or she will still be attached to the placenta by the umbilical cord. Many providers will immediately place the baby on your abdomen. If you are interested, ask if you can assist in clamping off and cutting the cord. For many couples, this can be an exciting and memorable moment.

After the baby is disconnected from the umbilical cord, he or she will be carefully examined and weighed and the Apgar score will be taken (see Table 10.1). The one-minute Apgar score was designed by Virginia Apgar to determine which babies might need resuscitation. Basically, it is a quick test to evaluate your baby's physical condition. The second score is taken at five minutes to see how the baby responded to the resuscitation. The scores assess five factors that are added together to calculate the total Apgar score.

Table 10.1: Apgar Scoring

Apgar Sign	2	1	0
Heart Rate (pulse)	Normal (above 100 beats per minute)	Below 100 beats per minute	Absent (no pulse)
Breathing (rate and effort)	Normal rate and effort, good cry	Slow or irregular breathing, weak cry	Absent (no breathing)
Grimace (responsiveness or "reflex irritability")	Pulls away, sneezes, or coughs with stimulation	Facial movement only (grimace) with stimulation	Absent (no response to stimulation)
Activity (muscle tone)	Active, spontaneous movement	Arms and legs flexed with little movement	No movement, "floppy" tone
Appearance (skin coloration)	Normal color all over (hands and feet are pink)	Normal color (but hands and feet are bluish)	Bluish gray or pale all over

The highest score is 10 and the lowest is 0. In general, a score of 7 or above is indicative that the baby is in good health and does not need any specific extra care.

If you plan to breast-feed, ask your provider when the best time is to begin.

Now go ahead and enjoy the first few minutes with your newborn baby!

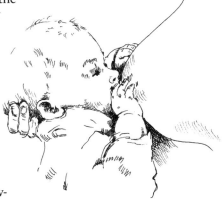

Figure 10.1: Breast-feeding

Episiotomy: An episiotomy is a surgical incision made in the perineum to enlarge the vaginal opening before the baby's head emerges. Unlike in the 1980s, when this book was originally published, in the United States today, episiotomies are rarely performed. Sometimes episiotomies are performed prophylactically to prevent potential problems, such as fetal distress, shoulder dystocia, or if a baby is being born with the assistance of forceps or vacuum-assisted delivery.

Prior to having an episiotomy, you will have an injection of local pain relief into the area. There are two types of episiotomies: a medio-lateral episiotomy, which is a cut that slants away from your rectum, and a median episiotomy, which is a cut made directly back toward the rectum. Your obstetrician will decide which is best for you. After the baby is delivered, your obstetrician will stitch up the surgical incision or cut.

Some studies have shown that regular perineal massage during the final weeks before labor may decrease the need to have an episiotomy. After the thirtieth week, the massage can be done for about ten minutes a day. You should speak to your practitioner, midwife, or doula about the exact method recommended for you.

One woman recounts her experience with her first child:

> "Either it was the pineapple I craved throughout my pregnancy, which made us think the baby was Polynesian, or the bulk prenatal pills, but this was going to be a big baby. After almost three hours of pushing and the baby barely crowning, the doctor gave us the choice of either using the vacuum and an episiotomy or a cesarean section. We opted for the latter, given it was the best choice for myself and the baby. After his birth, the doctor told me Zackary was caught in my pelvis and turned in the wrong direction. The doctor told me I 'would have never gotten him out on my own.' I looked the doctor square in the eye and told him, 'Thank goodness this isn't 1906!'"

Third Stage of Labor

The third stage of labor refers to the delivery of the placenta and the fetal membranes. Most women say that this is the easiest stage of labor because all the hard work is behind them. Many do not even notice the extra push they give when delivering the placenta.

However, the interval between your baby being born and the delivery of the placenta may feel like an eternity. When the umbilical cord is outside of you, you might feel a gush of blood from your vagina, which means that the placenta has separated from the uterine wall and will soon be delivered. After all the birth products (such as the placenta, umbilical cord, and fetal membranes) are delivered, they will be carefully examined.

During this stage, there is usually a great deal of commotion in the delivery room, as the staff prepares to receive your baby and make sure he or she is in optimal health. Typically, this stage lasts less than ten minutes, but it can last up to thirty minutes. If the physician sees that this stage is lasting too long or there is too much bleeding, he or she may want to remove the placenta manually or by a D&C. Only in rare situations is a blood transfusion required. The good news is that your uterus begins to contract during this stage and you should no longer feel pain.

After the third stage of labor is complete, your provider will carefully examine your pelvic area for any evidence of birth injury. If you have any torn skin, it will need to be repaired.

Problems with Labor

Sometimes labor does not progress normally and the medical team will have to intervene to maintain the health and well-being of both you and your baby. Below are descriptions of some of the most common interventions used today.

Labor Induction

Artificial labor induction is performed to initiate uterine contractions when they do not occur in a natural and timely manner. The decision about whether to induce should be a joint one that you make with your physician. It is important that he or she informs you of all the options and risks.

Reasons Labor Is Induced: Generally, the decision to induce labor is made when either your life or your baby's life is at risk or if your labor does not progress on its own. The reason for breaking the water is that this stimulates the release of prostaglandins in your body, which in turn encourages your uterine contractions to begin. Once uterine contractions begin, it is a signal to your baby that it is time to be born.

Some centers may offer you an elective induction for the purposes of convenience, but in general, this procedure is not recommended. Some of the most common reasons that your labor might be induced include:

- uterine infection
- carrying a large baby
- placenta has separated from the uterus
- Rh factor complications
- water breaking prior to the start of contractions
- baby is overdue (beyond forty-two weeks)
- delivery of a previous baby weighing more than 9 pounds
- problems with the baby's position
- intrauterine growth restriction (IUGR)
- maternal complications (diabetes, lung disease, kidney disease, obesity, high blood pressure, herpes outbreak)

Methods of Induction: Once the decision to induce has been made, the next decision is to decide exactly when. The most favorable time to have an induction is when the cervix is at least 50 percent effaced and 3 or 4 centimeters dilated. This means that it is time for your baby to be born.

There are two methods of induction: mechanical and with the use of medication.

After thirty-nine weeks, induction can be done mechanically by the surgical stripping of the fetal membranes. This procedure dates back to the early 1800s. The practitioner inserts his finger into the cervix until he feels the fetal membranes between the baby and the wall of the uterus. There are many disadvantages to this procedure—it is uncomfortable for the woman and the results of this type of induction are not predictable and therefore it is rarely used today.

An amniotomy is an artificial rupture of the membranes using a thin plastic hook to make a small tear in the membranes surrounding your baby. It will feel as if you are having a vaginal examination, and then you will feel a gush of fluid leak from your vagina. This technique has been used since the early 1900s, but it has many risks and contraindications.

More recent studies indicate that artificially rupturing the membranes (AROM) does not necessarily shorten the time of labor.

Today, induction with the use of medications is most often the method of choice. Prostaglandin may be applied in either gel or suppository form and inserted into the cervix. This stimulates dilation and effacement and helps the cervix "ripen." After this is done, you will be observed for the next few hours to see if your cervix is softening. Sometimes a second application may be necessary. At the time of this writing, this medication has not been approved for safe use during pregnancy because of its many side effects.

If your labor still does not progress, the practitioner will begin an intravenous infusion of oxytocin (Pitocin) to stimulate your labor. This is a safe and effective way to induce labor and it is about 80 percent effective.

While any of these induction techniques are being used, you and your baby will be continually monitored with electronic monitors. If after eight to twelve hours of the intravenous oxytocin your labor has still not progressed, your practitioner may let you rest and allow some time for your labor to progress naturally. If labor does not happen naturally, a cesarean delivery may be necessary.

Forceps Delivery

If your labor does not progress or there are severe complications during labor, your practitioner might suggest further intervention, such as a forceps delivery. Only qualified medical personnel should use forceps delivery as an option.

Forceps delivery is done only when the cervix is completely dilated in the second stage of labor. The forceps are shaped like a pair of spoons that are attached like salad tongs. Each spoon is placed on either side of your birth canal to cradle the baby's head. The forceps help the baby maneuver its way through the birth canal. Using forceps is one way to avoid cesarean delivery. A small complication of this procedure is that the baby may have a red mark or bruise on either side of the head. The good news is that it usually disappears within the first few days of life.

Vacuum-Assisted Delivery

Instead of using forceps, your provider may choose to use a vacuum extractor to help your baby to be born. The indications and risks are the same as for forceps, but it is just a different instrument. A plastic cup is placed against the baby's head. This creates a suction to gently pull the baby down through the birth canal. While this is being done, you will be instructed to continue pushing. This procedure is slightly more risky to the baby than is forceps delivery. Sometimes a bump may appear on the side of the baby's head, but it usually disappears within a few days.

Prolapsed Cord

A prolapsed cord refers to the umbilical cord slipping into the birth canal after the membranes rupture and before the baby is born. This rare event is more commonly seen with babies in the breech presentation. A prolapsed cord may also occur in multiple pregnancies before the delivery of a second or third baby. This emergency situation requires immediate delivery, usually by cesarean section. (For more information, see Chapter 5.)

Shoulder Dystocia

Shoulder dystocia is a complication of labor whereby one or both of the baby's shoulders become stuck in the mother's pelvis after the baby's head is already in the birth canal. There is no warning of this complication. However, some studies have shown that certain women are more prone to developing shoulder dystocia and they include those in the following categories:

- diabetics
- maternal obesity
- long active phase of labor
- prior shoulder dystocia
- previous baby weighing more than 9 pounds
- assisted second stage of labor with forceps

The practitioner will suspect shoulder dystocia if your baby's head is out and the shoulders do not follow. Shoulder dystocia is rare, occurring in 0.2 to 2 percent of all vaginal deliveries, that is an emergency situation. It can create a scary scenario in the delivery room.

With shoulder dystocia, there is a 20 percent risk of fetal bone fractures. In 40 percent of cases there is also a risk of nerve injury, such as brachial plexus injury (the nerves that go from the neck to the arm), to the baby. This is not permanent. Ninety percent of the time, it resolves within six months.

Pain Management in Labor

There are many ways to manage pain during labor and many were probably discussed with you during your childbirth education classes. For the most part, these methods include both nonmedication and medication modalities.

Nonmedication Methods

There are many ways to manage labor without the use of medications, and today, many women are leaning in this direction.

Mind-Body Connection: One of the best ways to approach labor is by relaxing your mind and your body in preparation for the big moment. If you are anxious, studies show that your chance of experiencing more pain during labor is increased. Anxiety also has a tendency to slow down the laboring process. At this time, the art of positive thinking has many added benefits. It is important for you to listen to your body's messages and tune into what your body needs and wants.

To prepare yourself for labor, there are many natural techniques that you can try. The natural techniques for coping with the physical and psychological aspects of labor include listening to relaxing music, hypnosis, visualization, massage, meditation, journaling, and other methods suggested by an experienced childbirth coach.

In addition, efficient breathing techniques can help you focus on your labor and achieve a rhythm of relaxation, inhalation, and exhalation. The premise for many of these techniques involves opening up your body and using imagery to prepare yourself for the birth of your baby. Visual imagery involves imagining your cervix as an ever-widening circle of ripples on a still pond or as a flower bud opening up.

Medications

The type of medication used to manage your labor depends on your personal preferences, in combination with how your labor is progressing. Everyone experiences labor differently and no two women are the same. Even though you might have made the decision prior to labor about your pain relief preference, the circumstances of your experience may make it necessary to change your plan. There is no reason to be a superhero and endure the pain when the relief is available to you, just for the asking.

Below is a list of the most common pain relievers used during labor.

Analgesics and Narcotics: The most common pain-relieving medications used during labor are meperidine (Demerol), nalbuphine (Nubain), fentanyl (Sublimaze), and butorphanol (Stadol).

These medications can be given at any time during labor, but they are usually given early when you are less than 7 centimeters dilated. Most practitioners prefer not to give these medications just before the baby comes out because they have a tendency to make the baby sleepy.

These medications are given either as an intravenous drip or as an intramuscular injection into your buttocks or thigh. Even though they will help to diminish your discomfort, they will not stop your ability to push. Typically, the effects of these medications last anywhere from two to six hours. Their main disadvantage is a tendency to make you feel a bit drowsy.

Epidural (Regional): Epidural anesthesia is the pain reliever chosen by about two-thirds of women in labor. Before you are given your epidural, the staff will begin an intravenous infusion to provide you with extra fluid. An epidural is sometimes called regional anesthesia, because it numbs only a specific portion of the body. It is usually given when you are at least 3 centimeters dilated. The injection is given into the membrane surrounding your spinal cord (dura) and the epidural catheter is left in place so the anesthesiologist can give you more medication if you happen to need it.

Epidurals are very safe and effective. In rare cases, some women experience what is called a spinal headache after receiving an epidural. This is due to a small leakage of cerebral spinal fluid. If you experience a small spinal headache, you will be given analgesics and be advised to rest.

Spinal Block (Regional): This regional block is commonly used for cesarean delivery. It is usually given in a single dose just before your delivery. Unlike the epidural catheter, the needle is removed immediately after the medication is given. Similar to the epidural, it is injected into the spinal fluid around the spinal cord. It takes only a few seconds to work and lasts for about two hours. Similar to the epidural, some women may experience a spinal headache with a spinal block. However, this is extremely rare because the needle is so much smaller than the one used for an epidural.

Paracervical Nerve Block: A paracervical nerve block is a local anesthetic injected through the vagina and into the cervical nerves to decrease the pain of cervical dilation. It is rarely used today.

Pudendal Nerve Block: A pudendal nerve block is used for vaginal deliveries. It involves the insertion of a medication into the wall of the vagina to decrease pain during the second stage of labor. It may be used if you are having a forceps delivery, vacuum delivery, or an episiotomy and usually lasts from a few minutes to an hour. The main disadvantage of this medication is that it may hinder your ability to push during labor.

Early Baby Care

The birth of your baby will be one of the most magical moments of your life. If your baby does not need immediate emergency care, the healthcare providers will hand your baby to you just after birth. Your baby will then be dried off and kept warm by being wrapped in soft baby blankets. A hat will be immediately placed on your baby's head because babies lose heat through their heads.

After your initial contact with your baby, he or she will be taken for routine care, such as the application of eye ointment to prevent infection and a vitamin K shot to ensure normal blood coagulation. These should both be done during the first hour after birth. In the United States, these two procedures are required by law.

Newborns are usually quite alert during the first hour of life, and if you plan to breast-feed, most hospital staff will try to give you your baby to nurse so he or she can get the valuable nutrients provided by your colostrum, the thin, yellow liquid that precedes your breast milk. When your baby is latched on properly, his or her lips will pout out and cover nearly your entire areola. This is an amazing feeling; some mothers describe it as feeling like a suction cup on your nipple. If your baby has difficulty latching on, it sometimes helps to change positions. The three most common positions for nursing are the cradle position, side-lying position, and the football hold. If you still have trouble getting your baby to latch on after changing positions, you might want to ask for the assistance of a lactation specialist.

Keep in mind that for some women breast-feeding comes easy, but others experience frustration, cracked nipples, clogged nipples, or an infection. If you fall into this category, be sure to solicit the assistance of your lactation specialist; they will have ideas to help you overcome the difficulties.

Screening Tests

There are certain screening tests that are routinely done on all newborns. Many abnormalities may be detected by a small blood sampling taken from either the baby's arm or a tiny cut in its heel. Below are some of the disorders that may be detected in the newborn's blood in the early hours of life.

Cystic Fibrosis: This genetic disorder causes the body to produce abnormally thick mucous secretions affecting mainly the pulmonary and gastrointestinal tracts. If detected early, children can live long and have a good quality of life.

Phenylketonuria (PKU): This test is done to ensure that your baby does not have the genetic disease that results in retaining excessive amounts of PKU. An excess amount of PKU can affect normal brain development. This condition is a rare genetic disease.

Congenital Hypothyroidism: This test is done to detect if your baby has a thyroid hormone deficiency that could slow down both the baby's growth and development. If untreated, it can lead to mental retardation.

Galactosemia: All newborns are tested for galactosemia. If this deficiency is detected, the newborn will be unable to metabolize galactose, which is a sugar found in milk.

Homocystinuria: Homocystinuria is a condition caused by an enzyme deficiency. If detected in the newborn, it can lead to eye problems, mental retardation, and skeletal abnormalities.

Sickle-Cell Disease: This inherited disorder causes the cells to change shape or to sickle during stressful times, such as during infection or low oxygen levels. This makes it difficult for the red blood cells to move through the body.

Medium-Chain Acyl-CoA Dehydrogenase (MCAD) Deficiency: This rare hereditary disease is caused by the lack of this enzyme, which is needed to convert fat to energy.

Biotinidase Deficiency: The neonatal blood test checks for the lack of the enzyme biotinidase, which is necessary for the body to use and recycle the B vitamin, biotin. With early diagnosis and treatment, the effects of the disease can be prevented.

Circumcision

Circumcision is the surgical removal of the foreskin of a boy's penis. Today, most American families consent to have their sons circumcised in the hospital setting within the first few days of life. According to the National Hospital Discharge Survey, circumcision was performed on 56.1 percent of all newborn boys in the United States in 2006. The decision to circumcise is a personal one and depends on the parents' values.

The procedure is performed either by the obstetrician, pediatrician, or nurse-midwife. In religious Jewish families, it is usually performed by the rabbi at home on the eighth day of life in a special ceremony. The procedure is performed in the presence of close family and friends, and the event is called a *bris*.

A circumcision takes about five or ten minutes to perform. Analgesics should always be used during the procedure. Sometimes a cream is used or more commonly, a local analgesic may be injected into the area. After the circumcision is completed, Vaseline will be applied to the penis so that the diaper does not irritate or cause friction to the surgical site. Complications from a circumcision are rare but may include infection and bleeding.

Many believe that circumcisions should be performed for both cosmetic and hygienic reasons. Studies have shown that the advantages of having a circumcision include prevention of urinary tract infections in newborns, a decrease in cervical cancer for future sexual partners, a decrease in penile cancer in adult men, and it may decrease the spread of sexually transmitted diseases, particularly HIV and HPV.

In 2005 the American Association of Pediatrics declared that "existing scientific evidence demonstrates potential medical benefits of newborn male circumcision; however, these data are not sufficient to recommend routine neonatal circumcision. In circumstances where there are potential benefits and risks, yet the procedure is not essential to the child's current well-being, parents should determine what is in the best interest of the child. To make an informed choice, parents of male infants should be given accurate and unbiased information and be provided the opportunity to discuss this decision. If a decision for circumcision is made, procedural analgesia should be provided."

Cord Blood Banking

The umbilical cord blood is the blood that remains in the umbilical cord and placenta after your baby is born. Usually this blood is discarded. However, this cord blood has an abundance of stem cells that can potentially contribute to the development of the body's tissues, organs, and systems.

Some couples decide to bank their baby's blood as a type of insurance because it can be used to treat certain future diseases of the child itself, or those of a parent or sibling. Some families may choose to save the blood and then donate the sample to a blood bank or possibly another family. If you decide to bank your baby's cord blood, this blood is saved in a banking site outside the hospital.

Retrieving the cord blood is simple, safe, and painless, and is done in less than five minutes. The cost of cord blood banking ranges from $900 to $2,100.

For more information, you should check with the American Association of Blood Banks at (866) 384-0476.

Postpartum

Although you will be delighted that your pregnancy, labor, and delivery are behind you, the postpartum time can be both trying and tiring. You will probably have some aches and pains and generally feel exhausted. It is important for you to give yourself time to get into your baby routine and be patient about watching the slow return of your energy.

Six weeks after your baby is born, your practitioner will ask you to make an appointment for an office visit. During this visit, he or she will examine your breasts and also do a pelvic exam to make sure that everything has returned to normal. If you are due for your annual Pap smear, it will also be performed at this time. This is also a good time to discuss any issues about contraception. You might also want to talk about how you feel about having your new baby at home and any emotional issues you may be encountering. Remember to bring a list of questions, because sometimes in the commotion of the appointment you may forget the concerns you had at home.

Postpartum Survival Guide

- Be sure to get good nutrition and adequate rest. (You should sleep when the baby sleeps.)
- Identify and ask for the things you need.
- Arrange for lots of help from your mother, father, mother-in-law, sister, brother, friend, or doula. Allow yourself to be cared for while you and your partner attend to the baby.
- Accept and express both positive and negative feelings.
- Talk with your partner about the changes you are both going through.
- Ease into new routines—let the baby lead the way.
- Keep expectations realistic: Newborns "only" sleep, eat, and poop, but they do so every hour. It takes more time and energy than most people realize.
- Take time for yourself: a warm bath, a nature walk, a good book, meditation, listening to music, talking with a friend—whatever you find rejuvenating.
- Give yourself credit. Mothering is a difficult job, and it takes time to find your rhythm.
- Hook up with both new and experienced parents for support, guidance, and feedback.
- Where possible, postpone other major life changes, like moving or changing jobs.

(Source: ©2006 by Melisa M. Schuster, LMSW; (734) 302-0033; www.melisaschuster.com)

Postpartum Depression

Having a baby can bring on a range of powerful emotions for women. Even though the initial reaction is typically glee, some women may become depressed for the first time in their lives. The depression can range from mild to severe. It is important to understand what postpartum depression is, who gets it, and how it is diagnosed. It is also a good idea to understand other psychological events that may also be associated with the postpartum period, including postpartum obsessive-compulsive disorder, postpartum panic disorder, postpartum posttraumatic stress syndrome, postpartum bipolar disorder, and postpartum psychosis.

What Is Postpartum Depression?

[The following section is adapted from an essay by Pec Indman, EdD, MFT.]

Often the term *postpartum depression* (PPD) is used to describe mood and anxiety disorders that occur within the first year after a baby is born. There are five postpartum mood/anxiety disorders. Postpartum depression is the most common.

The *baby blues* occurs in up to 80 percent of new moms. This is a *normal* response to the hormonal changes, the sleep deprivation, and adjustments that occur immediately after birth. We don't consider the blues to be a mood disorder. The blues usually begins around day three postpartum, and should be gone within two to three weeks. With the blues, mood is up and down, and women sometimes find themselves bursting into tears for no reason. But overall, there is a positive outlook. It differs from postpartum depression in timing (only occurring in the first three weeks) and severity (it is mild and goes away without treatment).

Postpartum depression occurs in 15 to 20 percent of all new moms. Many have a stereotype of a depressed person being curled up in a ball with the blanket pulled up over her head, crying. That's not really how it looks for most women with postpartum depression. What new mother has the time to hide in bed? Some call it postpartum depression/anxiety because many women experience both depression and anxiety.

Who Gets Postpartum Depression?

Women who have a history (or family history) of depression or anxiety, a previous incident of postpartum depression, a history of abuse, depression during pregnancy, marital/relationship problems or social isolation; women who have a sick baby; and teenage moms are all at an increased risk of postpartum depression. Women who have severe mood changes before their periods or while taking the birth control pill are also at an increased risk of developing postpartum depression.

Postpartum depression can begin at the birth of the baby, or it can occur at any time within the first year of the baby's birth. Sometimes sudden weaning or a first menstrual period can trigger its onset.

Diagnosing Postpartum Depression

The signs and symptoms of postpartum depression vary from woman to woman. Here are some of the most commonly seen symptoms:

- sadness (sometimes comes in waves—women feel "up and down")
- guilt (often women feel like they aren't good moms)
- irritability; less patient than normal
- sleep problems (difficulty falling asleep or staying asleep)
- appetite changes (may eat more or less than usual)
- lack of feelings toward baby
- worrying about every little thing
- lack of fun or pleasure
- feeling overwhelmed or unable to cope
- lack of focus and concentration and difficulty making decisions

Postpartum Obsessive-Compulsive Disorder (OCD)

About 3 to 5 percent of new moms get postpartum obsessive-compulsive disorder. Women who have a history of OCD or a family history of OCD have a higher probability of getting OCD during their postpartum period. Women who describe themselves as "worriers" or "anal" (having a high need for order and things being "just right") also have an increased incidence of being obsessive-compulsive at this time.

The word *obsessive* refers to repetitive thoughts. *Compulsions* refer to the behaviors people do to avoid or minimize the anxiety produced by the obsessive thought. In the movie *As Good As It Gets*, Jack Nicholson portrayed a character with severe OCD.

During the postpartum period, some women get obsessively worried, often about things happening to their baby. Sometimes women have frightening thoughts or even mental pictures of something bad happening to their baby; often the pictures may be about the mom herself hurting the baby. These images or pictures can seem vivid and horrifying. Unlike women with psychosis, who are not in touch with reality, women who have these images during postpartum are typically in touch with reality. These women know they do not want to hurt their babies. Women with postpartum OCD are horrified, "How could I have these thoughts? I love my baby. I would never hurt her. I feel like a monster."

These thoughts or images may just pop into your mind and at times can be quite repetitive. Sometimes women have behaviors, or compulsions, that help them feel more secure. They may do things such as hide the kitchen knives or avoid being alone with the baby. If you show any of these symptoms, it is important to bring it to the attention of your physician.

Postpartum Panic Disorder

About 10 percent of new mothers experience panic disorder. Some have had panic attacks before and sometimes even during pregnancy.

Symptoms of postpartum panic disorder include episodes of extreme anxiety or worry, rapid heartbeat, tight chest or shortness of breath, choking feelings, dizziness, restlessness, and irritability. Panic attacks can happen without any specific triggers, even in the middle of the night. Many women in the middle of having an attack feel a sense of doom or that they are going to die. They also worry about when the next attack will occur.

Postpartum Posttraumatic Stress Disorder (PPTSD)

Posttraumatic stress disorder can occur after giving birth. PPTSD is seen in about 1 to 6 percent of women. Symptoms include recurrent nightmares, extreme anxiety, reliving past traumas, or avoidance of reminders of the trauma (for example, the hospital). Women with PPTSD often feel that they were abandoned, not well cared for, and stripped of their dignity during the birth process. Another common feeling is that their voices were not heard and that there was poor communication during the labor and/or delivery. Some women with PPTSD believe that their trust was betrayed; they feel a sense of powerlessness and lack of protection by their caregivers. If you feel any of these symptoms, make sure to bring it to the attention of your provider.

Postpartum Bipolar Disorder

Bipolar disorder is often incorrectly diagnosed as depression. It is not uncommon for those with bipolar disorder to suffer more than ten years with an incorrect diagnosis, and as a result receive inadequate treatment. Women taking medication for bipolar disorder are sometimes told by their physicians to stop taking their medication before getting pregnant. Some, but not all, medications used for bipolar treatment can cause birth defects. Unfortunately, up to 80 percent of women who stop their medication will have symptoms during their pregnancy. Postpartum bipolar disorder puts women at risk for a manic or psychotic episode. Women with bipolar disorder need to work closely with a psychiatrist trained in reproductive mental health. Sometimes medications are needed to treat postpartum bipolar disorder and their benefits usually outweigh their risks.

Symptoms of a postpartum bipolar episode can include a decreased need for sleep and severe and rapid mood swings. In many cases, the woman has a family history of bipolar disorder.

Postpartum Psychosis

Postpartum psychosis is considered a medical or psychiatric emergency. There is an increased risk of a woman hurting herself, her infant, or her other children. Symptoms of postpartum psychosis can include:

- difficulty relaxing
- incoherence
- decreased appetite
- paranoia and confusion
- difficulty sleeping
- hearing or seeing things others do not (hallucinations)
- inability to differentiate reality from hallucinations
- delusional thinking (lack of touch with reality)
- manic behavior (hyperactivity, impulsive behavior)

The symptoms listed above tend to come and go.

All of these postpartum mood disorders are treatable with medication and rarely go away without the assistance of medication. If a new mother is not well, the family is not well. We now know that untreated maternal illness can cause long-term consequences for the infant, as well as other children in the home. Postpartum mood disorders can also contribute to marital/relationship stress and discord.

Women who have any of the symptoms described in this section, should be aware that:

> *You are not alone.*
>
> *You are not to blame.*
>
> *You will be well again.*

It is important to seek treatment from someone trained specifically in postpartum depression and postpartum mood disorders. To learn how to screen a potential therapist, visit http://www.pecindman.com.

Some good resources include: Postpartum Support International at http://www.postpartum.net or call (800) 944-4PPD, and http://www.Med EdPPD.org.

Suggested Reading

Bennett, Shoshana, PhD, and Pec Indman, EdD, MFT. *Beyond The Blues, A Guide to Understanding and Treating Prenatal and Postpartum Depression.* California: Moodswings Press, 2006.

Misri, Shaila. *Pregnancy Blues: What Every Woman Needs to Know About Depression During Pregnancy.* New York: Delacorte Press, 2005.

Nonacs, Ruta. *A Deeper Shade of Blue: A Woman's Guide to Recognizing and Treating Depression in Her Childbearing Years.* New York: Simon & Schuster, 2006.

Journaling Corner

Now that you are in the last stages of your pregnancy, how do you feel about having a new baby?

If you have other children at home, how have you prepared them for your new arrival?

Describe how you knew that you were in labor and your initial reaction.

Write about your labor and any complications you had.

Describe the birth of your baby and the events in the labor and delivery room.

Cesarean Birth

Nothing is worth more
than this day. — J. W. VON GOETHE

During the first two decades of the twentieth century, delivery by cesarean section (C-section) made up 1 to 3 percent of all deliveries. In the 1930s, when hospitals became the primary birthplace, the number began increasing. From the mid-1960s to mid-1970s, the rate increased 12 to 20 percent annually. Current statistics indicate that the number may continue to rise. In North America, cesarean deliveries now account for approximately 27 percent of the 3.9 million babies born each year. In institutions specializing in high-risk pregnancies, the rate may be even higher.

Years ago, cesareans were performed only when the life of the mother or the child was in serious jeopardy. Today, cesareans are not exclusively emergency procedures—they are much more common and one of the reasons is the increased use of the nonreassuring fetal testing (fetal nonstress test), which alarms the physician that the baby might be in danger. Since the 1970s, the fetal monitor has been an invaluable tool in identifying fetal distress through monitoring of the baby's heart rate.

Because of the increase in cesarean births many children are born both alive and healthy. There has been a definite decrease in fetal mortality and a significant decrease in infant deaths.

Reasons for Cesarean Delivery

Below is a summary of the most common indications for cesarean birth:

- repeat cesarean due to previous surgery on the uterus
- placenta previa, to prevent excessive maternal bleeding that may affect the fetus
- abruptio placenta, to prevent rapid blood and oxygen loss to the baby as a result of the placenta separating

- herpes infection, to prevent passing it on to the baby through the birth canal

- severe preeclampsia, to prevent fetal complications

- nonreassuring fetal tests detecting problems

- abnormal fetal position, such as breech or transverse presentation, making it impossible for the baby to pass through the birth canal

- diabetic mother, if the disease results in a very large baby or poor blood flow to the placenta

- prolapsed cord, to prevent loss of oxygen to the baby

- cephalopelvic disproportion (CPD), if the baby's head is too large to pass through the birth canal

- failure of labor to progress or if oxytocin has not been effective

- problems with forceps or vacuum delivery

Emergency Cesareans

Whether you are a high-risk mother or not, it is a good idea to be prepared for the possibility of having a cesarean, because surprises can occur. Emergency cesareans are done only after a definitive diagnosis is made. A woman will have an emergency cesarean if there is pelvic disproportion (the baby is too big to fit through the birth canal), fetal distress (e.g., due to the umbilical cord wrapping around the fetus's neck, placental insufficiency, low oxygen, or infection), maternal distress, such as abruptio placenta, maternal heart problems, or preeclampsia. Although time will be of the essence, it is important that you ask for a brief explanation for the surgery. It is also your prerogative to request a second opinion.

One second-time mother talks about how easy her first delivery was and how her second was high-risk right from the beginning:

"In addition to being diagnosed with gestational diabetes, my baby was in distress when I was in labor. I was on the fetal monitor, and after twelve hours of labor, meconium was found in the amniotic fluid and my baby's heart rate dropped whenever I had a contraction. Changing positions did not alter his status. The fact that my baby's cord was around his neck made my entire delivery an emergency situation. Before I knew it I was being shaved for a cesarean.

I just was not prepared for it. No one ever mentioned the chances of me having a cesarean, especially since the labor with my daughter went so well."

Risks of Cesareans

Cesareans are much safer now than they were in the past. Today, there is a better understanding of anesthesia and postoperative recovery. The percentage of women who have complications as a result of cesarean delivery is low in comparison to the number of healthy mothers and babies undergoing the procedure. You should be aware of some possible complications, including infection, peritonitis (an inflammation of the membrane covering the abdominal wall), urinary-tract infection, and side effects from anesthesia. Pneumonia and thromboembolism (a blocked blood vessel due to a blood clot) are other problems that rarely occur today thanks to early mobilization following surgery and the increased number of cesareans performed under epidural anesthesia instead of general anesthesia.

Hemorrhage from a cesarean is rare today, but it is a risk that accompanies any operation and if this happens, you will need a blood transfusion. The uterus has numerous blood vessels and is particularly susceptible to hemorrhage. In the past, hemorrhage was frequently fatal. In large hospital centers today, though, hemorrhage is usually effectively treated with medications and intravenous therapy. The chance of uterine hemorrhage is one of the major reasons home deliveries are not recommended.

Repeat Cesareans

Having had a cesarean once does not necessarily mean you will always have to have a cesarean. The need for subsequent cesareans will depend on the reason for the first one. If, for example, you had a cesarean because of a small pelvis, chances are that your second pregnancy will also be a cesarean. If you had a cesarean because your baby was in a breech position and your second baby is not, then you may be able to have a normal vaginal delivery. The American College of Obstetricians and Gynecologists (ACOG) estimates that one in three of all cesareans are repeat cesareans.

Following a previous cesarean, some physicians allow a trial vaginal labor, but often this remains a matter of professional judgment. Other practitioners may opt for a repeat cesarean birth because of the potential of a ruptured uterus or old incision, particularly if labor is going on for too long. However, the risk of these problems is very low during trial labor—between 0.5 and 1.5 percent for women who have had a previous low transverse incision. Trial labor is a personal and professional decision to be made by the physician and the woman. You should discuss it with your physician early in your pregnancy.

In 1998 the ACOG developed guidelines for vaginal delivery after a previous cesarean. Some of the conditions recommended for considering a trial vaginal labor include the following:

- women who have had one prior low transverse incision from previous cesareans
- women with a clinically adequate pelvis (size)
- women who want a normal labor and delivery
- women with no other uterine scars or previous rupture
- a physician readily available throughout labor who is capable of monitoring labor and performing an emergency cesarean delivery
- the availability of anesthesia and personnel for emergency cesarean delivery
- the availability of a physician who is capable of evaluating labor and performing a cesarean

Most practitioners believe that if you have had two or more cesarean deliveries, your next baby should also be delivered by cesarean.

Vaginal Birth after Cesarean (VBAC)

If you had one cesarean, you can discuss the possibility of a vaginal birth after cesarean (VBAC) for your second pregnancy. You should make your desires known, and your practitioner should share a similar philosophy. Keep in mind, however, that there is a chance you will need to have an emergency cesarean. It is estimated that 60 to 80 percent of VBACs result in successful vaginal births. The advantages include a decreased chance of needing a blood transfusion, fewer infections, easier recovery, and no increased overall risk to the baby.

Here are some questions to ask your physician:

- What are your feelings toward VBAC?

- What are my chances of having a VBAC?

- Will you permit me to have a trial labor? If no, why not?

- What percentage of your patients have had successful VBACs?

Before Your Cesarean

Surgery is scary. No two people handle surgery or recuperation the same way, so what is suggested here should not be considered gospel. Any questions should be directed to your health-care team.

Preoperative Preparation

If your cesarean is prearranged, you will most likely go to the hospital the morning of your surgery. In some hospitals you will be admitted to the unit that you will be in after your baby is born—the postpartum unit. Remember to request the same room after delivery. Some women prefer private rooms, while others prefer not to be alone. Some first-time mothers find it interesting to talk with other mothers in order to share experiences. Others may feel that having a baby is a private event and may prefer to be alone with their baby and family during visiting hours.

Before your cesarean, your blood will be drawn. Your nurse or physician should explain what to expect before, during, and after your surgery. After the explanation, your surgeon will ask you to sign a consent form. Many health-care providers have probably explained the procedure many times before, so do not be shy about asking questions. It is your body, and you have a right to know. Make sure to get the provider's name in case you have a question after he or she leaves. Keep a notepad and paper by your bed to write down questions that come to mind. One woman said that she never had questions during the explanation of the surgery. She remarks:

> "My questions always arose late at night when the lights were off and I was trying to fall asleep. Reaching over to the bedside table to my grab my pen and writing pad saved me the agony of trying to remember the questions the following morning."

Meeting the Anesthesiologist

Either the day before or the morning of your surgery, your anesthesiologist will visit and ask you many questions about your medical history, including your previous experiences with anesthesia. He or she will also give you a consent form to sign for permission to administer anesthesia during your surgery. The anesthesiologist is the person who helps make delivery less painful.

The Shave

Before your cesarean, you may have to face having part of your pubic and abdominal area shaved. Some centers no longer require shaving the genital area; however, if your center still requires it, it is not an ordeal. The total area that is shaved depends on your surgeon's preference and the institution's surgical protocol. Some physicians request that any hair visible when the woman is lying on her bed with her legs together should be shaved. Others still request complete pubic shaving, but most do not require shaving at all.

What—No Food?

The evening prior to your scheduled cesarean, you will be told not to eat or drink anything after midnight or for at least eight hours prior to your scheduled surgery time. This is to avoid the possibility of regurgitating and aspirating the contents of your stomach during surgery. The nurses may hang a sign outside your room or above your bed that says, "N.P.O." Do not worry, it is not a secret code among the staff—it stands for *non per os* (which is Latin for "not by mouth"). This is to remind the staff not to leave you drinks or food.

Intravenous Therapy

Some hospitals have a policy to administer an intravenous solution, sometimes called intravenous drip, the night before or the morning of surgery. The solution is usually placed in a vein in your lower arm. Request that it not be put in the arm that you write with. This fluid is usually sugar water, or saline water if you are a diabetic. The solution will nourish you in the absence of food. If your mouth gets dry, ask your nurse for glycerin or lemon swabs to help lubricate and freshen your mouth. Ice chips are not usually allowed. The anesthesiologist may insert another intravenous drip into your arm when you are in the operating room. This will be used in case you need additional medication during surgery.

The Morning of Your Cesarean

On the morning of your cesarean, your nurse will ask you a few questions, such as:

- When did you last drink?

- When did you last urinate?

- Did you sign your consent forms?

- Does your family know you are going for a cesarean? Where can they be reached?

- Do you have any valuable items that you want to check at the nursing station?

- Have you removed all your piercings?

You will also be asked if you are wearing contact lenses or nail polish or have any artificial parts, such as dentures. All artificial parts and nail polish must be removed. The operating room staff must be able to see the natural color of your nails to ensure that you have adequate blood flow. If you have ever seen cold, poorly oxygenated hands, you know how blue they can become!

More recently, hospital employees have been reminding patients to remove all of their body piercings, even if they are not in private parts. This is because electrical burns can occur when the jewelry is exposed to an electrical current during cauterization. Cauterization is sometimes used during surgery to reduce or stop bleeding.

Anesthesia

Your type of anesthesia will depend on the hospital's policies and your preference. Under general anesthesia, you will be completely asleep. This type of anesthesia is not used during labor because it slows down the entire process. Epidurals and spinal anesthesia are typically used in cesarean delivery. They provide numbness in the lower half of the body but will allow you to remain awake. Regional anesthesia is sometimes used in delivery, but not in cesareans.

Epidurals

Epidurals are given through a tiny catheter or tube placed in your lower back by a needle. An injection is made in the middle of the back and the catheter is moved into the epidural space, the space around the spinal column. The anesthetic is dripped in carefully measured doses. Epidurals numb the area immediately around the perineum and lower uterus, belly to toes. They take between five and thirty minutes to become effective. When your legs feel warm, this is usually the first sign that this block is working. It usually remains effective for forty-five to sixty minutes. During your surgery, the anesthesiologist may add more through the tubing that remains in your lower back.

Epidurals can be useful if you have respiratory problems because they reduce the workload of the lungs. They are also used for diabetics, because epidurals reduce the demands on the body's metabolism.

Spinal Anesthesia

Spinal anesthesia is used during delivery to anesthetize the entire birth area (from the stomach to the toes). The anesthesiologist injects a single injection into the subarachnoid space around the spinal column. The needle is then removed. This type of anesthesia lasts about two and a half hours, which is more than long enough to perform a cesarean section. Spinals stop labor and the ability to bear down. Some aftereffects include headache, stiff neck, and backache. Spinals are frequently used for cesarean delivery.

General Anesthesia

General anesthesia is usually used in emergency C-sections or in unusual situations. Ideally, you should not eat for six to eight hours prior to having general anesthesia; however, in the event of an emergency, these guidelines will need to be modified. Studies have shown that babies born to mothers who have general anesthesia tend to be temporarily lethargic after birth and do not respond as quickly as babies born under epidurals. However, being asleep during an operation has its positive side; you do not hear or see what is going on around you. For some, the sounds of the operating room and the talk of the staff may be frightening.

Epidurals/Spinals vs. General Anesthesia

Epidurals and spinals are generally quite safe and may have many advantages over general anesthesia. Being awake for the birth of your baby can be one of the most exciting moments in your life. Another advantage is that in most modern teaching institutions, your partner is allowed to be with you when you have had this type of anesthesia. For some women, this is a very important consideration. It is incredible how your partner can make a difference by comforting you and holding your hand. If your partner accompanies you into the operating room, he or she will usually be seated right beside you. There is usually a drape that conceals your lower body so that neither of you sees the actual surgery, although some eager partners may stand up on their toes to see the birth of the baby on the other side of the curtain.

Another advantage of having an epidural or spinal, otherwise known as regional anesthesia, is that you can control your own breathing, therefore minimizing any lung complications that are sometimes a side effect of general anesthesia.

The Surgery

Cesareans should be performed only in hospitals with adequate supplies, medications, anesthesia, antibiotics, and blood transfusion equipment. It is also critical that any surgical procedure is done under strict sterile conditions so that both mother and baby are not at risk of developing infection. After being washed and swabbed with a special antiseptic solution, your lower abdomen will be covered with surgical "drapes" or cloths. The only area that is exposed is the area where the incision will be.

While you are in the operating room, most hospital centers today will apply pneumatic compression boots to your feet to stimulate circulation and reduce your risk of developing blood clots or deep vein thrombosis. The most likely time to develop blood clots is during surgery, while you are lying completely still. The boots work by the continuous application of a pulsatile compression to the soles of your feet.

The preparation for the surgery and the suturing of your incision will take more time than the actual birth itself. It may take only five to ten minutes from the time the incision is made for your baby to be born and about forty-five minutes to suture the six or seven layers of incisions.

If you elected to be awake during your cesarean, the moment your baby is born is an amazing one. It is exciting to hear their first cry. The nurses will immediately suction your baby's nose and mouth with a fine mucus catheter. When the baby is breathing well, you or your partner will be able to hold your child. While you are holding your baby, the physician removes the placenta and you are sewn back together, layer by layer. You will then be transferred to the recovery room.

Your Incision

After receiving your anesthesia, when your abdomen is numb and when you are in a deep sleep, your obstetrician will begin the surgery. In order for your baby to be born, two incisions must be made: one on your uterus and one on your skin. The only sutures that are visible are those on the outer layer. Today, surgical staples are most commonly used; however, some centers may also use clamps and/or other adhesives.

There are two different types of incisions that can be made on the uterus and the skin: a vertical (or classical) incision and a transverse (or bikini) incision (see Figures 11.1 and 11.2). The transverse incision is performed down low, near your pubic hairline. Vertical incisions are done less frequently today. Typically, they are done in the following situations:

- in an emergency to remove the baby more quickly
- in the event of placenta previa

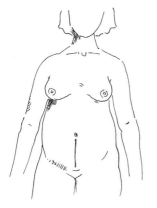
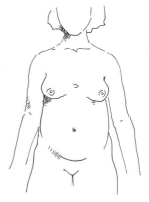

Figure 11.1: Vertical (classical) incision

Figure 11.2: Low transverse (bikini) incision

- in the event of premature delivery
- if you have a vertical incision from a prior cesarean

If your obstetrician decides to do a vertical incision on your uterus, you will be advised that for future pregnancies you have a repeat cesarean and not a VBAC, because these types of incisions are at more risk for reopening.

One of the primary concerns many women have is what their incision looks like. Today, cesarean incisions are smaller and less noticeable than they were years ago. More often than not, the incision is low, and is sometimes called a "bikini incision." As its name implies, you will be able to wear a bikini afterward without your scar showing.

After Your Cesarean

If the cesarean is your first experience with surgery, it might be frightening. It is a strange sensation to know that your skin will be cut and your insides exposed. If your cesarean is performed under emergency circumstances and you were prepared with prenatal classes, you may feel that all those hours of deep breathing and panting went down the drain. You may also feel a sense of disappointment and depression because you were unable to have a vaginal delivery. Some women find it very difficult to adapt to having given birth by cesarean and want to speak with other women who have had similar experiences. Local support groups can be sought out by speaking with the hospital's social worker or the nurses in your postpartum unit. For other women, these feelings of disappointment are less apparent, especially if getting pregnant was a problem.

The Recovery Room

You will likely be transferred to a recovery room while your baby goes to the nursery. In most centers, the babies are brought to the mother as soon as she is in the recovery room—usually within one hour after birth. La Leche League, for example, strongly advocates nursing as soon as possible after delivery. In some cases, if the woman is unable to hold her baby immediately, the husband or partner can be given the chance to get involved with the baby's immediate care. Many fathers feel great rewards by becoming involved.

In the recovery room or intensive care unit, the nurses will carefully monitor your vital signs, such as heart rate, breathing, temperature, and blood pressure. Your nurse will also check your lochia (vaginal discharge). Some women are surprised by how much bleeding they experience after a cesarean, although it is sometimes less than with a vaginal delivery. The bleeding may saturate about two to four sanitary pads. By about eight hours after delivery, it will seem like a normal menstrual flow.

The Exam

Your uterus may be very tender when touched, but the examination will not last long. The nurse will check to see if your uterus is contracting and returning to its original size. Oxytocin or its synthetic form, Pitocin, is sometimes given intravenously to help your uterus to contract. If it does not do so, this may be a sign of excessive bleeding.

The Urinary Catheter

Prior to going to the operating room, a urinary catheter will have been inserted into your bladder to monitor your urine output. This usually remains in place for anywhere from six to twelve hours after your cesarean. Initially the catheter is uncomfortable, and then it becomes more of a nuisance than anything else.

It may sting when you pass urine for the first time after the catheter is removed, so try not to be alarmed.

When Does the Anesthesia Wear Off?

If you had general anesthesia, you will probably sleep for a few hours in the recovery room after your baby is born. If you had an epidural, you will be awake but most likely drowsy. With epidurals, you are usually allowed to return to the postpartum unit when you are able to move your legs. They may seem numb and clumsy at first, but this is the first sign of the anesthesia wearing off. It is usually possible to move your legs about two hours after delivery, but this varies.

Deep Breathing and Coughing

Very soon after your cesarean you will be informed of the importance of deep breathing and coughing. This is especially important for women who have had general anesthesia. After lying in one position without moving for several hours, secretions will tend to accumulate in your lungs. Stagnant secretions are an ideal haven for bacterial growth, such as that which causes pneumonia.

"Huffing" is another way to loosen secretions in the lungs and may be more comfortable for you. Try exhaling forcefully through your mouth. Support your incision with your hand or a pillow during deep breathing and coughing exercises. Huffing should also make these important exercises more comfortable for you after your cesarean and in the weeks that follow. Deep breathing and coughing, walking, and drinking plenty of fluids are invaluable to help loosen unwanted secretions.

Pain and Discomfort

While in the recovery room, you will be given intravenous pain relievers. You may have two intravenous lines, one inserted before your cesarean and another one inserted by the anesthesiologist in the operating room. One is usually removed in the recovery room, the other a few days later when you are drinking and eating well. If your incision hurts, do not be shy about asking your nurse for a pain reliever.

Soon after your anesthesia wears off, you will start to feel your incision. It seems that every move you make is the wrong one. Some women have difficulty finding a comfortable position, and it may be tempting to not move at all—but do not do this, because it may increase your problems later. The most uncomfortable times are getting in and out of bed, and when you are doing your deep breathing and coughing exercises.

Since the first publication of this book, the use of patient-controlled analgesia (PCA) is available in some hospital settings. Basically, a PCA pump allows the new mother to self-administer pain medication intravenously as needed. Prior to having your cesarean, you will be told how to use this device. It is usually only needed for twenty-four hours following the delivery.

Eating and Drinking

Eating and drinking are not allowed until bowel function resumes, usually later in the day after delivery. Your abdomen will be examined with a stethoscope for sounds of bowel function. If sounds are heard, you will be able to drink and later to eat. Make sure to ask for glycerin swabs to relieve mouth dryness. Some hospitals will provide ice chips. Your first meal will be very light food—tea, clear broth, and/or Jell-O.

Gas Pains

Gas pains are common following cesarean birth because your bowel was manipulated during surgery in order to expose your uterus. Gas pains are usually worst on the third day after the cesarean, the time when bowel function returns to normal.

To relieve or reduce gas pains, lie on your left side and draw your knees against your chest; try breathing with your abdomen; try getting up and walking around. Sometimes hot liquids such as tea and broth might help relieve gas discomfort. One woman comments on gas pains:

> "They warned me about gas pains following my cesarean. They also told me that I should avoid gas-producing foods and carbonated beverages. It's funny, because one of the things that I found most soothing for my gas pains was ginger ale—I don't know if it was the ginger or the carbonation that was so soothing. All I know is that I drank an awful lot of it with great relief."

Getting Out of Bed

Most hospital units allow you to get out of bed after the anesthesia has completely worn off—about six or eight hours after your baby is born. In order to get your blood circulating, it is advised that you get out of bed, sooner rather than later. The first time you get out of your hospital bed, you may feel very uncomfortable. Two helpful tips are to ask for your pain reliever about half an hour before you get out of bed and to walk a little farther each time you get up. Remember, the more you lie still, the stiffer you become and the more uncomfortable it will be for you when you eventually start to move about. The first time you get out of bed, make sure that you have someone with you.

Everyone heals at different rates. You may feel wonderful one day and lousy the next. This is normal. Many women say that the third day after surgery is the most difficult; this is usually when the healing process begins. There are usually great improvements, however, the following day.

Breast-Feeding after a Cesarean

Whatever type of feeding method you choose for your baby, the fact that you had a cesarean should not interfere with your plans. During your last month of pregnancy, it is important to be fitted for a nursing bra and to bring this to the hospital with you. You can ask your nurse to bring your baby so you can breast-feed. If you are not up to it, do not feel guilty if you delay this first feeding.

Since the first edition of this book, the lactation consultant has joined the health-care team and is especially trained to assist mothers with many issues, including low milk production, latching difficulties, painful nursing, and inadequate weight gain. They are both teachers and counselors and can be a great resource for you.

If your hospital does not have one on staff, you may want to call the International Lactation Consultant Association for a referral. Their toll-free number is (800) 323-8750.

Positioning

Finding a comfortable nursing position is often a challenge following a cesarean delivery. It is normal to feel clumsy at first. Many women find lying in bed very uncomfortable and prefer to be seated in a chair with a pillow on their lap and the baby on top of the pillow. Others find holding the baby in a football hold with the baby's head cupped in their hand and feet directed toward their back, away from the abdomen, to be a comfortable position. Lying on your side may also be comfortable. Choosing a good breast-feeding position is a personal decision.

In most cases, you will be able to continue taking your pain relievers while breast-feeding, although some babies may become a bit drowsy as a result. If you need pain relievers, remind the hospital staff that you are nursing. Advil or Tylenol are good choices that will not interfere with breast-feeding and should not make you drowsy.

Recovery

Your recovery from a cesarean will depend on your individual recuperative powers, the type of anesthesia you were given, and the length of time you were in labor prior to your cesarean. One first-time mother who had general anesthesia says:

"I felt wiped out for so many days afterward that it took me a long time to get my feet on the ground. At the birth of my second child, I had an epidural, and, gee, what a world of difference! I was up and about that same evening. I felt alive and ready to begin mothering. If given a choice, I think all mothers should choose an epidural over general anesthesia. I didn't feel like I was hit over the head with a baseball bat."

Regardless of the type of anesthesia, the most difficult part about a cesarean is your personal recovery. Do not expect to go bouncing down the hall the same evening and be sitting in the lounge chatting with other mothers for hours on end. Avoid bringing stacks of books or knitting to the hospital, and do not plan on getting back to your daily swimming routine when you get home. Plan on being just a little more tired and maybe a little more irritable than usual. It is all normal. And remember the most important thing—it only gets better!

Going Home

Since the first edition of this book in the 1980s, it has become a federal law that following a cesarean, you must stay in the hospital for four days after your baby is born. Even if you feel better after three days, it is a good idea to stay and get the pampering and rest that you will need after surgery. If, however, you do request to go home after three days, a note will be made in your chart to that effect. Do not expect to be able to do too much right away at home. Your incision will be tender and you will be regaining your strength.

One mother who had twins by cesarean remarks:

"I had to learn to let the house go. I had the twins plus a twenty-month-old in diapers. My bed was unmade for the first six months. I actually spent the first month in the lazy chair with one twin breast-feeding and the other one at my feet. You just really have to take it in stride."

Lifting

It is recommended that you do not lift anything over 10 pounds for the first three weeks after your cesarean. If everything goes well, the usual recommended weight is under 10 pounds, and if you are lucky, that should include your baby! Try bending your knees when lifting your baby; this helps your legs do the lifting rather than your back or your abdomen. You will have more of a problem if there are other children at home. Your toddler may not understand why you can lift the baby and not him or her. He or she may show signs of regression. If you were also unable to lift your other children during pregnancy because of complications, there will not be much of a change, but if you did, you might have your hands full emotionally and physically. The best advice is to be patient and to try to get the toddler involved in the care of your new baby as much as possible. Ask him or her to do things like going to get a diaper or bringing the baby a toy. Like all of us, children love to feel needed.

If you can arrange to have help for the first few weeks, all the better. Some husbands or partners choose to take their vacation at this time, and it is a lovely way for the baby to start its first few weeks of life. One mother of a two-and-a-half-year-old came home to the same responsibilities she left behind. Her husband worked long, hard hours, and not only did she not have any family or professional help but she had a toddler, a baby, and a cesarean to contend with.

She comments:

> "People really don't understand what a cesarean birth involves. Mine was an emergency one and I was so naïve. I had no idea it would be like this. My attitude has changed now. Who cares if my house is messy or the laundry is not done? It is not humanly possible to do it all—my priorities have changed under the circumstances."

Climbing Stairs

If there are stairs leading to your bedroom, you will soon learn that they present a problem. If you have had a vertical incision, it is recommended that you do not climb stairs for one to two weeks. With a bikini incision, you can gradually do the stairs with assistance, taking one step at a time. Try slowly increasing your activity. Start going up and down once a day, then twice a day, and so on. The best advice is to listen to your body. If you have excruciating pain after activity, you are probably trying to do too much. Do not forget to ask your provider what is recommended, but in general, it is a good idea that for the first two or three weeks you economize on the number of times you go up and down the stairs.

Walking

If you have your baby during the warm weather, going out for walks can be refreshing for both of you. It will be a few weeks before you will be able to push a stroller, but you should make a habit of getting out each day. Mentally and physically, it is healthy for both you and your baby. Try walking a little bit farther each day; however, keep in mind that the more active you are, the more pain and bleeding you will have. If you are having a lot of pain, your body is telling you to slow down.

It takes about six weeks to fully recover from a cesarean. Sometimes it takes longer depending on the circumstances of your delivery. After that time, your incision is completely healed and you will safely be able to lift heavier objects. The six weeks pass very quickly, and before you know it you are well on your way to getting back into your normal routine—if there is such a thing for today's mother!

Journaling Corner

Was your cesarean expected or unexpected?

If your cesarean was unexpected, how did you handle it emotionally?

Describe your cesarean experience—how was the care, did it hurt, was your partner with you?

What was the most difficult part about having a cesarean? What advice would you give others who have to have a cesarean?

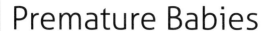

12 Premature Babies

Hope is the thing with feathers
That perches in the soul,
And sings the tune without the words,
And never stops at all,…

— EMILY DICKINSON

For those who have had a normal pregnancy, a premature baby may be an entirely unexpected event. For the high-risk mother, however, having a premature baby ("preemie") may have been a foreseen possibility from the beginning.

The experience of having a premature baby is not easy, whether or not you are prepared. Sometimes women find it difficult juggling their own needs, their baby's needs, and their family's needs. There may be sudden feelings of overwhelming responsibility and helplessness. These are all normal. The background information and tips on coping with a preemie offered in this chapter should take some mystery out of one of life's most intense moments.

What Is a Premature Baby?

A premature or preterm baby is one born prior to the end of the thirty-seventh week of gestation. In 2004, of the 4.1 million babies born in the United States, 12.5 percent were born prematurely.

A *small for gestational age* (SGA) baby is one that is smaller than average for its age. Unlike premature babies, SGA babies are well-formed and usually have fully developed internal systems, although there are often complications due to their small size.

Causes of Prematurity

It is not always possible to identify the reason that a baby was born prematurely. There simply may not be any more room inside the uterus for the baby to grow. Sometimes the baby is just ready to be born and therefore your water breaks.

Approximately 20 percent of preterm births occur because the health-care provider has decided to intervene by the induction of labor or with a cesarean delivery, due to either maternal or fetal problems or abnormalities. Examples include a woman who has poorly controlled diabetes or preeclampsia, or if the baby is very small and has had poor results from fetal testing, or if the mother has placenta previa.

The remaining 80 percent of preterm births are usually a result of one of the following reasons: early rupture of the membranes, infection, or unexplained preterm labor. A smaller group of babies are born prematurely as a result of maternal bleeding, abruptio placenta, or cervical insufficiency. There are also certain high-risk situations that may render you more susceptible to having a premature baby.

Multiple gestation is a common cause of premature labor, primarily because the uterus becomes overly distended and goes into labor. Approximately half of all multiple pregnancies end in preterm delivery.

Cervical insufficiency is a painless dilation of the cervix, and without a suture it will result in preterm delivery, sometimes in the second trimester. No contractions occur.

Certain environmental factors, such as an insufficient diet or a history of excessive smoking, drug, and alcohol use, may also result in your baby's early birth. Following an unsupervised weight-loss regime is never recommended during pregnancy. Women who are underweight or who weigh less than 100 pounds are at greater risk of having a premature baby. Alcoholic women often give birth to SGA infants, who may also be premature. Alcoholic women often have a poor diet; the direct consequences are fetal malnutrition and inadequate growth patterns. Women who receive little or no prenatal care may experience premature labor because of various undiagnosed complications.

Your baby's early arrival may be due to a combination of factors. It is normal to feel guilty and to ask yourself whether you did too much or if you did the wrong thing. Often what you imagine is worse than reality, so it is best to discuss your concerns with the professionals.

The Warning Signs

Ruptured membranes (breaking your water) occurs in approximately 20 to 30 percent of women experiencing premature labor. The most common signs and symptoms include a feeling of pressure and/or a thin mucus or blood discharge. However, premature labor is not always accompanied by warning signs. Many women are unsure that they are having a preterm birth, mainly because the symptoms are not as obvious. Some women notice a dull ache in their lower back and unusual sensations in their abdomen without experiencing any labor pains. You may find that you have mild abdominal discomfort similar to menstrual cramps. These may or may not be accompanied by abdominal pressure and diarrhea. If you have these symptoms or experience four to six Braxton Hicks contractions (painless contractions) in one hour that do not stop after rest, you should contact your physician.

Bleeding may occur as a result of abruptio placenta or placenta previa. In the former, the bleeding is due to the separation of the placenta from the uterus, which immediately deprives the baby of essential nutrients and oxygen. A cesarean may be necessary.

Once in the hospital, you will be monitored for contractions and your cervix will be checked for dilation. Today, most centers will check your cervical length by performing an ultrasound, in addition to also performing a fetal fibronectin test (see Chapter 7), to make sure that your baby is okay and that your water has not yet broken.

Your baby's health will also be evaluated using an electronic fetal monitor. Intravenous fluids or medications may be given to stop any contractions you may be having. It is possible that you will be sent home with medication and/or guidelines for restricted activity. If this happens to you, it is important for you to monitor your contractions at home. At 36 weeks, most women are instructed to stop taking any anticontraction medications and to resume their normal activities.

Characteristics of Prematurity

Obviously, the premature baby is at higher risk than the full-term baby. The sort of problems your baby may have depends on the extent of the prematurity and how advanced he or she is in their development. Most providers will try to keep your baby inside of you for as long as possible without risking your life or your baby's life. Your baby will mature better there than anywhere else—you are the best incubator.

Remember that each baby reacts differently to the stress of being born too early. Most important, remember that each baby has its own set of problems. Be fair to yourself and to your baby, and do not attempt to compare your baby to the baby in the next crib.

Appearance

Physically, the premature baby looks different from the full-term baby. The baby's skin will be very wrinkled, like that of an old person. Your baby's head will seem large in proportion to the rest of his or her body, and the arms and legs will be mere slender additions to a tiny body. Since there is little fat on the body of premature babies, they have difficulty maintaining their temperature. In the premature nursery, you may notice your baby being placed into a radiant warmer or incubator to keep him or her warm.

Preemies are also relatively inactive and may appear limp at times. This may be nature's way of conserving their energy for growth and development. In general, they sleep more in their early stages of life—sleeping is as important as eating for them. It is also common for preemies to be both restless and somewhat irritable. Your baby will probably respond when he or she hears your voice and sees you in front of him or her. Speaking and cuddling are very important at this time.

Your baby's needs are similar to yours. He or she needs to breathe, be warm, eat, drink, urinate, have bowel movements, and be loved. Any interruption or interference with any of these needs may present a problem for your little one.

Respiratory and Circulatory Systems

Because the lungs and respiratory muscles of premature babies are not adequately developed, your baby may have difficulty breathing on his or her own. Production of surfactant, the chemical that reduces the surface tension within the lungs, is necessary for babies to expand their lungs and breathe on their own. Under normal circumstances, the fetus produces this chemical by the twenty-eighth week of gestation, but only in sufficient quantities by around the thirty-fourth week. If premature delivery is anticipated, you may be given several doses of betamethasone, a corticosteroid that will help to promote your baby's lung maturity.

Since the original publication of this book in the 1980s, some institutions have been giving babies a form of therapy after birth to promote lung maturity and prevent respiratory distress syndrome (RDS). Surfactant is a substance that might be given in the form of a fine mist administered by mask or respirator. As the infant breathes, this mist enters the lungs.

Lung Maturity: During pregnancy your lungs breathe for both you and your baby. Your baby's lungs are basically not used. There is a short blood vessel called the ductus arteriosus that directs the blood away from the baby's lungs. In order for this vessel to remain open, a chemical called prostaglandin E circulates in the baby's blood. Normally, within twenty-four hours of birth this chemical decreases sharply, causing the ductus arteriosus to close. Once this happens, the baby's lungs are able to function on their own.

Sometimes in the preemie, the levels of this chemical do not decrease, and therefore, the ductus arteriosus remains open. This can result in a baby who is having respiratory and circulatory problems.

Heart Murmurs: If the ductus arteriosus is open and the blood flow becomes turbulent, your baby may have what is called a *heart murmur.* A murmur is like the sound heard when there is an obstruction in a quietly flowing stream. Heart murmurs occur quite commonly in the preemie and are often caused by this open duct. The duct usually closes as the baby matures; however, in some instances, treatment may involve giving oxygen or medications to slow down the production of prostaglandin E. In rarer cases surgery may be necessary.

Irregular Breathing: Irregular breathing is common among preemies. You may notice that your baby takes many short breaths, then a long breath, and then rests for a few seconds. Although this may be scary for you, as your baby's lungs mature, he or she will outgrow this type of breathing pattern. In the hospital, the staff will carefully monitor your baby's breathing patterns by observing the chest movements and counting the number of breaths per minute. The hospital staff will also detect whether your baby's breathing pattern is regular, labored, deep, or shallow. A special monitor may be used to identify a change of pattern in your baby's breathing.

Respiratory Distress Syndrome (RDS): Respiratory distress syndrome sometimes occurs when a baby is born early and the lungs have not yet produced surfactant. If time allows, you may be given steroids at least twenty-four hours prior to delivery in order to decrease the chance of RDS. In any event, immediately after birth, your baby will be given surfactant directly into the endotracheal tube leading into his or her lungs.

RDS is successfully treated with oxygen therapy, humidity, and sometimes medications. Sometimes a baby will need to be put on a respirator. Another special machine sometimes used to help your baby breathe is called a CPAP (continuous positive airway pressure). This can be administered in one of two ways—with nasal prongs (small tube in the nose) or with an endotracheal tube (through the mouth), which is then connected to a ventilator. This keeps positive pressure in the baby's lungs by never allowing the lungs to completely collapse.

Apnea: Apnea means not breathing. Because of an immature system, the premature baby sometimes forgets to breathe. This occurs in approximately one-third of babies born prior to the thirty-second week. Preemies who are at risk are monitored with special devices that sound an alarm to the nurses if they stop breathing. The nurse then stimulates the baby by tickling his or her feet, legs, or tummy, and this is usually enough stimulation to start the baby's breathing once again. Being present during one of these episodes may be frightening, but you should be confident that your baby is receiving the special care he or she needs. Your physician or nurse will tell you what to do should this happen when you go home.

Excessive Mucus: Excessive accumulation of mucus in the mouth and lungs is common in premature babies. If born prior to thirty-four weeks, the baby does not have an adequate cough reflex to remove the extra saliva that normally accumulates in the mouth. Eventually these secretions may enter the lungs, resulting in breathing difficulties and/or lung infections.

In certain instances, it may be necessary for a nurse to remove these secretions by suctioning, using a soft, thin tube passed through your baby's mouth into the throat. It can be disturbing for you to see your baby uncomfortable for a few moments, but the benefits of this procedure outweigh the consequences of not removing the secretions.

Jaundice: Jaundice is a yellowish discoloration of the skin and eyes that is caused by an accumulation of bilirubin in the bloodstream. Bilirubin is the normal end product when old red blood cells break down. In the mature system, the liver is responsible for removing this pigment, but in the newborn, the liver has difficulty ridding the body of all the bilirubin in the usual manner. More than 50 percent of newborns develop some jaundice, usually when they are a few days old. If your baby has excess bilirubin in his or her system, their skin will appear yellowish.

The bilirubin level is determined by taking blood samples from your baby's heel. Mild jaundice usually does not require treatment. If the levels are more elevated, your baby's jaundice may be treated with light therapy, intravenous antibodies, and, in rarer cases, with a blood transfusion. Your practitioner may also recommend feeding your baby more frequently. This increases the chance of the excessive bilirubin to be excreted in the stools. While any of these treatments are being initiated, be prepared for your baby to have loose, green stools.

If left untreated, high levels of bilirubin can lead to kernicterus, which is a rare form of damage to the brain centers of newborns. Today, this condition is uncommon because as soon as jaundice is detected, the baby will immediately be placed under light therapy to resolve the problem.

Anemia: Anemia is a deficiency of hemoglobin, the pigment found in red blood cells responsible for carrying oxygen throughout the body. The preemie often has fewer red blood cells than normal. If your baby is anemic, you may find that he or she is paler than usual. A blood test confirms anemia.

Anemia is treated with a transfusion of red blood cells that have been specially screened for HIV, hepatitis, and CMV. Your baby's blood type was determined at birth, and so immediate transfusion will be possible. Some very small babies may need more than one transfusion. You may find that following a blood transfusion, your baby becomes more alert and energetic, in addition to having a better appetite and better color.

Some preemies are discharged from the hospital with a prescription for iron supplements. These may cause your baby to be constipated and have dark stools. Speak with your neonatologist or pediatrician about what they recommend for constipation.

Digestive System

The digestive system in the preemie is also immature. You will notice when you feed your baby that you must do so very slowly, because the baby's stomach is very small. This is why frequent small feedings are often recommended.

Because of their immature systems, many preemies do not digest their food properly. This may cause them to have a distended abdomen. Spitting up, or regurgitation, is also common because of the immature swallowing reflex. Holding preemies in the upright position after feedings or elevating the head of the mattress and putting them on their stomach or left side in their crib will help prevent them from aspirating these secretions into the lungs, and it also decreases the gastric emptying time.

It is normal for a newborn to lose a few pounds during the first few weeks of life. This weight loss may last longer in the preemie. The preemie is usually maintained on intravenous solutions for a while and then is gavage fed (see below).

Feeding Problems: Feeding difficulties are probably among the most disturbing problems for parents visiting their newborn in the nursery. It may be frustrating for you when your little one either stops sucking or falls asleep while feeding. Eating is very tiring for your baby, and often feeding is done when the baby awakens by itself (demand feeding) so that your baby can get all the sleep he or she needs. Preemies, in general, are not demand feeders; however, they will not tell you when they are hungry. So in the beginning, feedings are usually given on a standard schedule. Do not be surprised if your baby falls asleep after or during feedings or if he or she has difficulty breathing after feeding.

One father comments:

> "I vividly remember feeding our daughter the first week of life when
> my wife was recovering from her cesarean. Sometimes I would go to
> my daughter's bassinet, change her, and pick her up, and she would
> still be asleep. My daughter had so little energy that the only way I
> could keep her awake during feeding time was undressing her and
> tickling her feet. Giving her 1 ounce of milk was a major task."

If preemies are born prior to thirty-three weeks of gestation, their sucking reflex will not have been adequately developed. They will therefore be given gavage feedings, which are formula or breast-milk feedings given through a tube passing through their nose or mouth into their stomach. This tube may be left in place continuously or taken out and replaced intermittently. The tube will not be uncomfortable for them because some preemies do not yet have a gag reflex (depends on the degree of prematurity). Tube-fed babies are usually given pacifiers to suck on while being fed, so that they learn to associate sucking with feeding. An intravenous solution may also be inserted through a vein to provide extra fluids and as a means of giving them any necessary medications.

Coordination of sucking and swallowing slowly begins to occur after the thirty-second week, but you may find that your little one continues to struggle until the thirty-fourth week. Some babies tolerate less food than others.

Necrotizing Enterocolitis: This rare inflammation, or swelling, in a section of the baby's bowel causes the baby's abdomen to become swollen. The condition usually requires surgery. It is most common in infants weighing less than 4½ pounds. The cause is unknown. The baby may have symptoms such as a distended, shiny abdomen, vomiting, and blood in the stool, sometimes accompanied by diarrhea. Successful treatment for this condition involves antibiotics and maintenance of adequate nutrition through intravenous therapy.

Breast-Feeding Your Preemie

Before your baby is born, you will have probably decided on your preferred feeding method. Breast-feeding provides a special emotional bond for mother and baby, thus making it a desirable feeding method. In addition, babies tend to tolerate breast milk more easily than formula, and even more important, breast milk contains special antibodies that help newborns fight infection, which is particularly helpful for the premature baby. Mother's milk also contains extra calories, proteins, and vitamins necessary for the baby's growth.

It is a good idea to speak with your lactation specialist or your La Leche League representative about the best plan for your and your baby. Some babies may not be ready to breast-feed while they are in the hospital. Whether your baby is ready and able to breast-feed will depend upon his or her gestational age and both your own and your baby's health status. For the most part, babies use more of their own energy to breast-feed. If your baby is too immature to suck on a bottle, many neonatal intensive care units (NICU) will keep your pumped breast milk in the refrigerator and feed the baby through a gastrointestinal tube. Your baby will most likely be fed every one to three hours.

Keep in mind that most babies do not develop the suck-swallow-breathe reflex until they are at about thirty-two weeks gestation. If your baby was born after this time, then chances are he or she will be mature enough to breast-feed. In any case, it is best to begin as early as possible.

Because of their immature systems and reflexes, breast-feeding the preemie will take a lot of persistence and consistency on your part. Finding the best position for breast-feeding is often challenging with the premature baby. You should have your nurse or lactation specialist help you with this. When starting to breast-feed, it is usually advised that you do so frequently, because the feeding sessions will probably be quite short. Typically, the preemie tires easily and does not take a lot of milk with each feeding.

Most authorities recommend feeding preemies at least every three hours, but maybe more frequently. It is important to be alert to their cues, and if they are hungrier more often, you should not hesitate to feed them. Some say that if the baby is awake it might be a cue that he or she is hungry. Other babies might show hunger by becoming fussy, smacking their lips, or trying to put their hands or fingers into their mouths.

My daughter, Rachel, was born one month early and I remember the biggest hurdle we had was that she fell asleep during her feedings. We would have to unwrap her and tickle her toes to get her to suck. Sometimes all she wanted to do was sleep and often after each feeding, I would be left with a lot of milk. Today, many centers recommend that you pump after each feeding in order to keep your milk production flowing.

When this book was initially published in the 1980s, my nurse suggested I use the manual pumping method, although the mechanical ones were also available. Today, however, it is more common to use a hospital-grade pump with a double collection kit. These pumps can be rented once you go home.

Careful hand and breast washing before you breast-feed or pump your breasts cannot be overemphasized. Prior to nursing, it is also important to massage your breasts. This is done by starting at the top, and pressing firmly on your chest wall while moving your fingers in a circular motion. This is best done all over the breast. Massaging helps to increase milk flow and relieve any problems with engorgement. Before beginning to massage, you can put warm washcloths on your breasts to relax them.

If you have chosen not to breast-feed your baby or if for some medical reason you are unable to do so, it is still important that you maintain skin-to-skin contact with your baby and hold him or her close to you as much as possible, particularly by using the kangaroo care hold, which is described later in this chapter.

Tips on Breast-Feeding Preemies

- Try to keep your baby nearby and feed him or her immediately after he or she awakens.
- Try keeping the drowsy baby awake by unwrapping some clothes, rubbing the soles of the feet, or stroking the throat under the chin.
- Nurse the baby before he or she becomes too hungry. The hungrier they are, the less patience they have for nursing.
- Express some milk before initiating nursing so that the baby can smell the milk.
- Apply warm compresses to the breast prior to feeding to stimulate milk flow.
- Ask your lactation specialist if you should use a breast shield.
- Give the bottle only after nursing. If that does not work because the baby is very hungry, offer a little bit before nursing to calm the stomach, and then nurse.
- Wean the baby from the bottle as soon as possible.
- Ask about using herbal preparations such as Brewer's yeast, fenugreek, or other herbs to increase milk flow.
- Join a support group or speak to other mothers of preemies to share ideas and concerns.

Your Emotions

Life with a premature baby is filled with feelings of fear and uncertainty and a sense of urgency. At times you will feel hopeless and helpless. You may find that during these times, your emotions fluctuate and it may be difficult to absorb all the information being given to you. Being a parent of a premature baby brings moments of tribulations and opportunities, usually in a different way than being a parent of a term baby. You will experience an avalanche of both positive and negative moments and feelings. You learn to take each minute and each day one at a time. You often wonder if your baby will survive. A baby's health status can change for better or worse within moments, as you will quickly learn.

One woman comments:

> "After the early birth of my baby at seven months, I really felt as if I had failed. I had a history of one stillbirth and felt like I was failing again. I really felt incapable of taking care of my daughter. Breast-feeding her in the nursery made me feel like I was contributing to her care. I believed it was so important to let her know that we loved her. I stayed in the nursery all day and my husband stayed there all night. At times the staff took it personally, thinking that we didn't have confidence in their care—but I really felt that it was the right thing to do. We felt she really needed us."

It is normal for you to go through a series of grief reactions following the birth of your preemie. You might think about the perfect baby you imagined during your pregnancy or you might have feelings of guilt for having borne a child one step short of "perfect." Some parents may feel depressed and even erroneously and prematurely begin planning for a life of rearing a child with a disability.

Having a baby in the neonatal intensive care unit can make a couple feel helpless, and they may experience feelings of a loss of control. It is important that you get as involved as possible in your baby's care and that you express your feelings to the hospital staff. Taking photos of your baby each day can help you feel involved, as well as participating in the diaper changes and feedings. Some couples are brought closer during these difficult times, while others find the strain too great and their relationship shatters. There are many factors that contribute to the strain felt by both parents.

Going home without your baby is likely to be disconcerting, and it will feel even more so if you live far from the hospital. When our baby was in the premature nursery, we rented an apartment near the institution so that we could visit frequently and could be there quickly in the event of an emergency. Visiting your baby is very important. Even at such an early age, the baby needs to know that someone cares and that there are special people there on a regular basis. Your voice will probably elicit a reaction from your baby because he or she has been hearing it since early in your pregnancy.

Your role as the parent of a preemie rests in conveying a sense of hope to your newborn, who despite his or her problems manages to pick up all the signals—good and bad—that you send out.

Most literature on premature babies focuses on the three aspects of the journey—coping with your feelings, developing your new identity as a parent of a premature baby, and managing your relationships. As soon as you recognize and are able to take control of these issues, your journey will become much easier.

One thing you should be aware of is that it is common for mothers of premature babies to get significantly more depressed a month or so after their baby is born. They may be overwhelmed with feelings of anger, guilt, sadness, and irritability, and they may cry uncontrollably. Even though the baby blues come and go for quite some time after your baby is born, you might want to seek professional help. The good news is that eventually you and your baby begin to adapt to your life together.

The Premature Baby and Stimulation

Long before his or her system has had a chance to mature, the premature baby encounters a great deal of handling, procedures, and stimulus. Even though most neonatal intensive care units try to minimize excessive stimulus, it is not always easy with all they have to do to keep your baby alive and healthy. Most centers today try to cluster care, thus allowing for longer periods of rest and sleep.

Babies express themselves through their physical behavior and body language. Using your own keen observational skills, you will soon be able to figure out when your baby has had too much stimulation. Some mothers say that their baby might look away when the stimulus gets too intense. Other babies may close their eyes, stick out their tongues, yawn, kick, arch their backs, or cry.

Here are some tips on handling premature babies during their waking hours:

- Use eye contact.

- Talk to your baby.

- When holding your baby, apply gentle yet firm pressure on the baby's back and chest with the open hand. This helps to calm the baby and it also blocks out other stimulus.

- Provide only one form of stimulation at a time and for a short period of time—they tire easily.

- Help your baby to bring his or her hands to the mouth, using a finger or pacifier.

- Place all objects approximately 8 inches away.

- If visiting is a problem, prepare a recording of your voice for the hospital staff to play.

- Close your baby's fist around a soft toy.

- If possible, change the position of the crib periodically for a different view.

- Remember, the best stimulation for your baby is seeing your face.

Kangaroo Care

Kangaroo care is a way of holding your baby so that there is skin-to-skin contact between the baby and the person holding him or her. The term was chosen to describe the similar method practiced by kangaroos and their young. During kangaroo care, the baby is held on the parent's bare chest (tummy to tummy) between the breasts. The baby's ear should be above the parent's heart, and the baby should only be wearing a diaper.

Kangaroo care is beneficial for both full-term and premature babies. Ask your provider if your baby is stable enough for you to begin kangaroo care. The actual practice of kangaroo care varies, but in general for preemies, it is usually practiced for two to three hours each day.

The best way to start is to have a shirt or hospital gown that opens in the front. Sit in a comfortable chair or rocker. Then have your nurse or family member place your baby gently on your chest with only a diaper on. Both your skins should be touching. It is a good idea to cover your baby's back with a light blanket or your gown. This is your time to relax together and allow your baby to enjoy the rhythm of your breathing and the sound of your voice. Some mothers may sing to their baby and others may hold their baby while reading. The important thing is that you are both bonding.

Today, more than 80 percent of neonatal intensive care nurseries advocate kangaroo care. Studies have shown that this technique results in numerous benefits for the preemie, including allowing the baby to fall into a deep sleep, shorter hospital stays, more rapid weight gain, less respiratory distress, and an improved rate of recovery.

Family and Friends

The birth of your premature baby will be considered a crisis in all your personal relationships. It is normal for it to affect everything you do. It is particularly difficult when the birth of a preemie comes without warning and you have no chance to prepare yourself.

Your partner will play a major role in your ability to cope with your premature baby. If you stand together and support each other rather than becoming angry and resentful, it will be much easier.

I remember how supportive my husband was during this time. We had a two-year history of infertility problems, and so the birth of our first daughter was wonderful beyond words. We put all our energy into helping her survive those first critical weeks of life. My husband was my "Rock of Gibraltar." In addition to being my replacement in the nursery, he made an effort to be with my daughter as much as possible, and especially made it a point to be there at feeding time to give her bottles. We learn a lot about our family during these difficult times. We learn whom we can depend on when we need them, who is there and who is not.

Siblings are sometimes allowed to visit the premature nursery. Fostering this early interaction is important. Depending on the age of your other children, it may be difficult for them to understand the crisis situation. Explain as much as you think they will understand without overwhelming them. If you are at home and want to visit your newborn, find alternative care for your other children, especially if they have any type of infection—even if it is just a common cold. Preemies are vulnerable to any type of infection because their immune system is underdeveloped.

Grandparents of preemies are usually encouraged to visit when the parents are at the baby's bedside. If it is their first grandchild, they may also be feeling a large amount of stress. In many instances, the grandparents feel even more excluded if there are other children at home and they are not directly involved in their care either.

Researchers have noted that grandparents feel triple grief, as they grieve for their new grandchild, for the infant's parents, and for themselves. Although they have this triple stress, in general, they are more understanding of the necessary restrictions on visiting, and they deal more easily with these limitations than do the parents. In some instances, such as in the case of single parents, grandparents may play a large role in offering support to the mother.

Outcome

Today, the prognosis for babies born prematurely is much better than it was years ago. Their health and survival depends on many factors, including any complications incurred during their first days of life and the type of care they receive. Many cities have high-risk units specializing in the care of these vulnerable infants. The presence of highly trained professionals helps to give parents confidence that everything is being done to ensure the best possible outcome for their baby.

In general, the shorter the gestation, the less chance there is for survival and the more obstacles the preemie will confront. Babies weighing more than 3 pounds, 6 ounces, with good respiratory patterns and good muscle tone, have a good chance of survival.

Most obstetricians will want to see you two weeks after your baby is born just to make sure that all is going well. This visit is a good time to ask any questions or express concerns about this baby and/or future pregnancies. It might be a good time to ask for the name of a consultant whom you can speak with prior to getting pregnant again, particularly if you had a very premature baby. If your premature delivery was due to a uterine abnormality, your specialist might recommend a surgical suture or the use of medications to prevent another premature delivery. More recent studies suggest a shot of progesterone (250 mg) be given each week, beginning at sixteen to twenty weeks and continuing to thirty-six weeks. Progesterone has been shown to prevent preterm birth in about one out of three women. Researchers are unclear exactly how it works, but it is the first medication in forty years shown to prevent preterm birth.

Baby's Homecoming

Bringing your baby home will probably be one of the most exciting yet apprehensive days in your life, second only to learning you were pregnant. Knowing that your little one has survived the trauma and the potential dangers of early birth gives you an enormous amount of strength. On the other hand, it can also be overwhelming and daunting, particularly after having spent days, weeks, or months in the hospital and having an entire medical team to help and support you.

It is normal to feel scared and unsure about your parenting abilities. It is important that you ask all the pertinent questions about caring for your baby and also obtain the telephone numbers for the hospital, your pediatrician, and a local community agency, which you can use to ask any questions as they arise. Some women find it helpful to join local support groups to share the experiences of parenting a premature baby. This also decreases the sense of isolation parents feel during these first difficult months of their baby's life.

Before taking your baby home, you might want to consider taking a course in CPR and make sure you are comfortable with all aspects of your baby's care. Remember to ask as many questions as possible and to have a contact number in case you have more questions once you arrive home.

Coming home with your baby will also have a dramatic effect on your family life. Having had your baby in the premature nursery will seem like a dream. Running back and forth to the hospital and attending to your household probably gave you little time to think about anything else. Once at home with your baby, you will realize that the experience of having a premature baby is physically and emotionally exhausting. It is normal for frustrations and anxieties to come to the forefront. Speak openly with your partner and request the same from him. Venting frustrations rather than exhibiting generalized anxiety will prove healthier in the long run.

Equipment needed at home for the premature infant is similar to that for term babies, with a few exceptions. Items such as disposable preemie diapers are available in certain areas. The manufacturer of Pampers has a premature-size diaper. Call Procter & Gamble toll-free at (800) 543-4932 or access them online at www.pg.com to see where you can purchase these diapers in your area. Speak with other mothers of preemies about where to buy preemie clothes or check out the Internet for product information and suggestions.

Most car seats are designed for larger infants; however, you can adapt a standard car seat by placing rolled towels on either side of your baby's head for additional support. Look for companies specializing in your baby's needs. Children's Medical Ventures, for example, has designed the Wee Fit Seat Insert for car seats that is specifically for preemies. Other companies sell car beds that lay flat, allowing a premature baby with respiratory problems to breathe more easily. Some studies have shown this not to be effective, so it is important that you speak with your provider prior to purchasing this bed. Be aware of air bag warnings and recalled products. And by all means, resist the temptation to hold your baby in your arms while driving.

The first few days at home are the most difficult. You may find that the care you give your newborn is more tiring than you might have expected. If this is the case, perhaps a community agency or a visiting nurse can give you a hand. It takes a while for you and your baby to get used to each other. You will learn all the normal sounds that your baby makes during the night, and your baby will begin to adjust to his or her new home.

One woman says:

> "I was both terrified and delighted to take my baby home from the hospital after she had been there for four weeks. I kept thinking about the day that I saw her stop breathing in the nursery because she had mucus in her throat. I was well prepared should it happen at home, but I was quite overprotective for the first little while. We protected her from all dangers, including an abundance of visitors. We were very strict as to who could visit, and those who visited had to be very careful and wash their hands before coming near the baby. In the end, all the precautions paid off because now, at the age of six, she is a happy and bright little girl who makes both her parents very proud."

Here are some resources where you can buy clothing for premature babies:

Preemiewear specializes in clothing for preemies or low-birth-weight babies. To order a free catalog in the United States, call (800) 992-8469.

Tiny Bundles offers unique, handmade preemie clothing, diapers, and pacifiers. To order a free brochure call (619) 451-9907 or write to 11438 Ballybunion Square, San Diego, CA 92128.

Death and Dying

The possibility of your baby's death may have been on your mind from the very beginning. This is a realistic and a normal concern, since about half of all infant deaths that occur during the first month occur among premature babies. About half of the deaths in preemies occur during their first day of life, so if you have already passed the first day, your baby's chances of survival are that much greater.

Many parents of dying children feel the need to be by the child's side right until the end, while others have difficulty coping with the emotional impact, finding it all too intense. If your child dies and you feel like hugging and cuddling it, you should be encouraged to do so. The tubes and apparatus are usually removed after death, so they should not interfere. Ask the hospital staff for special tokens of your baby, such as name tags, armbands, or a lock of hair. If you haven't given your child a name, you may want to. Most nursery staff will give you an opportunity to spend time with your baby. No matter how short your baby's life has been, a bond has been formed between you, a special bond that will live with you forever.

Sometimes siblings have a difficult time adapting to the loss. They may need extra love and attention at this time. On the next page I have included a relevant cartoon from *Frogs Have a Baby: A Very Small Baby*, by Jerri Oehler, RN, at Duke University Medical Center.

Future Pregnancies

Before you leave the hospital or on your first visit to the pediatrician or obstetrician, you may still have many unanswered questions about why your baby was born prematurely and if it could possibly happen again. It is important for you to voice your concerns. The risk of having another preemie is high, especially for women who have uterine abnormalities.

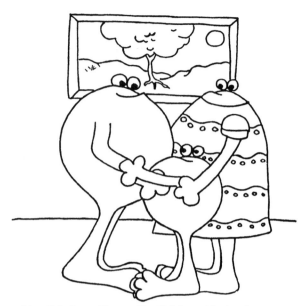

We will be here with you. It will take awhile to stop hurting and feel better. We love you and will take care of you. It's important to know that there will always be someone to love you and take care of you.

Most authorities agree that you should wait at least three months before becoming pregnant again, especially if the premature birth resulted in the death of your baby. If you had a cesarean delivery involving a vertical uterine incision, you should wait six months or longer.

Some women choose to change physicians and/or hospitals, while others prefer to stay with the old and familiar. This is up to the individual, and you should discuss your concerns with both your partner and your provider.

Depending on your situation, you may be categorized as high-risk in subsequent pregnancies. Make sure you understand what this means and whether you are in the same or a similar risk category as during your previous pregnancy. Although high-risk pregnancies are not something most women want to repeat, there is no doubt that the second time around is much easier, as you will know more about what to expect.

Journaling Corner

Discuss the events leading up to your baby's arrival and your feelings throughout.

Having a premature baby is like embarking on an unexpected journey. What are your fears and expectations as you embark on your journey?

What types of things do you wonder about your premature baby?

Discuss any feelings of hopelessness that you may have.

Do you feel less prepared to be a parent of a premature baby than a normal baby, and how/why?

Discuss your support systems that will help you navigate through your journey.

Special Concerns During Pregnancy

A mother's love endures through all.   — Washington Irving

This chapter discusses a number of concerns and issues relevant to pregnancy that do not necessarily fit into any particular chapter in this book but are nevertheless very important. It is intended to be a general overview of these subjects, and you are encouraged to seek additional assistance and information, as needed.

The Pregnant Single Parent

Some women unexpectedly become single mothers as a result of the death of a spouse from either illness, an accident, or war. Others might become single mothers because of a divorce. However, there is another group of women who call themselves "single mothers by choice."

For the most part, these are women who have decided to have or adopt a child knowing that they will be the sole parent. According to the support group Single Mothers by Choice (SMC), these mothers come from varying backgrounds, and many are career women in their thirties and forties. Some have decided that after establishing their careers, they want to become mothers. Others have always had a strong mothering instinct and, as their biological clock ticked on, they choose not to wait for marriage or finding Mr. Right before starting their families. Many of these women want "to have it all"—a career, the single life, and children.

Women may become mothers in numerous ways. Some may become pregnant accidentally, some intentionally, others choose artificial insemination, and others may choose to adopt.

Over the years, there has been a definite increase in single motherhood: 18 percent between 1980 and 1985. In 1990 one hundred and seventy thousand single women over the age of thirty had given birth.

One woman describes her decision to become a single mother:

"Shortly before my thirty-ninth birthday, my divorce was finalized. Irregular periods, which I thought were a response to stress, prompted a trip to my gynecologist's office. I remember sitting on the exam table wrapped in the paper gown when a smiling Dr. C. [Christie] entered the room. He asked me how I was doing—how marriage was treating me. I burst out crying. I'd been going to Dr. C.'s office for many years. During each annual exam, we discussed my desire to have children.

"Dr. C. had previously shown me a chart that displayed the increase in genetic defects with maternal age. The changes over age forty were dramatic. He used the word *perimenopausal* in response to my irregular periods. I used the shoulder of my paper gown to wipe my tears. He handed me a tissue. He shared that a few of his patients, single women, had used fertility treatments to become pregnant. The thought of becoming a single mother had never crossed my mind. I naïvely asked how these patients had gotten sperm. 'From sperm donors,' he replied. I sat stunned and silent, letting the information sink in, and within a few minutes I knew that I would do the same. The world suddenly opened up to me and offered possibilities I hadn't envisioned while pursuing the traditional route to marriage and family.

"My appointment with the fertility specialist was on my thirty-ninth birthday. After two miscarriages, I birthed my daughter at the age of forty-two—no easy feat, but worth it all. My mother had died when I was thirty-three, and my father was ill with diabetic complications. With the birth of my baby, I felt an instant connection to my ancestors. The compelling yearning for motherhood was finally fulfilled. I've never regretted my decision."

Even though you have made the decision to become a single mother, it does not mean you need to go through the pregnancy experience alone. Even though a partner is the most common choice for sharing the ups and downs of the pregnancy experience, there are other people who could share in your journey. It is important to seek the support of loved ones, other than a partner. For example, a close friend or relative can be there for you both emotionally and physically in your time of need. This person can attend the prenatal classes with you and be there on-call in the event of an emergency. If you do not have someone close who can share in the experience with you, you might want to seek the assistance of a national or local support group of single mothers. If they do not have someone in their group who can stand by your side, perhaps they can refer you to someone who can. A helpful group is called Parents Without Partners (see Appendix A).

By securing adequate outside support, you can minimize one of the risks often related with single mothering—depression. According to a recent study, single mothers have a 40 percent higher chance of becoming depressed than do coupled mothers. The two main reasons are the increased amount of stress from managing a child alone and the decreased amount of social support. As one single woman says, "No matter how hard you try, life for the single mother is love, duty, hard work, and little sleep."

In addition to the emotional stressors of being a single parent, there are also medical stressors. A study in England showed that children under the age of four are more likely to die if they are born to single mothers and mothers who are under the age of twenty.

One important thing to remember if you are a single mother is to make provisions for your child or children in case something happens to you. It is a good idea to speak with your attorney about preparing a last will and testament indicating who will become the guardian of your child or children in the event of you being struck by a debilitating disease or even death.

Teenage Pregnancy

Teen pregnancy rates in the United States have declined steadily from 1991 to 2005—from 60 out of 1,000 teenagers in 1991 to 40.5 out of 1,000 in 2005. However, in 2006, the teen pregnancy rate increased in all races and ethnicities to about 42 out of 1,000. Ideally, it would be best to prevent teenage pregnancies through educators in the schools or through families, employers, and community policy makers. However, if a teen does find herself pregnant, it is critical she receives adequate prenatal care and nutritional counseling.

Profile of a Pregnant Teen

For the most part, teenagers do not plan on becoming pregnant. Statistics have shown that more than 80 percent of teen pregnancies are unintended. Whether intended or not, even if the news of being pregnant is initially exciting, teens are quickly overwhelmed.

Early in their pregnancy, pregnant teens will be forced to come face-to-face with the reality of their situation. For starters, they may need to decide if they want to keep the baby or put it up for adoption. If they decide to keep the baby, they need to think about their living situation after the baby is born. Teens are not used to making such long-term plans and this can be particularly challenging for them. They also need to make some serious decisions about the balance between mothering, work, and school. It is most helpful if they are surrounded by a good support system.

According to Child Trends Inc and The National Center for Health Statistics (2008), 84 percent of teen births occurred outside of marriage, in comparison to 58 percent of those between the ages of twenty and twenty-four.

Issues Associated with Teen Pregnancy

Although it is possible for teens to have normal pregnancies and deliver healthy babies, they will need to be closely followed by the medical, psychosocial, and nutritional teams because they are at an increased risk for developing problems during their pregnancy.

When pregnant for the first time, a teen is often seen as being high-risk for a subsequent pregnancy and should be counseled so that she does not become pregnant again.

Some of the risks that the provider and the families of teens need to be aware of include:

- Teen mothers are less likely than their older counterparts to seek adequate prenatal care.

- Teen mothers have a higher incidence of poor eating habits and often fail to take prenatal vitamins.

- Teen mothers are less likely to gain adequate weight during pregnancy, resulting in low-birth-weight babies.

- Teen mothers are more likely to drop out of school.

- Teen mothers are associated with lower family income at some point.
- Teen mothers are at risk of pregnancy complications such as preterm birth and preeclampsia.
- Teenage mothers have a risk of having babies with structural abnormalities, such as gastrothesis.

There are many support groups and associations that can provide assistance to the teen mother and her family. Some of these can be found on the Internet or in Appendix A of this book. For example, groups such as The Healthy Teen Network (formerly The National Organization of Adolescent Pregnancy and Parenting, Inc.,) located in Bethesda, Maryland, is dedicated to making a difference in the lives of teens and their young families.

Questions Teens Can Ask Themselves about Their Pregnancy

- How do you feel about your pregnancy?
- Do you know who the father of your baby is?
- If your pregnancy was unplanned, how do you plan to prevent any future unwanted pregnancies?
- If your boyfriend asked you to participate in a DNA paternity test, how would you feel? Would you allow the test to be performed on you and your baby?
- Who has been the most supportive during your pregnancy?
- How will having your baby affect your life after the baby is born? Will you have to move? Change jobs? Drop out of school?

(Adapted from *The Unplanned Pregnancy Book for Teens and College Students* by Dorrie Williams-Wheeler.)

Domestic Violence

Pregnancy is supposed to be a joyous time marking the beginning of a new life, a time of peace and safety. For many women, however, it becomes a time of turbulence and fear. In some cases, pregnant women find additional emotional strength during pregnancy and this inspires them to seek help for their abusive relationship, whereas they might not have done so before.

Incidence of Domestic Violence

Domestic violence is the leading cause of death among pregnant women, ranking above accidents and medical complications of high-risk pregnancies. It also tends to escalate during pregnancy. The reason may have to do with the woman's increased vulnerability, but also the stress of the pregnancy on the relationship. Often, women who are hit or abused think that it might be a one-time isolated incident, where in fact, it might be a sign of the beginning of a problem in the relationship. If a partner strikes once, he is likely to do it again.

Years ago, while working as a volunteer in a domestic violence facility, one of the first things I learned was that domestic violence crosses all racial groups and economic barriers. It occurs in wealthy, middle-class, and lower socioeconomic homes.

In general, women of all ages are at risk for violence, but the incidence of abuse peaks during the reproductive years. According to the Centers for Disease Control and Prevention, at least 4 to 8 percent of pregnant women (over three hundred thousand per year) are abused during pregnancy. Women whose pregnancies were unwanted or unintended are four times more likely to be abused while pregnant. In relationships that were abusive prior to pregnancy, the partner may have forbidden the woman to use contraception as a form of control and dominance. The pregnancy might also trigger some negative emotions or jealousy from the father-to-be, causing him to lash out.

The Abusive Pattern

Many times women in already abusive relationships believe that pregnancy will favorably improve their partner's behavior, but more often than not, pregnancy has the opposite effect and it places an extra strain on an already strained relationship. There is a certain pattern or cycle to domestic violence, which may be identified below:

- Rising tension in a relationship is often the result of a minor argument or disagreement.
- The increasing tension builds over hours, days, or months.
- An event will trigger an abusive event that might be physical, verbal, or sexual.

- This event is followed by a period of calm, sometimes referred to as the honeymoon phase. This is the time the abuser might buy gifts or schedule special events for the woman.

- As time goes on, this cycle evolves and more incidents occur. The tension increases again and the cycle repeats itself. One or both partners think maybe things will get resolved and the abuse will subside, but it usually does not.

The Danger of Abuse

Domestic abuse during pregnancy is dangerous both for the mother and her unborn child. Studies have shown that most of the abuse during pregnancy is directed toward the abdomen, breasts, and genitals, all very dangerous areas for the pregnant woman. These strikes can result in miscarriage, low-birth-weight babies, premature labor, fetal injury, and fetal death. Those who have worked with the victims of abuse know how women frequently deny that they are in an abusive relationship. Often, they need assistance to identify that they are in that type of relationship (see the bulleted list below).

There are additional risks to the pregnant woman who is abused during labor. For example, the partner may control the woman's decision to not have an epidural or other interventions recommended by the hospital staff. Women react differently to this type of control. Out of fear, some pregnant women may become increasingly quiet, while others may scream or cry in response to her partner's difficult demands on her.

The effect of domestic violence after the baby is born is also very dangerous because the partner can use the mother's relationship with her baby as a weapon and might even deny her access to her own baby.

Often, the abusive situation does not change after the baby is born. As a matter of fact, it might become exacerbated. According to the National Clearinghouse on Family Violence, the abuser might increase the amount of abuse and also begin using the woman's relationship with her baby as part of the abuse by doing any or all of the following:

- denying her access to her newborn baby

- demanding sex soon after childbirth

- blaming her because the infant is the "wrong" sex

- not supporting or helping her after she comes home with the baby
- sulking or trying to make her feel bad for the time she spends with the baby
- putting down her parenting ability
- threatening to abduct or actually abducting the baby
- telling her she will never get custody of the baby
- making her stay at home with the baby
- preventing her from taking a job or making her take a job
- making or threatening to make false child abuse accusations against her
- withholding money (e.g., for supplies for the baby such as formula, food, diapers)
- blaming her for the baby's crying or other problems

What to Do

Being exposed to either physical or emotional violence can have severe health ramifications for the pregnant woman. If you are in a physically or emotionally abusive relationship, you should seek immediate help. It is important for you to know that you are not alone and that it is not your fault. In order to protect you and your unborn child, it is important that you seek the help you need. Today, medical professionals are bound by confidentially agreements and none of the information you share with them can be released without your permission. You should be aware, however, that some states have laws that require mandatory reporting of any abusive situations. These states include California, Kentucky, New Mexico, New Hampshire, and Rhode Island.

There are numerous organizations that support abused women, but a good place to start is with the National Coalition Against Domestic Violence. The staff may be able to direct you to a local group. In a crisis situation, you can call its 24-hour hotline at (800) 799-SAFE. The organization may also be accessed online at http://www.ncadv.org. Don't wait. The time to save you and your baby-to-be is now!

Many organizations have made donations to support abused women. One is the Mary Kay Ash Charitable Foundation, which has contributed millions of dollars to women's shelters across the United States. Since 2000 the foundation has reportedly awarded more than $11 million in grant money to shelters for women and children in all fifty states.

Sometimes hearing the stories of others who have survived domestic abuse can place your own life into perspective, give voice to your innermost feelings, and encourage you to seek help. One such book describing four generations of abuse is called, *Color Me Butterfly: A True Story of Courage, Hope, and Transformation* by L. Y. Marlow (2007).

If you suspect that you know a woman who is a victim of domestic violence, it is important that you bring it to the attention of the authorities. Here are some observations that might lead you to seek help:

- unexplained bruising or damage to the abdomen or breasts
- frequent use of addictive substances (i.e., alcohol, cigarettes)
- recurring complaints of psychosomatic illnesses
- refusal to seek medical care out of fear
- inadequate weight gain
- exacerbation of chronic illnesses
- recurrent vaginal, cervical, or kidney infections

History of Sexual Abuse

Sometimes women who have had a history of sexual abuse or rape, either as children or adults, find that being pregnant allows old emotions to resurface. There is no doubt that the pain and hurt of such experiences have long-lasting effects and sometimes women do not understand the magnitude of the pain until they become pregnant. The issues associated with a history of abuse may be triggered by either pregnancy, labor, and/or delivery. The unconscious memories may come to the forefront and bring back an array of unpleasant flashbacks.

During these times, it is important to think positively and to relax and remember that pregnancy should be a happy time for you.

Here are some tips that might help you:

- Prepare a birth plan.
- Share your history with your partner and health-care provider. Tell them about situations that might be uncomfortable for you.

- Give yourself permission to be afraid and concerned.

- Try to separate your past issues from your current pregnancy.

- Find a doula (birth assistant) for moral support.

- Love yourself and trust that you will also survive this experience.

- Keep a positive attitude.

Trauma During Pregnancy

According to a recent study by Dr. Andrew K. Chang at the Albert Einstein College of Medicine, 6 to 7 percent of all pregnant women experience some type of trauma. Motor vehicle accidents and domestic violence are the leading causes of trauma during pregnancy.

The most common time for trauma during pregnancy is during the last trimester, which is when the trauma can cause the most harm for the mother and fetus. About 0.3 to 0.4 percent of these pregnant women will encounter the type of trauma that necessitates hospitalization.

When a trauma occurs during the first trimester, the uterus is still small and most often protected by the pelvic bones. Sometimes the trauma will not affect the pregnancy at all. However, if the trauma is severe, a miscarriage could ensue. If the trauma occurs during the second or third trimesters, the consequences tend to be more severe. Even a small trauma can adversely affect the growing fetus, resulting in situations such as abruptio placenta, preterm labor, premature rupture of the membranes, uterine rupture, fetal injury, or fetal death. Sometimes it takes a few days for any of the above conditions to occur, but they typically manifest within the first twenty-four hours.

It is common for the pregnant woman to have uterine contractions following an injury, although it does not always result in preterm labor.

If you are more than twenty-four weeks pregnant and have been in a car accident, it is a good idea to visit your physician just to make sure everything is okay. He or she will want to make sure that you are not bleeding and are not having premature contractions. If your accident involved a direct hit to your abdomen, you will likely have an ultrasound and be asked to stay in the hospital for twenty-four hours of monitoring.

Many pregnant women ask if they should wear a seat belt, and the answer is always yes because it protects you and your baby. It is important to wear a seat belt, whether you sit in the front or backseat of the car. The placement of the seat belt is critical. It should be worn in the same way that a nonpregnant person wears one. The only difference is that the lap strap should go under your belly, across your hips, and as high as possible on your thighs. The shoulder strap should be positioned between your breasts and off to the side of your belly and above your uterus. Sometimes it is necessary to adjust the shoulder strap to make sure it fits in a way to protect you and your baby from injury. Some women like positioning a small pillow on their lap between the steering wheel and their expanding belly (for a diagram see Figure 2.3 on page 74).

Most physicians will tell you that it is fine to drive for the duration of your pregnancy, except of course if you are taking narcotics.

Prenatal care has come a long way. In the seventeenth century, a woman had a one in six chance of dying in childbirth and only one of every five children lived to see their first birthday.

Today, if the pregnant woman is diligent about seeking appropriate medical care, her high-risk situation can be appropriately identified and managed in a timely manner. In doing so, she will minimize her risk of problems. Studies have shown that the vast number of high-risk pregnancies will end in a healthy outcome. Even though the responsibility for identifying and managing high-risk conditions lies primarily with the health-care provider, it is important for couples to be well-informed about their situation.

We hope that this book helped to inform and educate you, your family, and your friends about your high-risk pregnancy, thereby improving your chances of a favorable outcome. However, keep in mind that this book is not a substitute for attaining quality health care but rather should complement it. Now enjoy the journey of your pregnancy!

Glossary

abruptio placenta. An emergency situation characterized by the premature separation of the placenta from the uterus.

adhesions. Scar tissue normally formed by the body following surgery, infection, inflammation, or disease.

adrenal glands. Endocrine glands above the kidney that secrete important hormones such as epinephrine and cortisone.

AFP. An abbreviation for *alpha fetoprotein*. A protein normally produced by the fetus's liver but produced in excess in the presence of certain fetal abnormalities.

amniocentesis. A prenatal procedure in which a small amount of the amniotic fluid that surrounds the fetus is removed for analysis.

amniotic sac. The sac containing the fetus and the "bag of water" or amniotic fluid.

androgen. Male hormone, such as testosterone, produced by the testes and responsible for male characteristics.

anencephaly. Born without a brain or spinal cord.

anoxia. An abnormal lack of oxygen.

antibody. A protein manufactured by the immune system that reacts against specific foreign substances (antigens).

Apgar score. A simple method of quickly assessing the health status of a newborn.

APLAS. An abbreviation for *antiphospholipid antibody syndrome*. An autoimmune disorder of blood coagulation.

apnea. The temporary absence of respiration.

ART. An abbreviation for *artificial reproductive technologies*, which includes all treatments or procedures that involve the handling of human eggs and sperm for the purpose of helping a woman become pregnant. Types of ART include in vitro fertilization, gamete intrafallopian transfer, zygote intrafallopian transfer, embryo cryopreservation, egg or embryo donation, and surrogate birth.

bacteriuria. Bacteria in the urine.

beta-thalassemia. A type of hereditary anemia occurring in populations bordering the Mediterranean and Southeast Asia.

betamethasone. A cortisone-like hormone sometimes given to women in premature labor to promote fetal lung maturity.

bilirubin. A byproduct of the normal breakdown of red blood cells.

blighted ovum. An egg that does not develop properly.

bloody show. Bleeding from the vagina, which is a sign of being in labor.

bradycardia. A slower-than-normal heartbeat.

Braxton Hicks contractions. Painless contractions that are usually normal.

breech position. Fetal position in which the buttocks and/or feet are down prior to delivery.

cephalic position. Fetal position where the head is down.

cerclage. A suture placed around a cervix characterized by cervical insufficiency to prevent miscarriage. See also **Shirodkar procedure.**

cervical insufficiency. The inability of the cervix to remain closed during pregnancy, resulting in spontaneous abortion. (formerly called incompetent cervix)

cervix. The lower end of the uterus, which connects the uterus to the vagina.

cesarean delivery. The surgical delivery of a baby through an incision made in the mother's abdomen.

chlamydia. A bacterial sexually transmitted infection.

chromosome. The part of the nucleus of a body cell that contains the parents' genetic material in twisted strands called DNA.

cleft lip. A congenital fissure of the lip; also called a **harelip.**

congenital. To be born with; or existing before or from birth.

corpus luteum. A body formed on the ovary following ovulation that secretes progesterone to prepare the body for pregnancy.

Crohn's disease. A type of inflammatory bowel disease.

crowning. The appearance of the baby's head at the entrance of the vagina during delivery.

CVS. An abbreviation for *chorionic villus sampling.* An analysis of chorionic tissue early in pregnancy to detect chromosomal abnormalities.

cytomegalovirus. A common virus that infects people of all ages. It is the most common type of uterine viral infection.

D&C. See **dilation and curettage.**

dilation and curettage. Also called a D&C. A procedure in which the interior of the uterus is scraped to diagnose a disease, empty uterine contents, or correct vaginal bleeding.

doula. A person who is specially trained to help a woman handle labor.

echocardiogram. A type of ultrasound of the heart. Sometimes referred to as an echo.

eclampsia. Preeclampsia accompanied by seizures or coma.

ectopic pregnancy. A pregnancy implanted outside the uterus, such as in the fallopian tubes, abdomen, cervix, or ovaries.

effacement. The thinning and shortening of the cervix during labor.

ejaculation. The emission of semen from the male urethra during climax.

embryo. The name given to the product of conception from the time of implantation until the eighth week. It is then called the **fetus.**

endometriosis. The abnormal growth of endometrial tissue outside the uterus.

endometrium. The inner membrane lining of the uterus.

epidural. A pain medicine used during labor that helps to numb the lower body.

epididymis. The duct system responsible for sperm maturation and their ability to fertilize an egg. It is responsible for sperm transfer.

episiotomy. An incision made in the perineum during delivery to prevent lacerations and to facilitate delivery.

estriol. A form of estrogen that increases during pregnancy.

estrogen. A female hormone responsible for female secondary sex traits.

fallopian tubes. A pair of tubes that retrieve and carry the egg from the ovaries to the uterus for implantation; fertilization occurs here.

fertilization. The union of the egg and the sperm, marking the beginning of pregnancy.

fetal distress. A critical condition of the fetus, usually during labor, in which the fetus's life may be in jeopardy.

fetal fibronectin test (fFn). A test sometimes given if a woman goes into preterm labor.

FISH test. Also known as the fluorescence in situ hybridization test. A test that helps to identify whether the fetus's chromosomes are normal or abnormal.

folic acid. A vitamin that can help protect the baby from some birth defects.

forceps. Metal device that is sometimes used during delivery to protect the baby's head and assist it through the birth canal.

FSH. An abbreviation for follicle-stimulating hormone. The hormone released by the pituitary gland that triggers ovum development or sperm production.

fundus. The upper, rounded, muscular, and contracting part of the uterus.

gamete. A sexual cell. It is an unfertilized egg or a mature sperm cell.

gene. The hereditary factor in the chromosome that carries characteristics from one generation to another.

genetic counseling. The advice offered by experts in genetics on the detection, consequences, and risks of recurrence of chromosomal and genetic disorders.

German measles. See **rubella.**

gestational diabetes. Diabetes that occurs only during pregnancy.

GnRH. An abbreviation for gonadotropin-releasing hormone. A hormone secreted by the hypothalamus that stimulates the pituitary to release FSH and LH hormones.

gonorrhea. A sexually transmitted infection caused by a bacterium.

gynecologist. A physician specializing in female reproduction, pregnancy, and often birth.

habitual aborter. A woman who has miscarried three or more times.

high blood pressure. When the force of blood against the blood vessels is elevated.

health-care provider. A person who gives you medical care. It can be a physician, nurse, nurse practitioner, midwife, or another trained professional.

HELLP syndrome. A name used to describe one of the life-threatening manifestations of severe preeclampsia.

high-risk pregnancy. A pregnancy in which there is a chance of a problem developing that might jeopardize the life or health of mother and/or baby.

hormone. A chemical substance secreted by an organ that initiates or regulates activity in another part of the body.

hCG. A hormone produced by the placenta early in pregnancy. It is used as the basis of pregnancy tests.

hyaline membrane disease. A lung disorder of premature infants caused by lack of surfactant production; a respiratory distress syndrome.

hydatidiform mole. Also called *molar pregnancy.* An abnormal development of the placenta that results in a benign or malignant tumor.

hydrocephalus. Excessive fluid in the skull.

hyperemesis gravidarum. Severe morning sickness.

hyperglycemia. High blood sugar.

hypoglycemia. Low blood sugar.

hypoxia. An insufficient amount of oxygen.

hysterectomy. The removal of the uterus.

hysterosalpingogram. An X ray done in the infertility investigation in which dye is injected to view the female anatomy.

IBD. An abbreviation for *inflammatory bowel disease.* A condition that causes a chronic inflammation in the digestive tract. The two most common types are ulcerative colitis and Crohn's disease.

implantation. The attachment of the fertilized ovum in the uterus.

induction. The process of causing or producing, as in the induction of labor with medications to stimulate uterine contractions.

intrauterine transfusion. A procedure in which blood is introduced into the fetus's abdomen; used for severe maternal-fetal blood incompatibilities.

IUGR. An abbreviation for *intrauterine growth restriction.* A reduction in fetal growth for reasons such as infection, inadequate placenta, or exposure to teratogens.

IVF. An abbreviation for *in vitro fertilization.* A process in which eggs are extracted from a woman and fertilized with a man's sperm, and the embryo is transferred to the uterus for development.

jaundice. Yellow discoloration of the skin due to elevated bilirubin (formed from the breakdown of red blood cells).

kangaroo care. A way of holding a baby so that there is skin-to-skin contact between the baby and the person holding it.

Kegel exercises. Exercises involving contracting and relaxing the muscles of the pelvic floor.

kernicterus. Damage to the newborn brain as a result of increased levels of bilirubin.

labor. The process of giving birth, divided into three stages ending with complete cervical dilation, delivery, and the expulsion of the placenta.

LH. An abbreviation for luteinizing hormone. A pituitary hormone that stimulates the secretion of progesterone in women and testosterone production in men.

L/S ratio. An abbreviation for lecithin/sphingomyelin ratio. A chemical test on the amniotic fluid to detect fetal lung maturity.

lupus. A chronic inflammatory disease of many systems in the body, occurring predominantly in young women.

luteal phase. The time from ovulation to menstruation.

magnesium sulfate. A medication used to treat preeclampsia and sometimes to prevent premature labor.

malpresentation. An abnormal fetal position.

meconium. The first feces of a newborn infant. If seen during pregnancy, it usually indicates fetal distress.

menstrual cycle. The monthly menstruation cycle starting with the first day of menses and ending on the first day of the next menses. Ranges from twenty-five to thirty-five days.

MFPR. An abbreviation for multifetal pregnancy reduction. A procedure done to reduce the number of fetuses in a pregnancy.

midwife. A person who delivers infants. A certified nurse-midwife is a registered nurse who has graduated from a nurse-midwifery program and has taken a certification exam.

miscarriage. A pregnancy loss prior to the twentieth week, most often in the first trimester; a spontaneous abortion.

molding. The process in which the fetal head changes to fit the pelvis during labor.

moxibustion. An Oriental medicine therapy using moxa, a mugwort herb.

neonatal. Pertaining to the first four weeks of life.

neonatology. The field of pediatrics concerned with the care of the newborn infant. Often pertains to high-risk newborns.

neural tube. The part of the developing baby that becomes the brain and spinal cord.

neural tube defects. A group of malformations caused by abnormal development of the nervous system.

nonstress test. A test assessing fetal heart rate and its response to spontaneous movements or contractions.

obstetrician. A physician who specializes in female reproduction, pregnancy, and birth.

oligohydramnios. An inadequate amount of amniotic fluid.

oncologist. A physician specializing in cancer care.

ovary. Female reproductive organ that stores and releases eggs with ovulation and secretes hormones such as estrogen and progesterone.

oviduct. The tube through which the egg passes from the ovary; the fallopian tube.

ovulation. The release of an egg from the ovary.

oxytocin. A hormone that stimulates uterine contractions.

oxytocin challenge test. A test of fetal well-being in which the mother is given small amounts of oxytocin while the fetal heart rate is monitored.

Pap smear. A screening test to detect abnormal cells in the cervix.

paracervical nerve block. A local anesthetic injected through the vagina and into the cervical nerves to decrease the pain of cervical dilation.

perinatal. Before, during, and immediately after birth.

perinatology. Specialty of obstetrics dealing with the care of high-risk mothers and their babies; maternal-fetal medicine.

pelvic rest. A treatment recommended in some in high-risk pregnancies involving keeping the pressure off the pelvis. This means no sex, orgasms, lifting, or long time spent on feet or walking.

perineum. The area between the vagina and the rectum.

PID. An abbreviation for *pelvic inflammatory disease.* The inflammation of the pelvic organs, especially caused by bacterial infection.

Pitocin. A synthetic form of oxytocin.

pituitary gland. The master endocrine gland located at the base of the brain; it secretes various hormones and oversees complex chemical interactions.

PKU. An abbreviation for phenylketonuria. A hereditary deficiency of the liver enzyme needed to convert phenylalanine into a usable form.

placenta. A vascular organ in the pregnant uterus from which the fetus receives its nourishment. It forms the communication between mother and child.

placenta previa. Placenta implanted in the lower part of the uterus so that it partially or totally covers the cervical opening.

polyhydramnios. An excessive amount of amniotic fluid.

postmaturity. Pregnancy continuing after the fortieth week.

postnatal. Occurring after birth.

post-term. A fetus of a gestational age more than forty-two weeks; also called postmature.

preeclampsia. A hypertensive disorder of pregnancy without seizures or coma.

premature. Born after the twentieth week and prior to the thirty-seventh week of gestation.

presentation. The position of the baby in the uterus.

preterm. See also **premature.**

progesterone. A hormone responsible for preparing the uterus for implantation. It is secreted by the placenta during pregnancy.

progestin. See **progesterone.**

prolactin. The pituitary hormone that in high amounts stimulates milk production.

prolapsed cord. A serious condition whereby the umbilical cord slips into the birth canal after the membranes rupture and before the baby is born.

prostaglandins. Hormones used to induce labor.

prostate gland. A male gland near the bladder that contributes to ejaculation fluid; it is prone to infections that may affect male fertility.

pudendal nerve block. Local anesthetic given into the pudendal nerves on both sides of the perineum.

pulmonary hypertension. An increase in blood pressure in the pulmonary artery.

quickening. Fetal movement perceived by the mother.

recurrent miscarriages. Having had three or more unexplained miscarriages during the first trimester. See also **habitual aborter.**

respiratory distress syndrome (RDS). See **hyaline membrane disease.**

retrolental fibroplasia. A condition caused by high oxygen concentration given to premature infants; it results in blindness.

Rh factor. An antigenic substance present in the red blood cells of most people. Those having the factor are called Rh-positive and those who do not are called Rh-negative.

RhoGAM [Rh(D)]. An immunizing agent given to Rh-negative women following birth to prevent production of antibodies in any Rh-positive babies they may have in the future.

risk factor. A known reason why something can go wrong.

rubella. A common childhood disease caused by the rubella virus.

saddle block. Local anesthetic given into the dura sac (outer membrane covering the spinal cord) that numbs the pelvic area for delivery.

selective reduction. The process of reducing the number of fetuses in a multiple pregnancy because of congenital abnormalities in one or more of the fetuses.

semen. The thick, cloudy secretion containing sperm discharged from the male urethra during sexual excitement; also called **seminal fluid.**

septate uterus. A congenital abnormality whereby the uterus is divided into two compartments.

SGA. An abbreviation for small for gestational age. A baby who weighs less than 90 percent of the average infant at the same stage of pregnancy or delivery.

Shirodkar procedure. See **cerclage.**

shoulder dystocia. When one or both of the baby's shoulders get stuck in the mother's pelvis after the baby's head is delivered.

shunt. A hole or passage allowing fluid to pass from one part of the body to another.

sickle-cell anemia. A hereditary type of anemia caused by malformed red blood cells.

sperm. Male reproductive cell produced by the testicle.

spermatic cord. The cord suspending the testes. It is composed of veins, arteries, lymphatics, nerves, and the vas deferens.

spinal block. An injection into the lower back that numbs the body below the waist.

spontaneous abortion. See **miscarriage.**

STI. An abbreviation for *sexually transmitted infection.* Any infection transmitted through sexual contact, through the genitals, mouth, or anus; a venereal disease.

stillborn. The death of a fetus before or during delivery.

stress test. A now rarely used method of detecting fetal well-being by monitoring its response to contractions induced with oxytocin.

surfactant. A substance produced in the fetal lung necessary for lung maturity.

syphilis. A sexually transmitted infection caused by a bacterium.

Tay-Sachs. A congenital disease affecting the fat metabolism and the brain. Symptoms include progressive weakness, disability, blindness, and finally death.

teratogen. Any substance capable of causing malformations in a developing embryo.

testosterone. Hormone produced by the testicles that is responsible for male sex characteristics.

thyroid. A gland situated in the front of the neck that is essential to normal growth and metabolic processes.

toxoplasmosis. An infection transmitted through undercooked meat or cat feces.

trichomonas. A sexually transmitted infection.

trimester. Three-month period during pregnancy. There are three trimesters of pregnancy.

TTTS. An abbreviation for twin to twin transfer syndrome. A high-risk condition of identical twins who share the same placenta.

ulcerative colitis. A form of inflammatory bowel disease.

ultrasound. A noninvasive test using high-frequency sound waves to detect fetal well-being and diagnose defects. The baby's picture is seen on a computer screen.

uterine fibroids. Benign tumors on the outside, inside, or within the wall of the uterus, often changing the size and shape of the uterus.

uterus. The female reproductive organ responsible for bearing the fetus from implantation until birth; also see **womb.**

vagina. The muscular passage from the uterus to the outside of the body.

vas deferens. Carries sperm from the epididymis to the ejaculatory duct.

version. A procedure in which the fetus and uterus are manipulated in order to turn the fetus to a "head-down" position. Sometimes called, 'external rotation.'

viable. Capable of sustaining life; after twenty-eight weeks of gestation.

womb. See **uterus.**

X-linked inheritance. Inheritance through genes located on the X chromosome.

zygote. The developing ovum from the time of fertilization until implantation in the uterus.

Bibliography

Aaronson, L. S., and C. L. Macnee. "Tobacco, Alcohol and Caffeine Use During Pregnancy." *Journal of Gynecological and Neonatal Nursing* (July/-August,1989): 279–85.

Acupuncture Today. "Moxibustion." http://www.acupuncturetoday.com/abc/moxibustion.php (accessed 17 November 2008).

American Association of Critical-Care Nurses. "High Risk Neonatal Nursing." In *Perinatal Nursing.* Edited by K. W. Vestal and C. A. M. McKenzie. Philadelphia, PA: W. B. Saunders, 1983.

American College of Gynecologists and Obstetricians. *Women's Health Series: Exercise and Fitness.* 1984.

American Pregnancy Association. "Eating Disorders During Pregnancy." http://americanpregnancy.org/pregnancyhealth/eatingdisorders.html (accessed 4 August 2008).

American Pregnancy Association. "Natural Herbs & Vitamins During Pregnancy." http://www.americanpregnancy.org/pregnancyhealth/natural herbsvitamins.html (accessed 17 November 2008).

Arias, F. *High-Risk Pregnancy and Delivery.* St. Louis, MO: C. V. Mosby, 1984.

Asch, R., J. Balmaceda, L. Ellsworth, and P. Wong. "Gamete Intra-fallopian Transfer (GIFT): New Treatment for Infertility." *International Journal of Fertility* 30, no.1 (1985): 41–45.

Baby Center. "Meal Planning During Pregnancy." http://www.babycenter.com/0_meal-planning-during-pegnancy_1352495.bc#articlessection1 (accessed 1 January 2009).

Baby Center. "Toxoplasmosis During Pregnancy." http://www.babycenter.com/0_toxoplasmosis-during-pregnancy_1461.bc (accessed 17 November 2008).

Beckman, D. A., and R. L. Brent. "Mechanism of Known Environmental Teratogens: Drugs and Chemicals." *Clinical Perontology* 13 (1986): 649–87.

Berman, Michael. *Parenthood Lost: Healing the Pain After Miscarriage, Stillbirth, and Infant Death.* Westport, CT: Bergin & Garvey Trade, 2001.

Billingsley, J. "The Child Who Never Arrived: A New Look at Miscarriage." *Ladies Home Journal* (November 1980): pp. 33–38.

Bills, B. "Nursing Considerations: Administering Labor-Suppressing Medications." *Maternal Child Nursing* (1980): 252–56.

Bilston, Sarah. *Bedrest.* New York: HarperCollins, 2003.

Blackburn, S., and L. Lowen. "Impact of an Infant's Premature Birth on the Grandparents and Parents." *Journal of Obstetric, Gynecologic, and Neonatal Nursing* (1986): 173–78.

Blakemore, K., and M. Mahoney. "Chorionic Villus Sampling." In *Genetics and the Fetus*. Edited by A. Milunsky. New York: Plenum Press, 1986, 625–55.

Bobak, Irene, et al. *Maternity and Gynecologic Care*. St. Louis, MO: C. V. Mosby, 1989.

Boggs, K. R., and P. K. Rau. "Breast-Feeding the Premature Infant." *American Journal of Nursing* (1983): 1437–39.

Boston Women's Health Collective. *Our Bodies and Ourselves: Pregnancy and Childbirth*. New York: Simon and Schuster, 2008.

Brackbill, Y., and D. Young. *Birth Trap*. New York: Warner Books, 1984.

Brengman, S., and M. Burns. "Vaginal Delivery After C-section." *The American Journal of Nursing* (November, 1983): 1544–47.

Brewer, G. S., and T. Brewer. *The Truth About Diet and Drugs in Pregnancy: What Every Pregnant Woman Should Know*. New York: Penguin Books, 1985.

Brown, M. J., D. Bellinger, and J. Matthews. "In Utero Lead Exposure." *Maternal Child Nursing* 15 (March/April, 1990): 94.

Brucker, M. C., and N. J. Macmullen. "What's New in Pregnancy Tests." *Journal of Obstetric, Gynecologic, and Neonatal Nursing* (1985): 353–59.

Campbell, B. "Overdue Delivery: Its Impact on Mothers-to-Be." *Maternal Child Nursing* 11 (1986): 170–72.

Canadian Foundation for the Study of Infant Deaths. *Information About Sudden Infant Death Syndrome*. Toronto: Canadian Foundation for the Study of Infant Deaths, 1991.

Centers for Disease Control. "Chlamydia: CDC Fact Sheet." http://www.cdc .gov/std/Chlamydia/STDFact-Chlamydia.htm (accessed 17 November 2008).

Centers for Disease Control. "Genital Herpes: CDC Fact Sheet." http://www .cdc.gov/std/Herpes/STDFact-Herpes.htm (accessed 17 November 2008).

Centers for Disease Control. "Mother-to-Child (Perinatal) HIV Transmission and Prevention: CDC Fact Sheet." http://www.cdc.gov/hiv/topics/perinatal/ resources/factsheets/perinatal.htm (accessed 17 November 2008).

Centers for Disease Control (press release). "Rubella No Longer Major Public Health Threat in the United States." http://www.cdc.gov/od/oc/media/ pressrel/r050321.htm (accessed 17 November 2008).

Charlish, A., and L. H. Holt. *Birth-Tech: Tests and Technology in Pregnancy and Birth*. New York: Facts on File, 1991.

Chism, Denise. *The High-Risk Pregnancy Sourcebook*. Los Angeles: Lowell House, 1998.

Collins, C. "Gestational Diabetes." *American Baby* (June 1987): 45–46.

Cook, P. "Drugs and Pregnancy." New York: The American Council for Drug Education. Congress Catalog Card Number: 86–070944.

Cox News Service. "One-Year Study Will Involve Testing Georgia Newborns for Cocaine." *Orlando Sentinel* (March 14, 1991): A6.

Crout, T. K. "Caring for the Mother of a Stillborn Baby." *Nursing* (April 1980): 70–73.

Davis, L. "Daily Fetal Movement Counting." *Journal of Nurse-Midwifery* 32 (1987): 11–19.

DeVita, V., S. Hellman, and S. Rosenberg. *AIDS: Etiology, Diagnosis, Treatment, and Prevention*. Philadelphia: J. B. Lippincott, 1986.

Dorris, M. *The Broken Cord*. New York: Harper & Row, 1989.

Douglas, Ann, and John R. Sussman, MD. *The Unofficial Guide to Having a Baby*. New York: Wiley Publishing, Inc., 2004.

Dowsett, C. A. "Sudden Infant Death Syndrome." *Ladycom* (November/December 1984): 21–24.

Elias, S., and G. J. Annas. "Fetal and Gene Therapy." *Current Problems in Obstetrics, Gynecology and Fertility* 10, no. 3 (1987).

Epiro, P., ed. "When Sudden Infant Death Strikes." *Patient Care* 15 (March 1984): 18–42.

Erick, Miriam. *Managing Morning Sickness: A Survival Guide for Pregnant Women*. Boulder, CO: Bull Publishing, 2004.

Evans, Joel, M. *The Whole Pregnancy Handbook*. New York: Gotham Books, 2005.

Federal-Provincial Subcommittee on Nutrition. *Nutrition in Pregnancy: National Guidelines*. Ottawa: Health and Welfare Canada, 1987.

Freeman, R., and S. Pescar. *Safe Delivery*. New York: McGraw Hill, 1982.

Gilbert, Elizabeth Stepp. *High Risk Pregnancy & Delivery*. 4th ed. St. Louis, MO: C. V. Mosby, 2007.

Goldberg, J. "Can They Save This Baby?" *Reader's Digest* (January 1991): 1–15.

Govani, L. E., and J. E. Hayes. *Drugs and Nursing Implications*. Norwalk, CT: Appleton-Century-Crofts, 1985.

Greenfield, Marjorie. *The Working Woman's Pregnancy Book*. New Haven: Yale University Press, 2008.

Gwinn, Marta, et al. "Prevalence of HIV Infection in Childbearing Women in the United States." *The Journal of the American Medical Association* 265, no. 13 (1991): 1704–08.

Hales, D., and R. K. Creasy. *New Hope for Problem Pregnancies*. New York: Berkley Books, 1982.

Harms, Roger M. *Mayo Clinic Guide to a Healthy Pregnancy*. New York: HarperResource, 2004.

Harrison, L. L., and S. Twardosz. "Teaching Mothers About Their Preterm Infants." *Journal of Obstetric, Gynecologic, and Neonatal Nursing* 15, no. 2 (March/April 1986): 165–72.

Hemmer, M., M. Staquet, and A. Baert, eds. *Clinical Aspects of AIDS and AIDS-Related Complex*. Oxford: Oxford University Press, 1986.

Hillard, P. A. "Twins." *Parents* (December 1984): 142–44.

Holden, Triona. *Positive Options for Antiphospholipid Syndrome (APS)*. Alameda, CA: Hunter House Publishers, 2003.

Huggins, G. Interview with author (February 1988).

———. "When Your Baby Is Breech." *Parents* (September 1990): 150–51.

Institute of Medicine. "Nutritional Status and Weight Gain." In *Nutrition During Pregnancy* . Washington, DC: National Academies Press, 1990, 27–233.

Ilse, S. *Empty Arms: Coping After Miscarriage, Stillbirth, and Infant Death.* Maple Plain, MN: Wintergreen Press, 1985.

International Childbirth Education Association. "Smoking and Childbearing: Maternal and Fetal Complications." *International Journal of Childbirth Education* 10, no. 2: IR–7R.

International Food Information Council. "Listeriosis and Pregnancy: What's Your Risk?" http://www.ific.org/publications/brochures/listeriosisbroch .cfm (accessed 11 December 2008.)

Jason, Janien, and A. Van Der Mer. *Parenting Your Premature Baby.* New York: Henry Holt, 1989.

Jensen, M. D., R. Benson, and I. Bobak. *Maternity Care: The Nurse and the Family.* St. Louis, MO: C. V. Mosby, 1977.

Kinney, J. M. "Pediatric Surgeons Focus on Congenital Defects." *Association of Operating Room Nurses Journal* 39, no. 2 1984): 195–96.

Kitzinger, S. *Birth over Thirty.* Toronto: Penguin, 1985.

Klaus, M. H., and J. H. Kennell. *Parent-Infant Bonding.* St. Louis, MO: C. V. Mosby, 1982.

Knuppel, R. A., and J. Drukker. *High-Risk Pregnancy: A Team Approach.* Philadelphia: W. B. Saunders, 1986.

Koren, Gideon, MD. *Everyday Risks in Pregnancy & Breastfeeding.* Toronto: Motherisk Program, The Hospital for Sick Children, 2004.

Laberge, J. M. "Fetal Surgery: Considering the Fetus as Patient." *Canadian Family Physician* 32 (1986): 2099–2103.

LaCerva, V. *Breast-Feeding: A Manual for Health Professionals.* Garden City, NJ: Medical Examination Publishing, 1981.

Lauersen, N. H. *Childbirth with Love.* New York: Berkley Books, 1983.

Liebman, B. "Eating for Two." *Nutrition Action Health Letter* 14, no. 3 (1987): 1–4.

Lynch, M., and V. A. McKeon. "Cocaine Use During Pregnancy: Research Findings and Clinical Implications." *Journal of Gynecological and Neonatal Nursing* 19, no. 4 (July/August 1990): 285–91.

March of Dimes Foundation. Professionals and Researchers. "Chicken Pox in Pregnancy." http://www.marchofdimes.com/printableArticles/14332_1185 .asp (accessed 17 November 2008).

March of Dimes Foundation. Pregnancy and Newborn Health Education Center. "Spotlight on Exercise." http://www.marchofdimes.com/printable articles/159_515.asp (accessed 4 August 2008).

March of Dimes Foundation. Professionals and Researchers. "Illicit Drug Use During Pregnancy." http://www.marchofdimes.com/professionals/ 14332_1169.asp (accessed 28 August 2008).

Marlow, D. *Textbook of Pediatric Nursing*. Philadelphia: W. B. Saunders, 1977.

Marmet, C. *Manual Expression of Breast Milk: Marmet Technique*. Pamphlet no. 107. Franklin Park, IL: La Leche League, 1981.

Martel, S., A. Wacholder, A. Lippman, J. Broham, and E. Hamilton. "Maternal Age and Primary Cesarean Rates: A Multivariate Analysis." *American Journal of Obstetrics and Gynecology* 156, no. 2 (1987): 305–08.

Martin, J. A., B. E. Hamilton, P. D. Sutton, S. J. Venturea, F. Menacker, S. Kirmeyer, et al. "Births: Final Data for 2006." *National Vital Statistics Reports* 57 (7) (2009).

Merck. "Autoimmune Disorders in Pregnancy." http://www.merck.com/mmpe/sec18/ch261/ch261d.html (accessed 17 November 2008).

Michaels, E. "Inducing Labor in Pregnant Women." *Chatelaine* (February 1985): 18.

Mills, J. L., B. L. Graubard, E. E. Harley, et al. "Maternal Alcohol Consumption and Birthweight: How Much Drinking During Pregnancy Is Safe?" *Journal of the American Medical Association* 252, no. 14 (1984): 1875–79.

Milunsky, A. *Genetic Disorders and the Fetus*. New York: Plenum Press, 1986.

Moore, K. A. *Facts at a Glance*. Washington, DC: Child Trends Inc., 1990.

Moore, M. L. *Realities in Childbearing*. Philadelphia: W. B. Saunders, 1983.

———. "Recurrent Teen Pregnancy: Making it Less Desirable." *Maternal Child Nursing* 14 (March/April 1989): 104–09.

Murkoff, Heidi, and Sharon Mazel. *What to Expect When You're Expecting*. New York: Workman Publishing, 2008.

Naeye, R. L. "Coitus and Associated Amniotic Fluid Infection." *New England Journal of Medicine* 301 (1979): 1198.

Nance, S. *Premature Babies*. New York: Berkley Books, 1982.

Newsweek staff. "Making Babies after Menopause." *Newsweek* (November 5, 1990): 76.

Nursing Photobook. *Attending OB/GYN Patients*. Pennsylvania: Intermed Communications, 1982.

Osofsy, H., and J. Drukker. "Sexual Intimacy in Pregnancy." In *High-Risk Pregnancy: A Team Approach*. Edited by R. A. Knuppel and I. E. Drukker. Philadelphia, PA: W. B. Saunders, 1986, 187–199.

Palinski, C., and H. Pfizer. *Coping with Miscarriage*. New York: New American Library, 1980.

Paul, Annie Murphy. "Too Fat and Pregnant: The Maternal Risks of Obesity. *New York Times Magazine* (July 13, 2008): 19.

Pletch, P. K. "Birth Defect Prevention: Nursing Interventions." *Journal of Gynecological and Neonatal Nursing* 19, no. 6 (November/December, 1990): 482–87.

Public Health Education Information Sheet. *PKU*. White Plains, NY: March of Dimes Birth Defects Foundation, 1985.

Public Health Education Information Sheet. *Tay-Sachs.* White Plains, NY: March of Dimes Birth Defects Foundation, 1986.

Purvis, A. "Major Surgery Before Birth Time." *Time* (June 11, 1990): 55.

Rapp, R. "The Ethics of Choice." *Ms. Magazine* (April 1984): 97–100.

Redshaw, M. E., R. P. Rivers, and D. B. Rosenblatt. *Born Too Early.* London: Oxford, 1985.

Resolve, Inc. *The Emotional Impact of Miscarriage.* Belmont, MA: Resolve, Inc., 1986.

——. *Medical Causes of Miscarriage.* Belmont, MA: Resolve, Inc., 1986.

Reynolds, J. L. "Prenatal Diagnosis by Amniocentesis and Chorionic Villus Biopsy." *Canadian Family Physician* 32 (1986): 105–08.

Riccardi, V. *The Genetic Approach to Human Disease.* New York: Oxford University Press, 1977.

Roberts, F., and M. E. Pembrey. *An Introduction to Medical Genetics.* Oxford: Oxford University Press, 1985.

Roberts, Holly, MD. *Your Vegetarian Pregnancy: A Month-by-Month Guide to Health and Nutrition.* New York: Fireside Books, 2003.

Roberts-Worthington, B., J. Vermeersch, and S. R. Williams. *Nutrition in Pregnancy and Lactation.* St. Louis, MO: C. V. Mosby, 1981.

Romm-Aviva, Jill. *Naturally Healthy Babies and Children: A Commonsense Guide to Herbal Remedies, Nutrition, and Health.* New York: Celestial Arts, 2003.

Sala, D. J., and K. J. Moise. "The Treatment of Preterm Labor Using a Portable Subcutaneous Terbutaline Pump." *The Journal of Gynecological and Neonatal Nursing* 19, no. 2 (March/April 1990): 108–15.

Schwiebert, P., and P. Kirk. *When Hello Means Goodbye.* Portland, OR: Perinatal Loss, 1985.

Seligmann, J., and L. Wilson. "The Tiniest Patients." *Newsweek* (June 11, 1990): 56–57.

Shettles, L. B., and D. M. Rorvik. *How to Choose the Sex of Your Baby.* New York: Broadway Books, 2006.

Shortridge, L. A. "Using Ritodrine Hydrochloride to Inhibit Preterm Labor." *Maternal Child Nursing* 8, no. 1 (January/February 1983): 58–61.

Shosenberg, N. *The Premature Infant: A Handbook for Parents.* Toronto: The Hospital for Sick Children, 1980.

Simkin, P., P. J. Whalley, and A. Keppler. *Pregnancy, Childbirth and the Newborn.* Deephoven, MN: Meadowbrook Books, 1984.

Smith, J. "The Dangers of Prenatal Cocaine Use." *Maternal Child Nursing* 13, (May/June 1988): 174–79.

Squires, S. "A Cure for Killer Pregnancies." *Ladies Home Journal* (October 1990): 132.

Stenchever, M. A. "Habitual Abortion." *Contemporary OB/GYN* 21, no. 1 (1983): 162.

Stevens, K. A. "Individualized Prenatal Nursing Care of Pregnant Adolescents Makes a Difference." *Gynecological and Neonatal Nursing* (November/December 1989): 521–22.

Thompson, J. M., et al. *Clinical Nursing.* St. Louis, MO: C. V. Mosby, 1986.

Twomey, J. G. "The Ethics of In Utero Fetal Surgery." *Nursing Clinics of North America* 24, no. 4 (December 1989): 1025–31.

United States Department of Health and Human Services. *Rubella and Congenital Rubella Syndrome.* Washington, DC: U.S. Department of Health and Human Services, 1984.

———. "Aids in Women—United States." *Morbidity Mortality Weekly Report* 39, no. 47 (November 30, 1990): 845–46.

Urdang, L., and H. H. Swallow. *Mosby's Medical and Nursing Dictionary.* St. Louis, MO: C. V. Mosby, 1983.

Vento, M. "Where We Stand." *Health Watch* (March/April 1991): 49–56.

Williams, M. "Long-Term Hospitalization of Women with High-Risk Pregnancies." *Journal of Gynecological and Neonatal Nursing* 15, no. 1 (January/February 1986): 17–21.

Williams-Wheeler, Dorrie. *The Unplanned Pregnancy Book: For Teens and College Students.* VA: Sparkledoll Productions, 2004.

Wilson, B. A. "The Disease that Cries Wolf." *Health Watch* (March/April 1991): 59–63.

Winslow, W. "First Pregnancy After 35: What Is the Experience?" *Maternal Child Nursing* 12, no. 2 (March/April 1987): 92–96.

Wisniewski, L., and K. Hirschorn. *A Guide to Human Chromosome Defects.* White Plains, NY: March of Dimes Birth Defects Foundation, 1980.

Support Groups and Associations

Untited States

Getting Pregnant

Endometriosis Association
8585 North 76th Pl., Milwaukee WI 53223
(800) 992-3636   (414) 355-2200   www.endometriosisassn.org

National Dairy Council
10255 West Higgins Rd., Suite 900, Rosemount IL 60018-4233
(847) 803-2000   www.nationaldairycouncil.org

RESOLVE
1310 Broadway, Somerville MA 02144-1779
(617) 623-0744   www.resolve.org

High-Risk Pregnancy

American Diabetes Association
P.O. Box 25757, 1660 Duke St., Alexandria VA 22314
(800) DIABETES   (703) 549-1500   www.diabetes.org

American Foundation for AIDS Research (AmFAR)
120 Wall St., New York NY 10005
(212) 806-1600   www.amfar.org

Center for Study of Multiple Birth
333 East Superior St., Suite 464, Chicago IL 60611
(312) 266-9093   www.multiplebirth.com

International Twins Association, Inc.
6898 Channel Rd. NE, Minneapolis MN 55432
(612) 571-3022   (612) 571-8910   www.intltwins.org

Lupus Foundation of America
2000 L St. NW, Suite 710, Washington DC 20036
(202) 349-1155   www.lupus.org

Mothers of Supertwins (MOST)
P.O. Box 951, Brentwood NY 11717
(516) 859-1110   www.mostonline.org

Myasthenia Gravis Foundation of America
355 Lexington Ave., 15th Fl., New York NY 10017
(800) 541-5454   www.myasthenia.org

National Diabetes Information Clearinghouse
P.O. Box NDIC, Bethesda MD 20892
E-mail: ndic@aerie.com   www.diabetes.niddic.nih.gov

National Organization of Mothers of Twins Club, Inc.
P.O. Box 23188, Albuquerque NM 87192-1188
(800) 243-2276   (505) 275-0955   www.nomotc.org

Triplet Connection
P.O. Box 99571, Stockton CA 95209
(209) 474-0885   www.tripletconnection.org

Twin Services
P.O. Box 10066, Berkeley CA 94709
(510) 524-0863   twinservices@juno.com

Twins Foundation
P.O. Box 9487, Providence RI 02940-9487
(401) 274-8946   www.twinsfoundation.org

Twin to Twin Transfusion Syndrome Foundation
411 Long Beach Pkwy., Bay Village OH 44140
(440) 899-TTTS   www.tttsfoundation.org

Women and AIDS Resource Network (WARN)
30 Third Ave., Suite 25, Brooklyn NY 11217

Genetics and Birth Defects

Alcoholics Anonymous World Services, Inc.
P.O. Box 459, New York NY 10163
(212) 870-3400   www.alcoholics-anonymous.org

Alliance of Genetic Support Groups
4301 Connecticut Ave. NW, Suite 404, Washington DC 20008
(800) 336-GENE   (202) 966-5557   www.geneticalliance.org

American Board of Medical Genetics
9650 Rockville Pike, Bethesda MD 20814
(301) 571-1825   www.faseb.org/genetics

American Cleft Palate-Craniofacial Association
1504 East Franklin St., Suite 102, Chapel Hill NC 27514
(919) 933-9044   www.cleftline.org

American Council for Drug Education
164 W. 74th St., New York NY 10023
(800) 488-DRUG (3784)   www.acde.org

Association of Birth Defect Children
3201 East Crystal Lake Ave., Orlando FL 32806
www.birthdefects.org

Blind Children's Center
4120 Marathon St., Los Angeles CA 90029-3584
(800) 222-3566   (323) 664-2153   www.blindcntr.org

Cystic Fibrosis Foundation National Center
6931 Arlington Rd., Bethesda MD 20814
(800) 344-4823   www.cff.org

Federation for Children with Special Needs
95 Berkeley St., Suite 104, Boston MA 02116
(800) 331-0688 (in MA)   (617) 482-2915   http://fcsn.org

Healthy Mothers, Healthy Babies
409 12th St. SW, Suite 309, Washington DC 20024-2188
(800) 322-2588   (202) 863-2458   www.hmhb.org

Juvenile Diabetes Foundation International
120 Wall St., New York NY 10005-4001
(800) 533-2873   (212) 785-9500   www.jdfcure.org

March of Dimes Birth Defects Foundation
1275 Mamaroneck Ave., White Plains NY 10605
(800) 367-6630   (914) 428-7100   www.modimes.org

Maternal PKU Collaborative Study
Division of Medical Genetics, Children's Hospital Los Angeles
4650 Sunset Blvd., Los Angeles CA 90027
(323) 669-2152

National Down Syndrome Society Hotline
666 Broadway, 8th Fl., New York NY 10012
(800) 221-4602   www.ndss.org

National Foundation for Jewish Genetic Diseases
45 Sutton Pl. S., New York NY 10022
(212) 371-1030

National Genetics Foundation
555 W. 57th St., New York NY 10019
(212) 586-5800

National Institute on Alcohol Abuse and Alcoholism
5600 Fisher Ln., Rockville MD 20857
(301) 443-3860   www.niaaa.nih.gov

National Organization for Rare Disorders (NORD)
P.O. Box 8923, New Fairfield CT 06812
(203) 746-6518   www.rarediseases.org

National Society of Genetic Counselors
233 Canterbury Dr., Wallingford PA 19086-6617
(610) 872-7608   www.nsgc.org

Parents Helping Parents
3041 Olcott St., Santa Clara CA 95054-3222
(408) 727-5775   www.php.com

Parents of Down Syndrome Children
c/o Montgomery County Association for Retarded Citizens
11600 Nobel St., Rockville MD 20852
(301) 984-5792

Spina Bifida Association of America
343 South Dearborn, Suite 317, Chicago IL 60604
(312) 663-1562   www.sbaa.org

Turner Syndrome Society of the United States
1313 Southeast 5th St., Suite 327, Minneapolis MN 55414
(800) 365-9944   (612) 379-3607   www.turner-syndrome-us.org

United Cerebral Palsy Associations
330 W. 34th St., New York NY 10001
(800) USA-5-UCP (872-5827)   (212) 947-5770   www.ucp.org

Pregnancy Loss
Aiding Mothers and Fathers Experiencing Neonatal Death (AMEND)
4324 Berrywick Terr., St. Louis MO 63128
(314) 487-7582   www.amendgroup.com

American Sudden Infant Death Syndrome Institute
6065 Roswell Rd., Suite 876, Atlanta GA 30328
(404) 843-1030   www.sids.org

Bittersweet Beginnings (loss of multiple births)
5700 E. Greenwood Pl., Denver CO 80222-5700
(303) 759-3979

Center for Loss in Multiple Birth (CLIMB)
P.O. Box 1064, Palmer AK 99645
(907) 746-6123   www.climb-support.org

Compassionate Friends, Inc.
P.O. Box 3696, Oak Brook IL 60522-3696
(630) 990-0010   www.compassionatefriends.com

Firstcandle.org
1314 Bedford Ave., Suite 210, Baltimore MD 21208
(800) 221-7437   E-mail: info@firstcandle.org

Helping Other Parents in Normal Grieving (HOPING)
Sparrow Hospital
1215 East Michigan St., Lansing MI 48909
(517) 483-3873

Miscarriage, Infant Death, Stillbirth (MIDS, Inc.)
c/o Janet Tischler
16 Crescent Dr., Parsippany NJ 07054
(201) 263-6730   www.midsinc.org

Mothers in Sympathy and Support
P.O. Box 5333, Peoria AZ 85385-5333
(888) 455-6477   www.misschildren.org

National Council of Guilds for Infant Survival (SIDS support)
P.O. Box 3586, Davenport IA 52808
(319) 322-4870

National Sudden Infant Death Syndrome Resource Center
2070 Chain Bridge Rd., Suite 450, Vienna VA 22182
(703) 821-8955   www.circsol.com/sids

PEN Parents, Inc.
P.O. Box 8738, Reno NV 89507-8738
(702) 826-7332   www.penparents.org

Pregnancy and Infant Loss Center
1421 East Wayzata Blvd., Suite 70, Wayzata MN 55391
(612) 473-9372

RTS Bereavement Services
Gunderson/Lutheran Medical Center
1910 South Ave., La Crosse WI 54601
(800) 362-9567   www.bereavementprograms.org

SHARE: Pregnancy and Infant Loss Support, Inc.
St. Joseph Health Center
300 First Capitol Dr., St. Charles MO 63301
(314) 947-5616   www.nationalshareoffice.com

Sudden Infant Death Syndrome Alliance
1314 Bedford Ave., Suite 210, Baltimore MD 21208
(800) 221-SIDS   (410) 653-8226   www.sidsalliance.org

Wintergreen Press
3630 Eileen St., Maple Plain MN 55359
(612) 476-1303   wpress@aol.com

Labor, Delivery, and Postpartum
Circumcision Resource Center
P.O. Box 232, Boston MA 02133
(617) 523-0088   www.circumcision.org

International Lactation Consultant Association
1500 Sunday Dr., Suite 102, Raleigh NC 27607
(919) 861-5577   www.ilca.org

Lamaze International
1200 19th St. NW, Suite 300, Washington DC 20036-2422
(800) 368-4404   (202) 857-1128   www.lamaze-childbirth.com

Mocha Moms
P.O. Box 1995, Upper Marlboro MD 20773
www.mochamoms.org

Making Our Milk Safe (MOMS)
1125 High St., Alameda CA 94501
www.safemilk.org

National Association of Parents and Professionals for Safe Alternatives in
Childbirth (NAPPSAC)
Route 4, P.O. Box 646, Marble Hill MO 63764
(573) 238-2010   E-mail: napsac@clas.net

Postpartumcouples.com
www.postpartumcouples.com

Postpartum Support International
P.O. Box 60931, Santa Barbara CA 93160
(800) 944-4773   http://postpartum.net

Resources on Depression in Mothers
www.granitescientific.com/depressionfrontpage.htm

Cesarean Birth
Cesarean Support, Education and Concern (C/SEC, Inc.)
22 Forest Rd., Framingham MA 01701
(508) 877-8266

International Cesarean Awareness Network
1304 Kingsdale Ave., Redondo Beach CA 90278
(310) 542-6400   www.childbirth.org/ICAN

Premature Babies

Children's Medical Ventures
191 Wyngate Dr., Monroeville PA 15146
(800) 345-6443   http://chmv.respironics.com

ComeUnity Premature Baby Premature Child
www.comeunity.com/prematurechild

Prematurely Yours
6712 Townspoint Rd., Suffolk VA 23435
(757) 560-5574   www.prematurelyyours.com

Tiny Bundles
c/o Pattie Park
11468 Ballybunion Sq., San Diego CA 92128
www.tinybundles.com

Special Concerns

American Academy of Pediatrics
141 NW Point Blvd., Grove Village IL 60007
(847) 228-5005   www.aap.org

American College of Nurse-Midwives
818 Connecticut Ave. NW, Suite 900, Washington DC 20006
(202) 728-9860   www.birth.org

American College of Obstetricians and Gynecologists (ACOG)
409 12th St. SW, Washington DC 20024-2188
(800) 762-2264, ext. 199   (202) 638-5577   www.acog.org

American Medical Association (AMA)
515 North State St., Chicago IL 60610
(312) 464-5000   www.ama-assn.org

Association of the Care of Children's Health
7910 Woodmont Ave., Suite 300, Bethesda MD 20814
(800) 808-ACCH   (301) 986-4553   www.acch.org

Birthways
P.O. Box 12097, Berkeley CA 94701-3097
(510) 869-2797   www.birthways.org

Centers for Disease Control and Prevention (CDC)
1600 Clifton Rd., NE Building 1 South, Atlanta GA 30333
www.cdc.gov

Consumer Information Center
Room G-142, (XC), 1800 F St. NW, Washington DC 20405
(888) 8-PUEBLO (878-3256)   (800) 688-9889 (Federal Information Center)
www.pueblo.gsa.gov

For Teen Moms Only
P.O. Box 962, Frankfort IL 60423-0982
(815) 464-5465

Healthy Teen Network (formerly National Organization of Adolescent
Pregnancy and Parenting)
1501 Saint Paul St., Suite 124, Baltimore MD 21202
(410) 685-0410   http://healthyteennetwork.org

International Childbirth Education Association (ICEA)
P.O. Box 20048, Minneapolis MN 55420-0048
(612) 854-8660   www.icea.org

Krames Communications
1100 Grundy Ln., San Bruno CA 94066-3030
(800) 333-3032   www.krames.com

La Leche League International
1400 N. Meacham Rd., Schaumburg IL 60173-4048
(847) 519-7730   www.llli.org

Maternity Center Association
48 E. 92nd St., New York NY 10128
(212) 777-5000   www.maternity.org

National Cancer Institute
Cancer Information Services
Bethesda MD 20892
(301) 496-4000   www.nci.nih.gov

National Family Planning and Reproductive Health Association
1627 K St., 12th Fl., Washington DC 20006
(202) 628-3535   www.nfprha.org

National Health Information Center
P.O. Box 1133, Washington DC 20013
(800) 336-4797   www.nhic-nt.health.org

National Maternal and Child Health Clearinghouse
2070 Chain Bridge Rd., Suite 450, Vienna VA 22182-2536
(703) 356-1964   www.nmchc.org

National Women's Health Network
514 10th St. NW, Washington DC 20004
(202) 347-1140   www.nwhn.org

Parents Without Partners International, Inc.
401 North Michigan Ave., Chicago IL 60611-4267
(800) 637-7974   (312) 644-6610   www.parentswithoutpartners.org

Planned Parenthood Federation of America
810 Seventh Ave., New York NY 10019
(800) 829-7732   (212) 261-4300   www.plannedparenthood.org

Single Mothers By Choice
P.O. Box 1642, Gracie Square Station, New York NY 10028
(212) 988-0993   www.singlemothersbychoice.com

Single Parent Resource Center
31 E. 28th St., New York NY 10016
(212) 951-7030   www.singleparentusa.com

Women in Crisis, Inc.
360 W. 125th St., Suite 11, New York NY 10027
(212) 665-2018

Canada

Canadian Cerebral Palsy Association
Wellington St., Suite 612, Ottawa, Ontario, K1R 6K7
(800) 267-6572   www.ccpsa.ca

Canadian Council of the Blind
P.O. Box 2310, Station D, Ottawa, Ontario, K1A 8N5
(877) 304-0968   www.ccbnational.net

Canadian Cystic Fibrosis Foundation
2221 Yonge St., Suite 601, Toronto, Ontario, M4S 2B4
(800) 378-CCFF (2233)   (416) 485-9149   www.cysticfibrosis.ca

Canadian Deaf-Blind and Rubella Association
2652 Morien Hwy., Port Morien, Nova Scotia, B1B 1C6
(519) 538-3431   www.cdbra.ca

Canadian Diabetes Association
National Office
15 Toronto St., Suite 800, Toronto, Ontario, M5C 2E3
(416) 363-3373   www.diabetes.ca

Canadian Foundation for the Study of Infant Deaths
586 Eglinton Ave. E., Suite 308, Toronto, Ontario , M4P 1P2
(416) 488-3260   www.sidscanada.org

Canadian Hard of Hearing Association
2435 Holly Ln., Suite 205, Ottawa, Ontario, K1V 7P2
(800) 263-8068   (615) 526-1584   www.chha.ca/english.html

Canadian Hemophilia Society
100 King St. W, Hamilton, Ontario, L8P 1A2
(416) 523-6414   www.hemophilia.on.ca

Canadian Institute of Child Health
885 Meadowlands Dr., Suite 512, Ottawa, Ontario, K2C 3N2
(613) 224-4144   www.cich.ca

Canadian National Institute for the Blind
1931 Bayview Ave., Toronto, Ontario, M4G 3E8
(416) 480-7580   www.cnib.ca

Canadian Pediatric Society
100-2204 Walkley Rd., Ottawa, Ontario, K1G 4G8
(613) 526-3332   www.cps.ca

Canadian Rehabilitation Council for the Disabled
Easter Seals/March of Dimes National Council
90 Eglinton Ave. E, Suite 511, Toronto, Ontario, M4P 2Y3
(416) 932-8382   www.indie.ca/crc

Compassionate Friends National Center (Canada)
685 William Ave., Winnipeg, Manitoba, R3E 0Z2
(204) 787-4896   www.compassionatefriends.ca

La Leche League International
P.O. Box 700, Winchester, Ontario, K0C 2K0
(800) 665-4324   www.lllc.ca

Parents of Multiple Births Association of Canada
P.O. Box 234, Gormley, Ontario, L0H 1G0
(905) 888-0725   www.pomba.org

Teenie Weenie Preemie Wear
3-132 Moilliet St., Parksville, British Columbia
V9P 1K6   www.teenieweeniepreemiewear.com

Turner Syndrome Society of Canada
814 Glencairn Ave., Toronto, Ontario, M6B 2A3
(800) 465-6744   (416) 781-2086   www.turnersyndrome.ca

Index